Clinical Evaluation and Management of Spasticity

CURRENT CLINICAL NEUROLOGY

Clinical Evaluation and Management of Spasticity, edited by
David A. Gelber and Douglas R. Jeffery, 2002

Early Diagnosis of Alzheimer's Disease, edited by *Leonard F. M. Scinto and Kirk R. Daffner*, 2000

Sexual and Reproductive Neurorehabilitation, edited by *Mindy Aisen*, 1997

Clinical Evaluation and Management of Spasticity

Edited by

David A. Gelber, MD
Springfield Clinic Neuroscience Institute, Springfield, IL

and

Douglas R. Jeffery, MD, PhD
Department of Neurology, Wake Forest University School of Medicine, Winston-Salem, NC

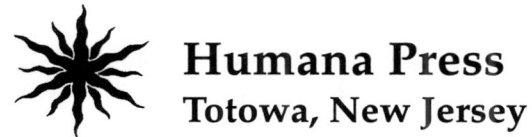

Humana Press
Totowa, New Jersey

© 2002 Humana Press Inc.
999 Riverview Drive, Suite 208
Totowa, New Jersey 07512

humanapress.com

All rights reserved. No part of this book may be reproduced, stored in a retrieval system, or transmitted in any form or by any means, electronic, mechanical, photocopying, microfilming, recording, or otherwise without written permission from the Publisher.

All authored papers, comments, opinions, conclusions, or recommendations are those of the author(s), and do not necessarily reflect the views of the publisher.

Due diligence has been taken by the publishers, editors, and authors of this book to assure the accuracy of the information published and to describe generally accepted practices. The contributors herein have carefully checked to ensure that the drug selections and dosages set forth in this text are accurate and in accord with the standards accepted at the time of publication. Notwithstanding, as new research, changes in government regulations, and knowledge from clinical experience relating to drug therapy and drug reactions constantly occurs, the reader is advised to check the product information provided by the manufacturer of each drug for any change in dosages or for additional warnings and contraindications. This is of utmost importance when the recommended drug herein is a new or infrequently used drug. It is the responsibility of the treating physician to determine dosages and treatment strategies for individual patients. Further it is the responsibility of the health care provider to ascertain the Food and Drug Administration status of each drug or device used in their clinical practice. The publisher, editors, and authors are not responsible for errors or omissions or for any consequences from the application of the information presented in this book and make no warranty, express or implied, with respect to the contents in this publication.

This publication is printed on acid-free paper. ∞
ANSI Z39.48-1984 (American Standards Institute) Permanence of Paper for Printed Library Materials.

Production Editor: Mark J. Breaugh.

Cover design by Patricia F. Cleary.

For additional copies, pricing for bulk purchases, and/or information about other Humana titles, contact Humana at the above address or at any of the following numbers: Tel.: 973-256-1699; Fax: 973-256-8314; E-mail: humana@humanapr.com, or visit our Website: humanapress.com

Photocopy Authorization Policy:
Authorization to photocopy items for internal or personal use, or the internal or personal use of specific clients, is granted by Humana Press Inc., provided that the base fee of US $10.00 per copy, plus US $0.25 per page, is paid directly to the Copyright Clearance Center at 222 Rosewood Drive, Danvers, MA 01923. For those organizations that have been granted a photocopy license from the CCC, a separate system of payment has been arranged and is acceptable to Humana Press Inc. The fee code for users of the Transactional Reporting Service is: [0-89603-636-7/02 $10.00 + $00.25].

Printed in the United States of America. 10 9 8 7 6 5 4 3 2 1

Library of Congress Cataloging in Publication Data

Clinical evaluation and management of spasticity / edited by David A. Gelber and Douglas R. Jeffery,
    p. ; cm. -- (Current clinical neurology)
  Includes bibliographical references and index.
  ISBN 0-89603-636-7
  1. Spasticity. I. Gelber, David A. II. Jeffery, Douglas R. III. Series.
  [DNLM: 1. Muscle Spasticity--diagnosis. 2. Muscle Spasticity--therapy WE 550 C6406 2002]
  RC935.S64 C545 2002
  616.8'3--dc21

2001039364

Preface

Clinical Evaluation and Management of Spasticity aims to be an authoritative resource for practitioners interested in learning more about the management of spasticity. Given the recent advances in treatment, there has for some time been a need for a text devoted entirely to this topic. This is the first such volume.

This book is divided into three sections, each intended to allow one to refer quickly to management strategies for specific neurologic diseases as well as specific treatment modalities.

The first section reviews basic concepts in spasticity, including the physiology and pharmacology of spasticity, the clinical evaluation of spasticity, and an overview of the clinical features and principles in the management of spasticity.

The second section outlines current treatments for spasticity. It covers such topics as physical and occupational therapy approaches, splinting and orthotics, electrical stimulation, orthopedic interventions, nerve blocks, use of botulinum toxin, specific medical interventions, including novel treatments such as tizanidine, and the use of intrathecal medications and neurosurgical interventions.

The final section reviews a coordinated approach to the treatment of spasticity and specific neurologic diseases, including spinal cord injury, multiple sclerosis, stroke, cerebral palsy, and traumatic brain injury. The chapters herein provide a framework for physicians to develop a care plan for patients with these disorders. Spasticity is often a poorly treated manifestation of many neurologic disorders, and it is our hope that this book will become the definitive reference to the management and treatment of spasticity, and will ultimately lead to the improvement of patient care.

David A. Gelber, MD
Douglas R. Jeffery, MD, PhD

Contents

Preface v

Contributors ix

    Part I Basic Concepts of Spasticity

1. Physiology and Pharmacology of Spasticity 3
   Robert R. Young
2. Clinical Features of Spasticity and Principles of Treatment 13
   Alex W. Dromerick
3. Measurement of Spasticity 27
   David C. Good

    Part II Treatment Modalities

4. Physical and Occupational Approaches 47
   Susan H. Pierson
5. Orthotic Management 67
   Géza F. Kogler
6. Electrical Stimulation 93
   Peter W. Rossi
7. Baclofen 103
   Eric P. Bastings and Amelito Malapira
8. Tizanidine 125
   David A. Gelber
9. Benzodiazepines 137
   Herbert I. Karpatkin and Mindy Lipson Aisen
10. Dantrolene 147
    Walter S. Davis
11. Alternative Pharmacologic Therapies 151
    Joni Clark
12. Nerve Blocks 159
    David S. Rosenblum

13 Botulinum Toxins 173
    Lauren C. Seeberger and Christopher F. O'Brien
14 Intrathecal Medications 187
    Randall T. Schapiro
15 Orthopedic Interventions for the Management
       of Limb Deformities in Upper Motoneuron Syndromes 197
    Mary Ann E. Keenan and Patrick J. McDaid
16 Neurosurgical Management 257
    Jose A. Espinosa

    Part III *A Coordinated Approach to the Treatment
    of Spasticity in Neurologic Diseases*

17 Management of Spasticity in Children
       with Cerebral Palsy 269
    *Carol Green, Daniel R. Cooperman, Susan E. Gara,
    and Carrie Proch*
18 The Evaluation and Treatment of Spasticity in Patients
       with Multiple Sclerosis 287
    Douglas R. Jeffery
19 The Development and Management of Spasticity
       Following Traumatic Brain Injury 305
    Patricia B. Jozefczyk
20 Spasticity in Spinal Cord Injury:
       A Clinician's Approach 353
    Kurt Fiedler and Douglas R. Jeffery
Index 369

Contributors

MINDY L. AISEN, MD • *Rehabilitation Research and Development, Department of Veterans Affairs, Washington, DC*
ERIC P. BASTINGS, MD • *Department of Neurology, Wake Forest University Baptist Medical Center, Winston-Salem, NC*
JONI CLARK, MD • *Department of Neurology, Southern Illinois University School of Medicine, Springfield IL*
DANIEL R. COOPERMAN, MD • *Department of Pediatric Neurology, Rainbow Babies Children's Hospital, Cleveland, OH*
WALTER S. DAVIS, MD • *Independent Practice, Charlottesville, VA*
ALEX W. DROMERICK, MD • *Department of Neurology, Washington University School of Medicine, St. Louis, MO*
JOSE A. ESPINOSA, MD • *Division of Neurosurgery, Department of Surgery, Southern Illinois University School of Medicine, Springfield, IL*
KURT FIEDLER, MD • *Department of Neurology, Wake Forest University School of Medicine, Winston-Salem, NC*
SUSAN E. GARA, OTR/L • *Department of Pediatric Neurology, Rainbow Babies Children's Hospital, Cleveland, OH*
DAVID A. GELBER, MD • *Springfield Clinic Neuroscience Institute, Springfield, IL*
DAVID C. GOOD, MD • *Department of Neurology, Wake Forest University School of Medicine, Winston-Salem, NC*
CAROL GREEN, MD • *Department of Pediatric Neurology, Rainbow Babies Children's Hospital, Cleveland, OH*
DOUGLAS R. JEFFERY, MD, PhD • *Department of Neurology, Wake Forest University School of Medicine, Winston-Salem, NC*
PATRICIA B. JOZEFCZYK, MD • *University of Pittsburgh Medical Center, Pittsburgh, PA*
HERBERT I. KARPATKIN, PT, NCS • *Rehabilitation Research and Development, Department of Veterans Affairs, Washington, DC*
MARY ANN E. KEENAN, MD • *Department of Orthopedic Surgery, Albert Einstein Medical Center, Philadelphia, PA*

GÉZA F. KOGLER, MD, CO • *Department of Surgery, Orthopaedics and Rehabilitation Division, Southern Illinois University School of Medicine, Springfield, IL*
AMELITO MALAPIRA, MD • *Department of Neurology, Wake Forest University Baptist Medical Center, Winston-Salem, NC*
PATRICK J. MCDAID, MD • *Department of Orthopedic Surgery, Albert Einstein Medical Center, Philadelphia, PA*
CHRISTOPHER F. O'BRIEN, MD • *CNI Movement Disorders Center, Colorado Neurological Institute, Englewood, CO*
SUSAN H. PIERSON, MD • *Drake Center, Cincinnati, OH*
CARRIE PROCH, PT • *Department of Pediatric Neurology, Rainbow Babies Children's Hospital, Cleveland, OH*
DAVID S. ROSENBLUM, MD • *Spinal Cord Injury and Neuro-orthopedic Division, Gaylor Hospital, Wallingford, CT*
PETER W. ROSSI, MD • *Medical Director, Roper Rehabilitation Hospital, Charleston, SC*
RANDALL T. SCHAPIRO, MD • *The Fairview Multiple Sclerosis Center, Minneapolis, MN*
LAUREN C. SEEBERGER, MD • *CNI Movement Disorders Center, Colorado Neurological Institute, Englewood, CO*
ROBERT R. YOUNG, MD • *Department of Neurology, Keck School of Medicine, University of Southern California, Los Angeles, CA*

I
BASIC CONCEPTS OF SPASTICITY

1
Physiology and Pharmacology of Spasticity

Robert R. Young

CLINICAL PHYSIOLOGY OF SPASTICITY

Spasticity is a movement disorder characterized by positive symptoms of abnormally excessive motor unit activity (dystonia, inappropriate co-contraction of antagonistic muscle groups, and hyperactive stretch reflexes and cutaneous flexor reflexes including a Babinski sign). Spasticity must be differentiated from the negative symptoms, i.e., a lack of normal motor function, which always accompany it. The negative symptoms, which include weakness or paralysis, unusual fatiguability, and lack of dexterity, are referred to in this chapter as "paresis." Together, these two major consequences of damage to the central nervous system (CNS) characterize a syndrome known as "spastic paresis" (1).

Spastic paresis is a common result of any injury of the CNS (infarct, hemorrhage, trauma, demyelination) that affects upper motor neurons (UMNs) or motor pathways at any level from the cerebral cortex to the spinal cord. It also results from spontaneous degeneration of motor pathways, as with motor-system disease.

Spasticity may, very rarely (e.g., some patients with hereditary spastic paraparesis), itself be thought to account for all of a patient's difficulty walking, but careful examination almost always reveals paresis as well as spasticity, even in those patients. The clinical significance of this inevitable coupling of spasticity and paresis is that even complete alleviation of spasticity, when that becomes possible, is unlikely to alleviate paresis, the most disabling symptoms afflicting these patients; paresis will not be "cured" until neuronal replacement therapies become feasible. Spasticity itself often produces pain and functional disability and must certainly be treated vigorously. However, the most serious restrictions of function affecting patients with CNS damage are owing to disconnections within the CNS, which produce negative symptoms.

From: *Current Clinical Neurology: Clinical Evaluation and Management of Spasticity*
Edited by: D. A. Gelber and D. R. Jeffery © Humana Press, Inc., Totowa, NJ

The details of each patient's spastic paretic syndrome are unique, to a greater or lesser extent, to that patient. The pathophysiologic components or subunits making up any one patient's spastic syndrome vary, presumably dependent on exactly how much of which CNS structures have been damaged. Some patients with cerebral lesions have tightly fisted, dystonic hands, whereas others are paralyzed but with relatively little spasticity. In patients with cerebral lesions, the spinal motor neurons and segmental interneurons that are reflexively most active produce a posture in which there is excessive contraction of antigravity muscles. The flexors of the upper limb and extensors of the lower limb are hyperactive. This posture is known as hemiplegic dystonia, and is one of the nonmobile forms of dystonia. In patients with lesions of the spinal cord, the flexor neuronal pools are hyperactive, producing flexion of the legs, the paraplegic posture.

With spasticity, muscles resting at mid-length are flaccid without electromyography (EMG) activity. Very slow stretch may meet with no resistance, unless fibrous intramuscular or periarticular contractures have developed. As the velocity of muscle stretch increases, stretch-reflex activity will be recruited in a velocity-dependent manner; the faster the stretch, the more resistance is felt. Patients with hemiplegia may also have rigid muscles (in which contraction is length-, rather than velocity-sensitive) in the same limb in which there are spastic muscles.

Patients with spinal lesions, but not those with cerebral lesions, have grossly exaggerated cutaneous reflexes. With spinal spasticity, completely non-noxious very light touch to the skin of the distal lower extremity can produce massive, prolonged reflex contraction of muscles that flex the hip, knee, and ankle (triple flexion). A small component of this stereotyped, non-coordinated withdrawal is dorsiflexion of the great toe, the Babinski sign, which also appears with cerebral lesions.

If trivial stimuli can produce gross flexor spasms in spastic patients, truly noxious, long-lasting stimuli (e.g., pressure sores, ingrown toenails, etc.), which would be painful if the patient could feel them, will obviously produce marked chronic increases in spasticity. Pain is also a consequence of spasticity; flexor spasms are often acutely painful while tonically contracting, dystonic muscles are chronically painful. Evidence that mechanisms underlying pain and spasticity overlap to a considerable degree derives from the observation that neurosurgical procedures are simultaneously effective in relieving pain and suppressing spasticity *(2)*. An example of a useful technique is the placement of microsurgical dorsal-root entry-zone lesions (DREZ-tomy), which destroy laterally placed small-diameter nociceptive fibers without affecting large-diameter fiber cutaneous or proprioceptive input.

The interval between CNS damage and development of full-blown spasticity varies widely, whereas the paresis produced is maximal immediately following an acute injury. With spinal lesions, areflexia and hyporeflexia—spinal shock—may last weeks. In the days before antibiotics, few patients with complete spinal-cord injuries survived long enough for extensor reflexes (tendon jerks) to return. With cerebral lesions, reflexes usually become hyperactive within a few days but grossly dystonic postures do not, with rare exceptions *(3)*, develop for a few weeks. This temporal evolution in the development of spasticity obviously reflects plasticity within the CNS; the exact nature of these plastic changes and the structures involved remain to be elucidated. If spasticity does not develop during the first 3 mo after an ischemic cerebral lesion, prognosis for recovery is poorer than in those who become spastic. Damage to the lentiform nucleus may be responsible for the persistence of flaccidity in that circumstance *(4)*.

In summary, spasticity is a multi-faceted syndrome, fractions of which develop at different rates, and it seems unlikely there will prove to be one unitary pathophysiology or abnormal neurochemistry underlying it or one pharmacotherapy that will alleviate it.

PATHOPHYSIOLOGY OF SPASTICITY

The negative symptoms of paresis result from: 1) lesion-induced disconnections of motor neurons and nearby interneurons from higher-level controls or 2) segmental damage to motor neurons and their axons. It is not yet clear which aspects of these negative symptoms may be owing to cocontraction of antagonist muscle groups, for example; that is, which symptoms may be because of spasticity, dystonia, or other excess CNS activity rather than to loss of function, pure and simple. At the present time, any "positive" causes of negative symptoms would be more amenable to therapy than those negative symptoms that require re-wiring of the CNS for their amelioration.

Spasticity is associated with increased muscle tone (increased tonic stretch reflexes evidenced by unusual resistance to movement at a joint) and with hyperactivity of phasic proprioceptive, cutaneous, and autonomic reflexes. Fibrous contractures within muscle or of periarticular connective tissue, which develop slowly as the spastic dystonic posture of a limb becomes fixed, produce increased resistance to passive stretch of muscle and thus are one cause of increased tone. More subtle are other changes within muscles that increase the thixotropic *(5)*, elastic, or other mechanical properties of relaxed muscles, stiffening these muscles even when they are without EMG activity; that is, when they are not contracting. These mechanical changes, which may include alterations in a muscle's normal resting length (e.g., reduction in the number of sarcomeres in fibers within that muscle), play a larger role in producing increased tone and dysfunction of spastic muscles *(6)* than was previously recognized, but it is unlikely they reach such a magnitude as to be responsible for serious spastic dysfunction; they certainly do not account for spastic hyperreflexia.

A more frequent topic of discussion than these intramuscular causes of increased tone are hyperactive stretch reflexes. When spastic muscles are stretched, there is a free interval at the beginning before stretch meets with increased resistance; in rigid muscles, there is no free interval. The greater the spastic increased tone, the shorter the free interval and the lower the stretch velocity necessary to produce a stretch reflex. There is good evidence that in spastic muscles, the length/velocity threshold that must be reached before a stretch reflex becomes active is abnormally low *(7)*. This suggests that spinal motor neurons innervating spastic muscles are more excitable than normal.

An older, much publicized, but now discredited hypothesis *(8)* involved hyperactive fusimotor outflow to muscle spindles, making them more taut than normal and more sensitive to stretch. This explanation for lower thresholds for spastic stretch reflexes arose from observations of reduced spasticity following perineural injections of local anesthetics that were assumed to block small-diameter fusimotor fibers but not larger-diameter alpha motor axons, an unlikely event in the clinical situation. Furthermore: 1) there is no evidence, from microneurographic recordings of human Ia afferents, of fusimotor hyperactivity in spastic muscles; and 2) Ia endings in normal relaxed human muscles are so exquisitely sensitive (intramuscular vascular pulsations produce pulse-synchronous bursts of Ia activity, for example) that it is difficult to imagine their being more sensitive in spastic muscles.

Spastic hyperreflexia must therefore be owing either to increased excitability of the lower motor neuron (LMN) itself, to increased excitatory/reduced inhibitory input to it, or both; that is, to increased excitability of segmental reflex arcs including stretch-reflex arcs and cutaneous-reflex arcs.

Because increased excitatory or decreased inhibitory input to motor neurons, whether from descending axons or segmental afferents, results in their depolarization (their resting potentials being brought closer to the threshold for firing), it is difficult to differentiate the effects of changes in synaptic activity from changes in intrinsic electrical properties of motor-neuron membranes. Although very little experimental data concerning such properties in spastic motor neurons have been collected, there is as yet no evidence for such intrinsic changes in neural membranes *(9)*. However, effects on motor-neuron excitability of neuromodulators, as opposed to synaptic neurotransmitters, have been described. For example, Hultborn and colleagues *(10)* showed that a depolarizing electrical pulse, when applied to a motor neuron, produces a much longer depolarization if serotonin is present extracellularly. Serotonin, released from axons descending from brain stem and acting as a neuromodulator, can thus produce significant and long-lasting effects on motor-neuron excitability when the neuron is activated by other, nonserotoninergic pathways.

Two other mechanisms whereby motor-neuron excitability might be altered are: 1) sprouting and regrowth of terminal excitatory axons onto areas of motor-neuron dendrites that had become bare owing to degeneration of descending fibers and 2) denervation hypersensitivity of those dendritic membranes. These mechanisms are also difficult to prove but, if they are involved, one of their hypothetical virtues is as possible explanations for the delayed, gradual development of hyperreflexia over a period of weeks following rostral damage.

In classical discussions of increased spinal reflexes, attention is usually focused on reduction in inhibition, in particular presynaptic, reciprocal, and recurrent types of inhibition. Delwaide *(11)* was among the first to demonstrate that in spastic patients, vibration applied to the Achilles tendon does not produce a reduction in the H reflex as it does in normal subjects. Vibration of muscles produces profound Ia afferent input, which should excite interneurons that act presynaptically to depolarize Ia terminals, reducing the amount of excitatory neurotransmitter they release when an impulse travels down them (presynaptic inhibition). Collateral branches from several types of descending motor fibers (e.g., corticospinal, rubrospinal, reticulospinal) end upon, and excite, presynaptic inhibitory interneurons, so damage to the CNS rostral to the motor neuron could render the presynaptic interneuron less excitable, thus reducing presynaptic inhibition, as Delwaide suggests, thereby increasing tendon jerks and stretch reflexes.

Impulses in Ia afferents from a given muscle excite its own motor-neuron pool (phasic and tonic stretch reflexes) and excite Ia reciprocal inhibitory interneurons leading to its antagonist muscle, the latter then becoming less excitable owing to reciprocal inhibition. In spastic patients, reflex spread is common with reflex-induced co-contraction of antagonist muscle groups, a failure of reciprocal inhibition. These Ia inhibitory interneurons are also activated by descending motor fibers, damage to which could also reduce this type of inhibition, resulting in spastic co-contraction *(12)*.

When motor neurons are activated, impulses going out the alpha motor axons to the muscle also, via recurrent axon collaterals, activate Renshaw interneurons at the segmental level; Renshaw cells are also activated by descending pathways. Renshaw activity then adds inhibition to the motor-neuron pool which was active but also inhibits local Ia inhibitory interneurons. This recurrent inhibition is reduced in spastic patients with supraspinal lesions (including those with motor-system disease) *(13)* but recurrent inhibition is actually increased in patients with spinal-cord injuries *(14)*. In this latter case, increased inhibition of Ia interneurons would add to the symptoms produced by reduction in reciprocal inhibition, as noted earlier. This example, in which recurrent inhibition may either be decreased or increased in spastic individuals, illustrates the importance of recognizing different types of spasticity, as defined by site of lesion and clinical appearance.

Similarly, reflex effects from Golgi tendon organ (Ib) afferents are unchanged after spinal-cord lesions in humans, whereas with hemiplegic spasticity, Ib inhibition is replaced by facilitation *(15)*. Spasticity is not one single disorder, does not have a single pathophysiology, and, until functionally complete neural regeneration is possible, will not have one optimal therapy for all patients.

In addition to reduction in presynaptic inhibition, reduction in reciprocal inhibition and either reduction or increase in recurrent inhibition, other probable causes of reflex hyperexcitability are loss of inhibitory descending (particularly reticulospinal) influences on unspecified segmental interneurons receiving input from cutaneous afferents and smaller-diameter sensory fibers (group II, III, and IV) from muscle. This may be particularly important for the genesis of hyperactive flexor reflexes.

PHARMACOLOGY OF SPASTICITY

Glutamate is the major excitatory neurotransmitter at ionotropic receptors in the cord and throughout the CNS. Gamma-amino butyric acid (GABA) is the major inhibitory neurotransmitter throughout the CNS and is especially important in spinal interneurons. Glycine is a postsynaptic inhibitory neurotransmitter and strychnine is a highly selective glycine receptor antagonist. Acute strychnine poisoning, in nonfatal doses, produces transient spastic paraparesis *(16)*. Acetylcholine is released from recurrent collaterals of alpha motor axons just as it is at their intramuscular terminals; it activates Renshaw cells. Noradrenergic pathways descend from the locus ceruleus to reach the dorsal and ventral horns of the cord; their functions there are poorly understood. Pain both accentuates spasticity and is caused by spasticity; substance P is co-released with glutamate from small-diameter nociceptive afferent fibers ending on spinal dorsal-horn cells. Enkephalin is located in nerve terminals in the same region of the superficial dorsal horn. Neuromodulators will probably prove to be as important as neurotransmitters in the neurochemistry of spasticity; serotonin was mentioned earlier and glutamate acts as a modulator at metabotropic receptors. Substance P enhances the postsynaptic actions of glutamate; diazepam does the same at $GABA_A$ receptors.

These neuroactive substances and their interactions outlined previously represent only a fraction of those known; the latter are surely only a small fraction of those that exist. Until the complete neurochemistry of the circuits involved in spasticity have been mapped out, rational therapy for the various aspects of the spastic paretic syndrome will not be possible, even if clinically useful agonists and antagonists for each transmitter and modulator could be manufactured. Meanwhile, trial and error and serendipity have been important in the recognition of therapeutically useful compounds.

Two pharmacologic agents act peripherally to block contraction of muscles, whether spastic or nonspastic. Dantrolene blocks release of calcium from sarcoplasmic reticulum, interfering with excitation-contraction coupling (17), and botulinum toxin A cleaves SNAP-25 in the presynaptic motor axon (18), interfering with release of acetylcholine. The former weakens all muscles in a patient and the latter weakens those muscles into which it is injected. Both can be useful, but within rather narrow clinical constraints. Weakening of all muscles is not often a useful strategy and botulinum toxin can be injected into only a few muscles at any one time. But if focal spasticity is troublesome, botulinum toxin can alleviate it. Emergency therapy for spasticity is rarely necessary but in such circumstances (e.g., abrupt intrathecal baclofen [ITB] withdrawal), dantrolene may be useful.

Three drugs have been proven safe and efficacious for treating spasticity and are widely used: baclofen, diazepam, and tizanidine (19). Baclofen, structurally similar to GABA, is a $GABA_B$ agonist, the metabotropic effect of which is to reduce influx of calcium into (and thus reduce the release of glutamate from) primary afferent terminals, reducing excitatory transmission. It is useful by mouth for treatment of painful spasms in patients with lesions of the cord and by intrathecal infusion for reduction of all types of segmental reflexes. However, it may increase paresis.

Diazepam and certain other benzodiazepines act at functionally coupled benzodiazepine-$GABA_A$ ionotropic receptors, enhancing chloride flow into neurons, hyperpolarizing and thus inhibiting them. This action of diazepam is only apparent when GABA is released onto these receptors (20). Diazepam is useful as adjunct treatment for spinal and supraspinal types of spasticity but causes sedation and reduction in mental acuity.

Tizanidine is an imidazoline derivative that has $alpha_2$-adrenergic agonist activity. It may work by enhancing noradrenergically mediated presynaptic inhibition; it may also have antinociceptive actions. Tizanidine reduces spasms in patients with spinal lesions; it produces less sedation than diazepam and less paresis than baclofen. Because they operate through different mechanisms, baclofen and tizanidine together are sometimes more effective than either alone.

Memantine, a noncompetitive NMDA receptor antagonist *(21)*, interferes with the excitatory effects of glutamate, and is currently being evaluated as an antispastic agent.

Vigabatrin, a GABA analog that inhibits GABA transaminase and prolongs the action of GABA, has been shown to have antispastic actions similar to baclofen in patients with spasticity of spinal origin *(22)*. Ivermectin, a GABA agonist used to treat onchocerciasis, reduces spastic dystonia and spontaneous spasms in patients with spinal-cord lesions *(23)* but is not available in the US. Gabapentin, which does not activate GABA receptors or alter GABA metabolism, has also been effective in treating patients with spasticity and pain of spinal-cord origin *(24)*.

L-threonine, the precursor naturally metabolized to glycine, has modest beneficial effects in patients with spinal spasticity *(25)*.

Nicotine, an agonist at nicotinic acetylcholinergic receptors, reduces recurrent inhibition *(26)*.

Opiates, which reduce pain by activating descending pathways inhibiting nociceptive neurons in the spinal dorsal horn, are excellent antispastic agents but, because of their addictive properties, are not used for the chronic treatment of spasticity.

Cyproheptadine, a serotonin antagonist, has been useful in the treatment of spasticity in patients with spinal lesions *(27)*.

These are examples of rational therapies based on what is known of spinal neurochemistry and pharmacology. As research proceeds, better drugs, with more specific actions and fewer side effects, will be devised.

SUMMARY

Spasticity is poorly treated by many primary caregivers. Such physicians give patients sleeping pills, rather than baclofen or tizanidine, in an attempt to compensate for painful nocturnal spasms that awaken them. They may also use pain pills, but rarely opiates or the drugs mentioned earlier. Knowledge of modern anti-spasticity therapies must reach those caregivers who are responsible for the long-term care of patients with spastic paresis. The various therapies outlined previously are certainly not ideal or universally effective but they are, in the proper circumstances and for the appropriate indications, very useful. Understanding of the physiology and pharmacology of spasticity should assist us all in improving patient care.

REFERENCES

1. Young, R. R. (1995) Spastic paresis, in *Diagnosis and Management of Disorders of the Spinal Cord* (Young, R. R. and Woolsey, R. M., eds.), W.B. Saunders, Philadelphia, pp. 363–376.
2. Sindou, M. (1992) Microsurgical DREZ-tomy for the treatment of pain and spasticity, in *Principles and Practice of Restorative Neurology* (Young, R. R. and Delwaide, P. J., eds.), Butterworth-Heinemann, Oxford, pp. 144–151.
3. Russell, W. R. and Young, R. R. (1969) Missile wounds of the parasagittal rolandic area, in *Modern Neurology* (Locke, S., ed.), Little Brown, Boston, pp. 289–302.
4. Pantano, P., Formisano, R., Ricci, M., et al. (1995) Prolonged muscular flaccidity after stroke: morphological and functional brain alterations. *Brain* **118,** 1329–1338.
5. Walsh, E. G. (1992) *Muscles, Masses & Motion.* Mac Keith Press, London, pp. 83–90, 154.
6. Rymer, W. Z. and Katz, R. T. (1994) Mechanisms of spastic hypertonia. *Phys. Med. Rehab.* **8,** 441–454.
7. Powers, R. K., Marder-Meyer, J., and Rymer, W. Z. (1988) Quantitative relations between hypertonia and stretch reflex threshold in spastic hemiparesis. *Ann. Neurol.* **23,** 115–124.
8. Hagbarth, K.-E., Wallin, G., and Lofstedt, L. (1973) Muscle spindle response to stretch in normal and spastic subjects. *Scand. J. Rehabil. Med.* **5,** 156–159.
9. Hochman, S. and McCrea, D. A. (1987) The effect of chronic spinal transection on homonymous Ia EPSP rise times in triceps surae motoneurons in the cat. *Abstr. Soc. Neurosci.* **12,** 186.
10. Hounsgard, J., Hultborn, H., Jesperson, B., and Kiehr, O. (1984) Intrinsic membrane properties causing a bistable behavior of alpha-motoneurons. *Exp. Brain Res.* **55,** 391–394.
11. Delwaide, P. J. and Olivier, E. (1987) Pathophysiological aspects of spasticity in man, in *Motor Disturbances* (Benecke, R., Conrad, B., and Marsden, C. D., eds.), Academic Press, London, pp. 153–167.
12. McLellan, D. L., Hassan, N., and Hodgson, J. A. (1985) Tracking tasks in the assessment of spasticity, in *Clinical Neurophysiology in Spasticity* (Delwaide, P. J. and Young, R. R., eds.), Elsevier, Amsterdam, pp. 131–139.
13. Katz, R. and Pierrot-Deseilligny, E. (1982) Recurrent inhibition of alpha-motoneurones in patients with upper motoneurone lesions. *Brain* **105,** 103–124.
14. Shefner, J. M., Berman, S. A., Sarkarati, M., and Young, R. R. (1992) Recurrent inhibition is increased in patients with spinal cord injury. *Neurology* **42,** 2162–2168.
15. Downes, L., Ashby, P., and Bugaresti, J. (1995) Reflex effects from Golgi tendon organ (Ib) afferents are unchanged after spinal cord lesions in humans. *Neurology* **45,** 1720–1724.
16. Nishiyama, T. and Nagase, M. (1995) Strychnine poisoning; natural course of a nonfatal case. *Am. J. Emergency Med.* **13,** 172–173.
17. Ward, A., Chaffman, M. O., and Sorkin, E. M. (1986) Dantrolene. A review of its pharmacodynamic and pharmacokinetic properties and therapeutic use in

malignant hyperthermia, the neuroleptic malignant syndrome and an update of its use in muscle spasticity. *Drugs* **32,** 130–168.
18. Gracies, J.-M. and Simpson, D. (1999) Neuromuscular blockers, in *Rehabilitation Pharmacotherapy* (Nance, P. W., ed.), W.B. Saunders, Philadelphia, pp. 357–383.
19. Nance, P. W. and Young, R. R. (1999) Antispasticity medications, in *Rehabilitation Pharmacotherapy* (Nance, P. W., ed.), W.B. Saunders, Philadelphia, pp. 337–355.
20. Polc, P. (1995) Involvement of endogenous benzodiazepine receptor ligands in brain disorders: therapeutic potential for benzodiazepine antagonists? *Med. Hypotheses* **44,** 439–446.
21. Bauer, H. J. and Hanefeld, F. A. (1993) *Multiple Sclerosis.* W.B. Saunders, Philadelphia, pp. 146–149.
22. Grant, S. M. and Heel, R. C. (1991) Vigabatrin. A review of its pharmacodynamic and pharmacokinetic properties, and therapeutic potential in epilepsy and disorders of motor control. *Drugs* **41,** 889–926.
23. Costa, J. L. and Diazgranados, J. A. (1994) Ivermectin for spasticity in spinal-cord injury. *Lancet* **343,** 739.
24. Dunevsky, A. and Perel, A. B. (1998) Gabapentin for relief of spasticity associated with multiple sclerosis. *Am. J. Phys. Med. Rehabil.* **77,** 451–454.
25. Lee, A. and Patterson, V. (1993) A double-blind study of L-threonine in patients with spinal spasticity. *Acta Neurol. Scand.* **88,** 334–338.
26. Shefner, J. M., Berman, S. A., and Young, R. R. (1993) The effect of nicotine on recurrent inhibition in the spinal cord. *Neurology* **43,** 2647–2651.
27. Nance, P. W. (1994) A comparison of clonidine, cyproheptadine and baclofen in spastic spinal cord injured patients. *J. Am. Paraplegia Soc.* **17,** 150–156.

2
Clinical Features of Spasticity and Principles of Treatment

Alex W. Dromerick

INTRODUCTION

Evaluating and treating the patient with spasticity is not easy. The clinician is typically presented with a patient who wants things that current treatments cannot usually achieve: more independence, more strength, and more coordination. Certain aspects, such as the control of painful spasms and the decrease of resistance to passive movement, can now be reliably addressed. However, the ever-increasing array of treatment choices forces the clinician to specify exactly what the goals of treatment are and to compare the possible benefits of treatment with the possible risks.

That entire books are written on the topic of spasticity testifies to the complexity and clinical importance of this disorder. The question of what, how and when to treat have been vigorously debated, and there remain few objective measures of the success of treatment. In this chapter, we will give a general overview of spasticity in neurologic disease and provide some guidelines for its rational treatment.

DEFINITION AND APPROACH TO THE PATIENT

> "Spasticity is a motor disorder characterized by velocity-dependent increase in tonic stretch reflexes ("muscle tone") with exaggerated tendon jerks, resulting from hyperexcitability of the stretch reflex, as one component of the upper motor neuron syndrome... [There are] other features of the upper motor neuron syndrome resulting from the release of flexor reflexes, such as flexor spasms...[and] the negative symptoms such as the pattern of weakness and loss of dexterity caused by withdrawal of the influence of descending motor pathways." *(1)*

Perhaps the most important thing that a clinician considering treating spasticity can remember is that what is really being addressed are the interlocking consequences of the upper motor neuron (UMN) syndrome. It is often difficult to dissect out what complaints of the patients are related to hypertonia and what symptoms are related to other consequences of the UMN injury. These other aspects of the UMN syndrome include muscle weakness, decreased dexterity, increased flexion withdrawal reflexes, and clonus. These symptoms can be seen following UMN damage from any cause *(2)*.

Another important consideration is that other neurologic impairments can also be seen in persons with the UMN syndrome. Many disease processes of the central nervous system (CNS) do not simply affect corticospinal tracts, but can also involve other sensorimotor subsystems. Central pain syndromes are common in persons with stroke or spinal-cord injury, and the pain in such cases may exacerbate the symptoms of spastic hypertonia. Hypertonia owing to spasticity may be accompanied by hypertonia owing to other causes, particularly dystonia. Dystonia, the co-contraction of agonist and antagonist muscles, has a mechanism and treatment that differs from hypertonia owing to spasticity. Tremor can also complicate both the diagnosis and treatment of hypertonia owing to spasticity.

A third consideration is that the patient may also be suffering from the complications of spasticity, particularly those involving the musculoskeletal system and skin. Often, these complications are quite treatable, and can form the focus of the efforts of the clinician. Fully addressing these complications may require the services of a multidisciplinary team of physicians, nurses, and therapists to optimally manage spasticity.

SYMPTOMS AND SIGNS OF THE UMN SYNDROME

Neurologic symptoms and signs are usually thought of as being "positive," that is, the presence of a new pathologic phenomenon, or "negative" the absence of some prior normal function. Table 1 outlines the symptoms of UMN injury, and their classification.

Positive Symptoms of the UMN Syndrome

The fundamental disruption in spasticity occurs in the stretch reflexes.

Phasic reflexes are those reflexes that are elicited by a tap on a muscle tendon or body. They are characterized by the force of tap needed to elicit a response, the speed and amplitude of the response, and the presence or absence of the spread of this response to adjoining or contralateral muscles. In UMN injury, tapping on a muscle tendon elicits a response that is faster, of higher amplitude, and that spreads to involve other muscle groups.

Tonic reflexes are manifested to the examiner as the resistance to passive movement across the joint. The classic impairment seen in spasticity is the "spastic catch" phenomenon. As discussed at length elsewhere, this velocity-dependent event causes triggering of muscle contraction, thus lead-

Table 1
Symptoms of Upper Motor Neuron Syndrome

Positive Symptoms
   Increased passive resistance to stretch
   Flexor spasms
   Clonus
Negative symptoms
   Weakness
   Incoordination
   Fatigability

ing to the passive resistance seen in spastic hypertonia. This phenomenon illustrates the properties of velocity dependency that are characteristic of hypertonia because of spasticity (3). A patient with spastic hypertonia may demonstrate little or no hypertonia if the limb is moved through its range of motion very slowly. As the examiner increases the velocity of movement of the limb, the limb begins to manifest the spastic catch. The spastic catch is usually followed by a slow relaxation. If the examiner continues to increase the velocity of passive movements, the limb can display so much hypertonia that further movement becomes impossible—a phenomenon called "blocking." Much less common is the "clasp-knife" phenomenon, where there is initial resistance to movement with a sudden relaxation and reduction in resistance. The clasp-knife phenomenon can be seen in any spastic muscle.

The degree of spastic hypertonia can vary throughout the day. Many people with spasticity find that there are certain times of day when their tone is relatively good and other times when tone can be quite problematic. Most patients attribute this to fatigue, but other exacerbators may play a role. Many patients find that their spasms or hypertonia are made worse in some positions and lessened with other positions.

Painful spasms, both flexor and extensor, are commonly seen. These involuntary contractions of muscle can be provoked by many causes, including position, cutaneous stimuli, the onset of sleep, pain, and infection. Painful in themselves, they may also interfere with sleep, make wheelchair seating or splinting difficult, and even cause further spasms because of autoinduction of a pain-spasm-pain cycle. Although most dramatic in persons with spinal-cord injuries, spasms can occur with any type of UMN injury, including stroke and other forms of brain injury. Such spasms can be so severe that they can throw patients from wheelchairs and break splints.

The pattern of spasms can change as time passes after the injury. For example, in persons with spinal-cord injury, the initial flaccid period is followed by a period of alternating flexor and extensor spasms. After 6–12 mo, the extensor spasms predominate *(4)*. These spasms can even be useful, because they can sometimes be induced by cutaneous stimulation of the groin or thighs, and be used by person with spinal-cord injury for standing during transfers.

Clonus is a series of rhythmic alternating contractions of agonist and antagonist muscles. This is a common involuntary movement after UMN injury *(5)*. Most commonly seen in the ankle, it can present in any skeletal muscle in the body. Clonus can be simply a curiosity to the patient and onlookers, or it can be disabling. It can prevent the functional use of an extremity, make splinting difficult, or be a distraction or embarrassment to the patient. Clonus is typically elicited only in certainly positions, usually a stretched position of the involved muscle. The contractions can usually be abolished by a change in position. It can be distinguished from a motor seizure by its positional nature, stereotyped appearance, and lack of spread to other areas of the body.

Co-contraction or synergy is another characteristic phenomenon in UMN injury. Persons with anything more than very mild spasticity often find it difficult to isolate the movements of a single muscle. Thus, when they attempt to flex the fingers, they find that they can do this only while simultaneously activating other muscles of the upper extremity. Most commonly in the upper extremity, finger flexion is accompanied by flexion at the wrist or elbow as well as internal rotation and adduction of the shoulder. Voluntary movements in the limbs can also be accompanied by contraction of trunk muscles, in the patient may often assume a twisted or flexed truncal posture. Notable but less troublesome are mirror movements, which are simultaneous movements of the same muscles on the contralateral side of the body. These are thought to represent changes in central motor function in response to acquired nervous-system injury.

Other causes of abnormal muscle tone can coexist with hypertonia owing to spasticity. Most troublesome and difficult to treat is dystonia, which is the simultaneous contraction of agonist and antagonist muscles. These contractions can be quite painful, and can thus exacerbate the hypertonia owing to spasticity. The combination of spasticity and dystonia can be the most challenging aspect of the clinical care of the patient.

Negative Symptoms of the UMN Syndrome

Weakness usually accompanies spastic hypertonia. Early after the injury, there is often a period of flaccidity, typically accompanied by areflexia. In persons with spinal cord injury, this is often referred to as "spinal shock" and in those with cerebrovascular disease, "cerebral shock." Regardless of cause, this period of flaccidity lasts from a few hours to a few weeks and then typically evolves into the hypertonic spastic syndrome.

Slowness and incoordination of voluntary movements are common complaints in persons with partially preserved motor function. It is important to remember that slowness and incoordination are not owing to the passive resistance to movement of spasticity, but rather the incomplete and disordered activation of motor units of UMN injury. In most cases, this condition is not treatable. One important exception can be when opposing muscle groups are unequally affected by spasticity (imbalance). For example, in the case when finger extensor tone is so severe that weekend finger flexors cannot overcome the resistance that the finger extensors generate, selective weakening of those finger extensors may allow the patient to develop a usable grip.

Fatigue is also a common complaint of persons with spasticity. Some of this may be because of the increased energy expenditures required to accomplish tasks such as walking or other motor activities. Some may be because of the mental fatigue associated with the requirement to more carefully consciously monitor movements. Patients, even those who seem to have made complete recovery from an UMN injury, often report that simple tasks require much more attention and concentration to accomplish. The contribution of decreased aerobic capacity because of reconditioning should not be overlooked. There may also be a central component, and the phenomenon of fatigue is particularly well known in multiple sclerosis (MS).

Clinical Consequences and Complications of Spasticity

While patients sometimes complain purely of stiffness in body parts affected by UMN injury, the hypertonia is typically embedded within multiple other phenomena.

Peripheral changes seen in the UMN syndrome may also contribute to the hypertonia of spasticity. The elastic and plastic properties of muscle also change with chronic spasticity, presumably making it more difficult for the patient with central weakness to execute muscle shortening and movement of a joint *(6)*. This change in the mechanical properties of the muscle can also contribute to examiner's perception of resistance to passive movement; it is not velocity-dependent.

Positioning of patients in braces, splints, and wheelchairs can be complicated by spastic hypertonia. The plantar flexor tone seen in the ankle may cause difficulties in proper seating of the heel into an ankle-foot orthosis. This tone may require the addition of unsightly straps or metal uprights, the use of more expensive custom-fitted orthoses, and even the use of expensive highly rigid materials such as carbon fiber. Spastic hypertonia may dictate the use of expensive, complex wheelchair seating systems simply to prevent further contracture or skin breakdown.

Skin breakdown can be common in persons with spastic hypertonia. Poor positioning in wheelchairs, splints, or while lying in bed may lead to skin breakdown over pressure points. Common pressure points include heels, malleolli, sacrum, greater trochanters, and elbows. Loss of range of motion may the associated with skin breakdown in intertriginous areas, particularly the groin and axilla.

Contracture, the permanent loss of range of motion of a joint, is made more likely by the presence of spastic hypertonia. Contractures are areas of stiffness and shortening of soft tissues caused by joint immobilization in severe spasticity, and they can develop within a few days of the onset of weakness *(7)*. Difficult, painful, and time-consuming range-of-motion exercises can discourage the patient's caregivers from fully executing the daily exercises necessary to prevent permanent loss of range of motion.

Changes in mechanical properties of muscle also occur with disuse and the muscle shortening typically seen in persons with spasticity. As the increased tone forces extremities into postures that allow chronic muscle shortening, certain changes in the mechanical and physiological properties occur. When a muscle is in a contracted position, the length of the sarcomeres shorten. Biomechanically, the muscle becomes less efficient because of the shortened lever arm.

UMN injuries do not often cause atrophy of the affected muscle groups. However, some disuse atrophy does occur within a few weeks of the injury. Atrophy may lead to poorly fitting braces and splints. Palpation of muscles often reveals some increased tautness in the affected muscle groups. Fasciculations are not present, but clonus often is.

Differential Diagnosis of Hypertonia

Extrapyramidal disease or injury can cause rigidity, a form of hypertonia that is not velocity-dependent. Both agonist and antagonist muscles are involved simultaneously, thus there is resistance to passive movement in all directions. In some cases, limbs passively placed in a new position may maintain that position; this is called waxy flexibility or lead-pipe rigidity.

Gegenhalten is a manifestation of corticospinal or extrapyramidal system injuries. In this case, spontaneous movements can be quite normal, but when the limb is touched or passively moved, the antagonist muscles stiffen in proportion to the force being applied.

Reflex muscle rigidity is usually seen in response to local pain or irritation. This condition manifests as a muscle involuntarily contracted in a sustained fashion. It can occur with any local injury, including injury to the muscle or soft tissue, cold, or arthritis.

Myotonia is an uncommon condition usually seen in inherited disorders such as myotonic dystrophy, paramyotonia, and myxedema. In this case, increased tone is seen as a result of voluntary contraction. In the "hand-grip" test, forceful squeezing of the finger flexors is followed by a very slow release of grip because the patient is unable to suppress muscle tone. A similar finding occurs if the muscle is struck with a reflex hammer: "percussion myotonia."

TREATMENT OF SPASTICITY

Goals of Treatment

The decision to treat spasticity should not be made lightly, and the need to prospectively specify the goals of treatment must be emphasized. All current treatments for spasticity entail costs in time, money, effort, or side effects. The clinician must be realistic about the ability of current treatments to improve the patient's complaints. To prevent misunderstanding, the limitations of current treatments should be reviewed with the patient before initiation.

The available data suggest that current treatments act primarily to ameliorate the positive symptoms of spasticity, including flexor spasms, passive resistance, and clonus. For patients whose symptoms concern primarily the positive symptoms of the UMN syndrome, current treatments can often bring relief, albeit at the price of significant side effects. For example, if the patient is having difficulty with nursing care or positioning of the limb owing to spasticity, then it is appropriate to attempt to decrease the spasticity to prevent complications such as contractures. Treatment of spasticity is also indicated if the patient is experiencing pain owing to spasticity or flexor spasms.

Frequently, the patient presents requesting improvements in the "negative" symptoms of the UMN syndrome, such as weakness and incoordination, which are not clearly related to hypertonia alone. One misconception about the weakness and incoordination seen with the UMN syndrome is that much of it is because of hypertonia, and that if the hypertonia were reduced, the patient would gain improved function. At best, this notion is controversial; most data suggests that weakness is owing to poor activation of motor units, not resistance of muscle to movement caused by hyperactivity of the stretch reflex *(8)*.

Control of Flexor Spasms

Flexor spasms are involuntary muscle contractions that are often painful. They occur in 15–60% of spinal-cord-injury patients, but also occur (less dramatically) in persons with cerebral injuries. The spasms of spinal-cord injury are said to respond better to certain treatments, particularly baclofen, than does spasticity of cerebral origin.

Facilitate Range-of-Motion Exercises and Splinting

One important reason to treat the passive resistance to stretch is to facilitate range-of-motion exercises. Range-of-motion exercises are important in preventing contracture, and anything that helps the patient execute these exercises can minimize or prevent the onset of contracture. Stretching may also decrease tone, at least for a few hours. Many people with spasticity encounter pain as a limiting factor in cooperating with range-of-motion exercises. Others find that simply getting the limb to relax to the point where stretching can actually begin is quite frustrating; people with acquired brain injuries often have low tolerance for frustration. Thus, interventions that reduce passive resistance can lead to better patient compliance with range-of-motion exercises, thus preventing the complications of contracture.

The goal of splinting is preservation of range of motion by maintaining a joint in a stretched position for several hours. Typically, the brace is designed to position the limb so that the joint in question is in the anatomically neutral or, if voluntary movement is preserved, the most functional position. The effectiveness of the splint is dependent on its ability to maintain the extremity in the splint, and oftentimes, straps are required to keep the limb properly seated in the splint. Reduction of hypertonia or decreases in the frequency and severity of spasms will facilitate the use of such splints and casts. Reduction of tone will also decrease the likelihood of skin breakdown at pressure points and decrease the pain associated with maintaining a prolonged stretch.

Appearance

Many persons with UMN injury object to some of the appearance changes associated with the UMN injury. In particular, ambulatory persons with UMN involvement of the arm often find that as they walk or engage in some other physical exertion, their arm will passively flex at the elbow. Some of these people feel that this passive flexion of the arm draws attention to their disability, and will request treatment for prevention. Both the clinician and the patient must consider risks and benefits of treatment.

Clinical Features

CONSIDERATIONS IN TREATMENT

Systemic vs Local Treatment

One major choice the clinician faces is the use of local vs systemic treatments. Local treatments are those directed at a specific muscle or nerve. These local treatments include botulinum toxin, phenol neurolysis, or alcohol neurolysis. These local treatments avoid systemic side effects such as sedation or confusion, hepatoxicity, or diffuse weakness. Local treatments can also be preferred when there are focal imbalances of agonist and antagonist muscle tone, or where intervention is desired on only a few muscles. Systemic medications have the advantage of affecting large areas, and are therefore useful in treating widespread conditions such as paraplegia or hemiplegia. Duration of action is shorter, in that systemic medications are fully metabolized within a few days.

Team Approach

Only rarely can spasticity be clinically managed by a single clinician, because the condition usually requires the skills of several disciplines, not to mention the cooperation of the patient and family. While the diagnosis and pharmacologic management of spasticity is initiated by the physician, other interventions will be initiated by therapists, nurses, and others. Management of splints, wheelchair seating, bladder-training protocols, and assistive technology will all be executed by nonphysicians.

Timing of Treatment

Treatment choice will often depend on the length of time the spasticity has been present. Early after a precipitating injury, the motor exam is often changing quite rapidly. The patient's needs in spasticity treatment are also changing quite rapidly. Thus, investing in expensive carbon-fiber braces in the first few weeks after a stroke or spinal-cord injury may not be the best use of resources. Similarly, the use of invasive treatments, including implanted baclofen pump or other surgical procedures, is rarely warranted in the first few months.

On the other hand, even persons months or years out from their injury may have changes in their spastic hypertonia that will require changes in their treatment. Spastic hypertonia can increase over time, requiring treatment that is more aggressive.

Why Not to Treat

Sedation is the most common side effect of oral medication for spasticity. Many persons with spastic hypertonia find that the sedation associated with most of the oral medications adversely affects their ability to function and leads to an overall reduction in their quality of life. In particular, persons with cerebral injuries are particularly prone to sedation. Dosages of medication must be quite low at first, often below the therapeutic threshold, and can only be increased slowly. Paradoxical agitation or confusion can result from mild to moderate sedation, limiting the total dosage. In such cases, peripherally acting treatments may be the best choice. Dantrolene is less sedating than the centrally acting benzodiazepines or gamma-amino butyric acid (GABA) agonists. Another attractive choice when sedation limits dosing is botulinum toxin.

Weakness is another common adverse event. Weakness is usually dose-dependent, and is particularly prone to occur with dantrolene. Of course, botulinum toxin has as its mode of action the weakening of muscles; generally the duration of toxin-induced weakness is several weeks to several months.

Cost of treatment can range from the rather inexpensive dantrolene or diazepam to the extremely expensive botulinum toxin. Particularly early after injury when motor function is changing rapidly, expenditures on expensive positioning devices or wheelchairs can be difficult to justify. Later, in the chronic phase, resources to pay for the newer, more expensive interventions may be lacking. Many persons requiring treatment for spastic hypertonia have chronic neurologic disease, and may have few resources to pay for on-going daily, expensive medications. The cost of treatments such as intrathecal baclofen can run into the tens of thousands of US dollars each year. The physician must consider the benefits of treatment and for the alternative uses of these resources.

Hepatotoxicity is particularly associated with tizanidine and dantrolene. Particularly as doses escalate, regular monitoring of liver function must be maintained. In particular, the cerebrally injured patient on anticonvulsants and the hyperlipidemic person on HMGCoA reductase inhibitors should be regularly monitored.

Incontinence can result from systemic treatment of spasticity. Some persons maintain their continence through the maintenance of sphincter tone. The use of systemic drugs to reduce tone may adversely affect sphincter tone, causing or worsening incontinence.

Not All Spasticity is Bad

Some consequences of spasticity can be useful. For example, in many persons with stroke, the weak affected leg is transformed into a "cane" by the extensor tone of spasticity. The use of this "cane" allows for transfers and ambulation. The flexed, adducted position of the hemiplegic arm keeps the arm in a safer position; the position also moves the arm closer to the center of gravity, improving balance.

Clinical Features 23

An even more dramatic example occurs in persons with paraplegia. Some paraplegics tap or pinch their thighs and groin to induce extensor spasms in their legs so that they can use their legs as "pillars of support." This maneuver allows the patient to bear weight for transfers even in the absence of voluntary leg-muscle activity. Abolishing such spasms would make the patient less mobile, not more.

Ablation of this tone will lead to the loss of the ability to transfer or ambulate. Similarly, persons with bladder-sphincter spasm may rely on that spasm to remain dry. Use of medications like dantrolene, which can cause sphincter weakness, may lead to urinary dribbling or incontinence where none existed before.

TREATMENT

Treatment options for spasticity will be discussed in detail throughout this volume, and only a bird's eye view will be described here.

A methodical, step-wise approach works well. Serial examination of the patient is essential. Tone can vary with position, and the patient should be examined in the same position at each assessment. An objective or semi-objective endpoint to assess treatment effect is helpful: such measurable things as range of motion, spasm frequency, pain scales, ability to seat properly in a brace or splint, or the Ashworth scale. Follow-up in the office or by telephone should be regular, and more frequent when treatment is being altered. Reports from caregivers are particularly important in persons with cerebral causes of spasticity who are cognitively impaired.

Exacerbating conditions should be treated aggressively. The first line of defense against spasticity is to remove those factors that exacerbate it. Table 2 outlines common exacerbators of spastic hypertonia. A careful history and physical examination can often elicit modifiable factors to improve the patient's clinical status. Perhaps the most common is pain, often related to the musculoskeletal complications of hypertonia. Contractures, prolonged positioning without frequent position changes, poorly fitting braces, and pressure points are all common causes of pain. Central pain syndromes can also contribute to exacerbating spasticity, and treatment of the syndromes can often reduce the symptomatic complaints of spastic hypertonia.

Wounds and infection can also worsen spastic hypertonia. Wounds owing to skin breakdown or other causes can increase hypertonia and spasms. Areas of skin breakdown or former intravenous catheter sites should be examined for infection. Urinary-tract infections are very common in persons with UMN injury, and often act to worsen hypertonia. Systemic infections, such as pneumonia or intra-abdominal infections, can worsen tone and spasms, and should be searched for carefully, particularly persons with quadriplegia

Table 2
Non-neurological Exacerbators of Spastic Hypertonia

Pain
Fatigue
Anxiety
Wounds
Fractures
Systemic infection
Ingrown toenail
Heterotopic ossification
Urinary retention
Constipation
Intra-abdominal processes:
    infection, obstruction, ischemia, inflammation

who may not be able to localize the location of infection. Similarly, other intra-abdominal processes such as constipation, gallbladder disease, urolithiasis, or intestinal obstruction can worsen spasticity.

Many patients report increases in tone, spasm, or clonus when they are tired or anxious. Most patients benefit from regular rest; advocates of complementary therapies also advocate relaxation regimens, meditation, and acupuncture.

Physical medicine and positioning interventions are a mainstay in the treatment of spasticity. Frequent and careful stretching maintains range of motion, reduces edema, and is said to reduce tone for several hours. Because of the temporary nature of stretching, further treatment is also instituted in most cases. Splints are used to preserve range of motion by maintaining anatomic position of joints for hours at a time. "Tone reducing" splints have not been systematically evaluated for efficacy superior to that of conventional splinting, but may play a role in certain individuals. Careful wheelchair seating minimizes pain and skin breakdown and therefore prevents exacerbation of spastic hypertonia. Cold compresses and ice bags are traditional treatments for tone, but probably useful only during therapy sessions in which range-of-motion exercises are performed. They may also be helpful for short-term exacerbations, but not longer-term management.

Systemic medications are useful for persons who do not respond to more conservative treatment, particularly persons with spinal-cord involvement. There are four major drugs used currently for spasticity management and each will be discussed elsewhere in detail. One of these, dantrolene, acts in the muscle membrane to decrease the force of muscle contraction. The other commonly used drugs, baclofen, diazepam, and tizanidine, work centrally.

Baclofen has been proven effective in spinal forms of spasticity where it reduces the frequency of flexor spasms and the pain caused by them. Diazepam is similarly effective but has the drawback of sedation in many patients. Tizanadine has similar efficacy to baclofen, and has the advantage of not causing weakness in clinical trials to date. Other drugs are occasionally still used for tone control, including anticonvulsants, antiarrhythmics, and clonidine. However, these second-line drugs have for the most part been replaced by tizanidine and botulinum toxin.

Intramuscular botulinum toxin and phenol neurolysis are useful for reducing tone in small numbers of specific muscles. They are not helpful for large-scale tone reduction in hemiplegia or paraplegia; systemic medications are cheaper, easier, and more effective. However, when the correction of a specific muscle imbalance can improve function, these interventions come to the fore. For example, an occasional patient will have persistent voluntary finger flexion, but this flexion is unable to overcome the spastic finger extensors. In such a case, selective weakening of the finger extensors may restore a gross grasp. For persons with inversion and plantar flexion posturing of the ankle, weakening of ankle invertors and plantar flexors may improve toe clearance and prevent "pistoning" of the heel out of an ankle brace.

Intrathecal medications are becoming more commonly used with the advent of implantable-pump technology and the demonstration of the effectiveness of intrathecal baclofen (ITB) in spinal-cord causes of spasticity. Use in persons with acquired brain injury such as traumatic brain injury or stroke is less well-studied, but is used occasionally by clinicians. Reserved for persons who fail oral medications and local interventions, intrathecal therapy requires a high level of commitment for monthly refills, monitoring for are infection, and adequate pump function.

Surgical procedures, especially dorsal rhizotomy, are being increasingly utilized, though data from randomized, controlled trials of these treatments are sketchy.

REFERENCES

1. Lance, J. W. (1980) *Symposium Synopsis*. Mosby, St. Louis.
2. Mayer, N. H, Esquenazi, A., and Childers, M. K. (1997) Common patterns of clinical motor dysfunction. *Muscle Nerve* **20,** S21–S35.
3. Landau, W. F. (1969) Spasticity and Rigidity, in *Recent Advances in Neurology* (Plum F., ed.), F. A. Davis, Philadelphia pp. 1–32.
4. Burke, D. (1988) Spasticity as an adaptation to pyramidal tract injury, in *Functional Recovery in Neurological Disease* (Waxman, S. G., ed.), Raven Press, New York, pp. 401–423.

5. Haerer, A. F. (1992) Corticospinal (pyramidal) tract responses, in *The Neurological Examination* 5th ed. J.B. Lippincott Company, Philadelphia, pp. 453–464.
6. Huffschmidt, A. and Mauritz, K. H. (1985) Chronic transformation of muscle in spasticity: a peripheral contribution to increased muscle tone. *J. Neurol. Neurosurg. Psychiatry* **48,** 676–685.
7. O'Dwyer, N. J., Ada, L., and Neilson, P. D. (1996) Spasticity and muscle contracture following stroke. *Brain* **119,** 1737–1749.
8. Sahrmann, S. A. and Norton, B. J. (1977) The relationship of voluntary movement to spasticity in the upper motor neuron syndrome. *Ann. Neurol.* **2,** 460–465.

3
Measurement of Spasticity

David C. Good

INTRODUCTION

Spasticity is generally defined as velocity-dependent increased resistance during passive movement of peripheral joints owing to increased involuntary muscle activity. However, the word spasticity is clinically used to describe a constellation of symptoms that arise secondary to the upper motor neuron (UMN) syndrome associated with a wide variety of neurological conditions. The clinically observed components of spasticity include increased resistance to passive movement, increased phasic-stretch reflexes, clonus, and flexor or extensor spasms (1–3). These features of spasticity clearly can impede functional motor activities. However, the UMN syndrome includes other important components including weakness, co-contraction of agonist and antagonist muscles, the presence of "pattern" movements (mass contraction of groups of muscles across joints when isolated movements are attempted), and lack of fine motor control. These other components of the UMN syndrome usually contribute more to motor impairment than spasticity. Spasticity is actually beneficial in certain situations. For example, increased extensor tone may facilitate standing in some patients. Theoretical benefits of spasticity include maintenance of muscle mass, reduction of edema, decreased risk of deep venous thrombosis (DVT), and prevention of bone demineralization in weakened extremities (1).

Spasticity is seen in neurological conditions affecting the UMN anywhere from the cerebral cortex to the spinal cord. Depending on the location of the neurological lesion, spasticity may accompany hemiparesis, paraparesis, or tetraparesis. Because spasticity can be associated with so many clinical conditions, has different components, and may vary in severity among individual patients, it is difficult to define in a comprehensive fashion. To complicate matters, the neurobiology of motor systems and the actual pathogenesis of spasticity remain somewhat of a mystery. There is a general consensus that the segmental spinal-reflex arc is a key underlying factor in many of the clinical manifestations of spasticity. Changes in alpha-motoneuron excitability and in spinal segmental-reflex function are widely thought to be caused by alterations in descending modulating pathways, including the dorsal reticulospinal tract and descending monaminergic pathways originating in the locus ceruleus *(4)*. The underlying mechanisms and the clinical characteristics of spasticity vary according to the causative disorder and location of the lesion *(2)*.

Spasticity must also be differentiated from rigidity *(2)*. Both include involuntary increase in muscle tone, but spasticity generally occurs only during muscle stretch (i.e., not at rest) and is usually accompanied by increased tendon reflexes and a Babinski's response. The relative resistance to passive movement usually differs when agonist and antagonist muscle groups across the same joint are stretched. In rigidity, muscle tone is increased even at rest, and tends to be present during passive range of motion in all directions across individual joints. The plantar reflex and tendon reflexes are usually normal. The prototype disease-causing rigidity is Parkinson's disease (PD). To complicate matters, some patients with the UMN syndrome exhibit features of rigidity. In fact, some muscles in the same limb may behave as though they are spastic, where others may appear rigid *(2)*. Thus, some patients with spasticity do have increased muscle tone at rest. In many persons with hemiplegia, the upper limb is held flexed and adducted, and the lower limb is extended. With paraplegia or tetraplegia, the lower limbs are flexed and adducted, as are the upper limbs, if they are affected *(2)*.

In summary, there is no single cause or single clinical manifestation of spasticity. Therefore, it is not surprising that no unitary measure of spasticity has gained complete acceptance.

Despite the multiple causes and manifestations of spasticity, and the fact that some aspects of spasticity can be beneficial to individual patients, the composite syndrome often has deleterious motor consequences. Flexion or extension spasms may interfere with transfers and clonus may cause loss of balance or slow gait. Flexor or extensor spasms of the lower extremities (and less often the upper extremities) may interfere with activities of daily living, including dressing and toileting. The relative imbalance of muscle groups across joints may result in abnormal positioning of limbs, which in turn impairs mobility. For example, excessive plantar flexor tone may contribute to foot drop during the swing phase of gait, and impair "push-off" at the end of the stance phase. Activities of daily living may be affected. Excessive adduction of the hips or flexion of the hip or knee may hinder dressing or toileting. Adduction and pronation of the shoulder, or flexion of the elbow, wrist, and fingers may impair dressing and other upper-extremity activities.

Measurement of Spasticity

Hygiene can be an issue in persons with excessive contraction of shoulder adductors and finger flexors. A frequent complaint is spasms or clonus in the legs preventing sleep. Imbalance of agonists and antagonists across joints also predisposes to fixed contractures and pressure ulcers.

COMPLICATING FACTORS IN THE MEASUREMENT OF SPASTICITY

As mentioned earlier, the clinical components of spasticity vary according to the causative factor and location of the lesion within the nervous system. However, many other factors contribute to the variability of spasticity, making it difficult to quantify. Clinicians are familiar with the temporal sequence of the development of spasticity following acute injury to the nervous system. With spinal cord conditions, the term "spinal shock" is widely used. After acute spinal-cord injury, muscle tone and reflexes are initially hypoactive, and features of the spasticity syndrome develop slowly over time. The same phenomenon is also seen with acute lesions of the brain, such as hemiparesis following stroke. Therefore, the severity of spasticity often depends on the time it is measured following the initial event.

Even in chronic conditions, there is considerable inter-individual and intra-individual variability. Among patients with similar degrees of weakness, the severity of tone, spasms, and clonus may vary considerably. A small percentage of patients following stroke (and to a lesser extent, spinal-cord injury) remain permanently flaccid. In a single individual, the manifestations of spasticity are affected by many factors. The position of the body or limb is an important variable. Environmental factors such as ambient temperature and time of day may also affect the severity of spasticity. Passive stretching of affected limbs usually results in decreased muscle tone and spasms for several hours. Increased fatigue, or increased body temperature (for example, associated with fever) frequently increase muscle tone and spasms. Finally, a common cause of increased spasticity is an acute nociceptive stimulus. Acute DVT, fracture, cellulitis, acute arthritis, sprains, pressure ulcers, and a host of other medical problems can worsen spasticity. In persons with spinal-cord dysfunction, spasticity can be aggravated by urinary-tract infections, renal or bladder calculi, fecal impaction, and acute abdominal conditions. Clinicians caring for persons with chronic neurological conditions should undertake a careful search for an underlying condition when an individual's spasticity worsens.

Even in chronic patients with no aggravating factors, spasticity may vary in severity. It is best to assess spasticity in a reproducible environment. For an assessment of spasticity to be reliable over time in the same individual, measurement should occur the same time of day, in the same position, and with the same degree of fatigue. It is best to avoid measuring spasticity shortly after a period of prolonged therapeutic stretching, unless the goal of measurement is to determine the effectiveness of this therapy.

REASONS TO MEASURE SPASTICITY

Some components of the spasticity syndrome are also useful diagnostically during a general physical examination. The presence of clonus, hyperreflexia, mass spasms, and alterations of muscle tone are useful components of the neurological examination to help localize and diagnose lesions of the central nervous system (CNS). However, by far the most important reason to measure spasticity is to assess the effectiveness of a therapeutic intervention.

From a clinical perspective, quantification of spasticity is necessary to evaluate the effectiveness of stretching and physical-therapy programs, oral medications, botulinum toxin injections, intrathecal baclofen (ITB) therapy, or any of the other commonly employed treatments for the spasticity syndrome. This is especially important for pharmacological management, where the dose of oral medication or rate of ITB infusion depends primarily on the objective measurement of muscle tone or spasm frequency.

Appropriate measures for spasticity are also important from a research perspective to better understand the underlying pathophysiologic mechanisms associated with spasticity, and to assess the effectiveness of new potentially beneficial treatments.

Spasticity may be evaluated clinically, or through the use of laboratory tests *(3)*. Clinical evaluation is usually quick, simple, and can be carried out in any environment. Laboratory assessment usually requires special equipment, but has the advantage of quantifying subtle manifestations, and can provide information regarding underlying pathophysiological mechanisms. Laboratory evaluation can be loosely grouped into biochemical and electrophysiologic techniques, although some types of evaluations utilize both. Although sophisticated testing may seem to be an improvement over clinical evaluations, the results do not correlate well with patients' signs and symptoms *(2)*.

ROUTINE CLINICAL EVALUATION OF SPASTICITY

As mentioned, part of the evaluation of spasticity occurs during performance of the general neurological examination. Strength is generally tested using the Medical Research Council (MRC) scale. Many persons with spasticity have superimposed weakness, and this is often the major factor causing disability. Knowledge of strength may therefore affect treatment decisions for spasticity. The deep tendon reflexes are commonly graded from 0

Table 1
Ashworth Scale

Grade	Description
0	No increase
1	Slight increase producing a catch when joint is moved in flexion or extension
2	More marked, but joint easily flexed
3	Considerable increase, and passive movement difficult
4	Affected part rigid in flexion or extension

(absent) to 4 (clonus). Strength and reflexes are both tested in the upper and lower extremities. Muscle tone is tested by asking the individual to relax, and passively moving individual joints. Spasticity should be differentiated from rigidity, but as previously mentioned, the two may co-exist. In persons with spasticity, there is usually a difference between resistance in one direction of movement as compared to the opposite direction. In addition, when a joint is moved rapidly, a "spastic catch" owing to activation of the phasic-stretch reflex is often felt. Some persons with spasticity exhibit the "clasped knife" phenomenon, where resistance is perceived through most of passive range of motion, but a sudden "release" is felt towards the end of range. Although described as a classic sign associated with spasticity, it is often lacking.

A great deal can be learned about the clinical effects of spasticity by watching the patient during functional activities. Do sudden movements precipitate mass spasms or clonus, compromising transfers or bed mobility? Does abnormal joint position owing to imbalance between agonist and antagonist muscles affect positioning, activities of daily living (ADLs), or ambulation? Observations of this nature may yield information highly relevant to the patient in everyday life.

For assessing the effect of treatment, more quantitative measures are often needed. The Ashworth scale is the most widely used semiquantitative clinical scale to assess spasticity (*see* Table 1). Ratings are based on the examiner's subjective assessment of resistance experienced when muscles are passively lengthened. The Ashworth scale was first developed in 1964 as a tool to assess the effectiveness of a drug to treat spasticity associated with multiple sclerosis (MS) *(5)*. As originally described, it is an ordinal scale that assesses muscle tone from 0 (no increase in tone) to 4 (affected part rigid in flexion or extension). It has been modified by the addition of an additional category between 1 and 2 (*see* Table 2) *(6)*. The Modified Ashworth

Table 2
Modified Ashworth Scale

Grade	Description
0	No increase in muscle tone.
1	Slight increase in muscle tone, manifested by a catch and release, or by minimal resistance at the end of the range of motion when the affected part(s) is moved in flexion or extension.
1+	Slight increase in muscle tone, manifested by a catch, followed by minimal resistance throughout the remainder (less than half) of the range of movement (ROM).
2	More marked increase in muscle tone through most of the ROM, but affected part(s) easily moved.
3	Considerable increase in muscle tone, passive movement difficult.
4	Affected part(s) rigid in flexion or extension.

scale has reasonably good inter-rater reliability for elbow flexors *(6)*, as well as a variety of other muscles in the upper and lower extremities *(7,8)*. Simultaneous Ashworth measurements and electromyography (EMG) showed positive correlation between Ashworth score and various EMG parameters *(9)*. Although it is quite subjective and divides spasticity into rather broad categories of increased tone, the Modified Ashworth scale has become the "gold standard" for semi-quantitative clinical assessment of spasticity, having been used in multiple trials of spasticity treatment *(10–13)*. A cumulative Ashworth score can also be calculated, and is the sum of individual scores for flexion and extension at major joints of each extremity. A score can be calculated for each limb, or a combination of limbs. Although the Ashworth scale is easy to obtain in a clinical setting, it is subjective and more or less dependent on the evaluator. Also, increased resistance to passive movement can be reflex-mediated (reflex hyperexcitability) and/or nonreflex-mediated (soft-tissue resistance). These are not differentiated by the Ashworth scale, but this is an important issue, because different causes of increased resistance may require different treatments.

Another clinical scale that attempts to integrate spasticity with gross categories of movement is the Oswestry scale *(14,15)*. This scale contains an even greater degree of subjectivity than the Ashworth scale, and its validity and reliability have not been reported.

Another common way to clinically assess components of spasticity is to calculate a "spasm score" *(10,16)*. This is obtained by visually or electronically recording the number of spasms observed during a given period of time, usually 1 h (*see* Table 3). Spasms can be one of the most troublesome

Table 3
Spasm Frequency Scale

Score	Criteria
0	No spasms
1	No spontaneous spasms (except with vigorous motor stimulation)
2	Occasional spontaneous spasms and easily induced spasms
3	More than 1 but less than 10 spontaneous spasms per hour
4	More than 10 spontaneous spasms per hour

features of the spasticity syndrome, affecting functional activities, as well as preventing sleep. Therefore, measurement of the number of spasms is potentially important. The spasm score can be quite variable because the number of spasms is very much affected by position, activity, and many other factors. Nonetheless, it has been frequently used as one of the outcome measures for therapeutic trials of medications for spasticity *(10,11,13)*.

BIOMECHANICAL EVALUATION

A number of biomechanical methods to measure aspects of spasticity have been devised. Some are relatively simple, and others are quite sophisticated, measuring torque-angle relationships during passive and active movements.

The pendulum test is a relatively simple test that has been used to quantify spasticity in knee muscles *(17–19)*. It is tested with the subject sitting on an examining table. The foot is dropped from the position of full knee extension, and electrogoniometric recording of motion and oscillation is performed *(see* Fig. 1). The test depends on the assumption that when the extended spastic limb is dropped, it behaves like a linear damped pendulum *(18)*. Damping is contingent on the level of spasticity in the quadriceps muscles. Unfortunately, the movement of the leg is not strictly pendulum-like, because unequal contributions are provided by flexor and extensor muscles, and the limb may not necessarily oscillate about the vertical *(20,21)*. Also, the results of the test depend not only on spasticity, but also the intrinsic mechanical properties of the individual leg *(20)*. Soft-tissue changes, including changes in the joint and muscle length, may affect the results *(20,22)*. Microcomputer-based systems are now available to better quantify the pendulum test *(23)*. Using automated devices, maximum velocity and acceleration of the first downward phase in rebound can be measured, and several indices can be calculated. The most valuable is R_2, which measures the angular excursion of the pendulum swing of the dropped limb as a fraction of

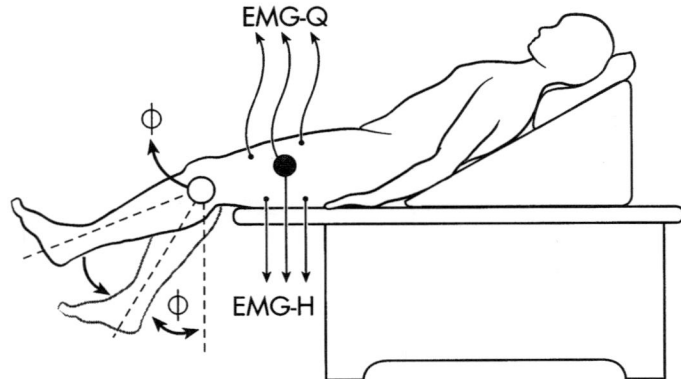

Fig. 1. Experimental set-up for the pendulum test for measuring spasticity at the knee joint. EMG-Q and EMG-H are recorded from the quadriceps and hamstrings bilaterally, and Ø is the knee angle.

the initial angle made by the suspended limb with the vertical *(23)*. If the swing overshoots the vertical, R_2 is greater than 1. If the swing is interrupted before the limb reaches the vertical, R_2 is less than 1, indicating spasticity (*see* Fig. 2). This measure has been used in several drug trials *(23)*. The pendulum test is able to distinguish between spasticity in hemiparetic patients and rigidity in patients with PD *(24)*.

Although the pendulum test has some intuitive appeal, and correlates with the Ashworth scale *(25,26)*, it requires technology not possessed by most clinicians *(26)*. Therefore, its value is greatest in a research setting.

Although the tendon reflexes are commonly assessed as part of the clinical evaluation, they are generally not quantified rigorously because of variations in tapping. To standardize the tendon jerk, investigators have developed instrumented hammers or have measured the impact force *(27,28)*. The amplitude of the associated limb motion, the muscle EMG, or the muscle-contraction force in response to tendon stretch can be measured *(3,29)*. The amplitude of the EMG response to tendon stimulation may be compared to the amplitude of the M-wave obtained in response to supramaximal motor-nerve stimulation as an estimate of the population of motor units activated by the stretch reflex *(3)*. When interpreting tendon jerk results in spasticity, it is important to note that large fluctuations occur in response to accurately quantified stimulation in normal individuals *(29)*. The position or angle of the joint as the tendon is struck is also an important variable that can affect results *(30)*. Zhang et al. *(28)* used an instrumented hammer to tap the patellar tendon. The tapping force was recorded and the quadriceps EMG and

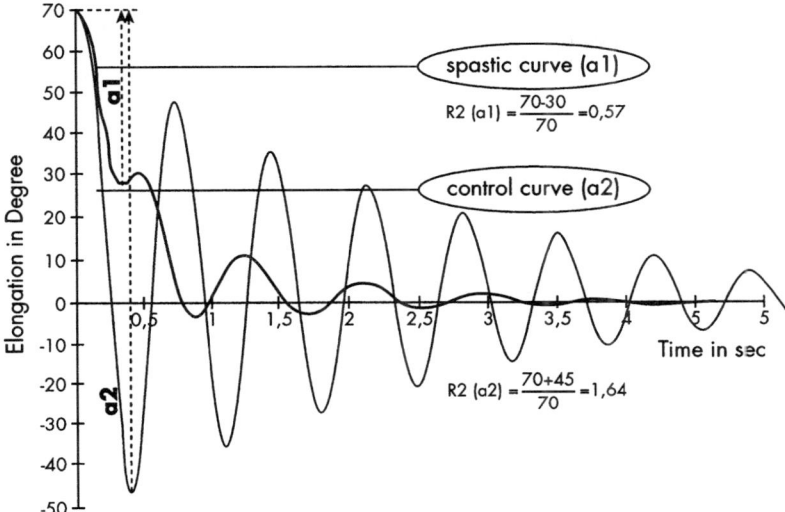

Fig. 2. Calculation of the index R_2 from the pendulum curve of a spastic and a normal leg. In the spastic leg, the first descending swing is interrupted by a quadriceps reflex (a_1) at 30°. In the normal leg there is an overswing to −45° (a_2). Calculation of R_2 is indicated in the two examples. Adapted with permission from ref. *(23)*.

knee-extension torque was recorded isometrically. A number of system measures were calculated including tendon reflex gain, contraction rate, reflex-loop delay, and threshold tapping force. Significant differences in these variables can be demonstrated between normal and spastic individuals. However, the technology involved in devices of this sort cannot be readily applied to the average clinical situation.

A number of mechanical recordings of muscle torque and angular stiffness have been used in the evaluation of spasticity (*see* Fig. 3) *(31–34)*. This technology utilizes sinusoidal analysis and Nyquist plots to characterize stiffness and viscosity in response to force applied across spastic joints. Zhang and colleagues have used similar technology to measure the relationship between muscle torque and joint angle at different velocities of movement *(35–37)*. Mechanical recording of this type requires even more complex equipment and therefore such techniques have been relegated to research laboratories.

The problem with all biomechanical spasticity measures is that they do not readily differentiate between reflex and intrinsic (soft tissue) contributions to muscle tone. Many authors feel that changes in both reflex and

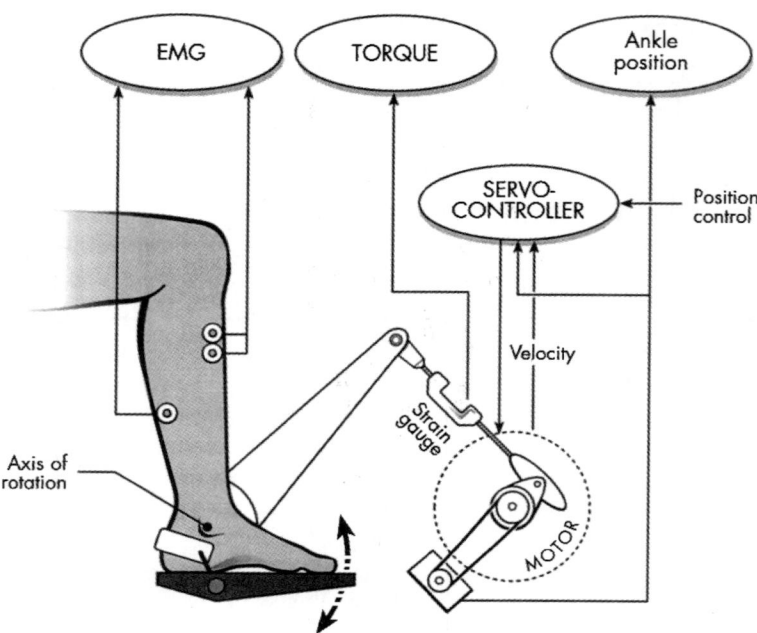

Fig. 3. Experimental set-up to measure torque, ankle position, and EMG activity in response to movement of the ankle joint by an applied external force. Torque is measured from a strain-gauge mounted on the arm from the pedal to the motor shaft. A potentiometer to measure ankle position is mounted on a separate shaft in connection with the motor shaft. Surface electrodes are used to measure EMG activity from the anterior tibialis and triceps surae muscles.

intrinsic mechanical stiffness are responsible for the increased resistance to passive movement in spastic limbs. Complex devices like those just described can provide important insights into research issues related to this topic *(35,37–40)*. Another example of the importance of this technology to research is the demonstration that resistance to stretch varies dramatically between passive conditions and during active spastic-muscle contractions, a finding that could have significant clinical ramifications *(41)*.

Although not practical in a general clinical setting, biochemical devices using sinusoidal movements to study torque-angle-EMG relationships have been used as tools to measure the effects of drug and other treatment approaches in patients with spasticity *(33,42)*.

ELECTROPHYSIOLOGICAL EVALUATION

Surface EMG recordings have long been used to quantify muscle contractions associated with spasticity *(43–45)*. Raw EMG signals are usually averaged and rectified for analysis. Simultaneous recordings are often made from multiple muscles, including agonist and antagonist groups. The onset and duration of contraction in response to a variety of self-initiated and induced movements may be recorded. Examples include muscle contraction in response to motor-nerve stimulation *(46–48)*, stimulation of sensory nerves *(49)*, or stimulation of the skin *(50)*. Novel techniques include calculating the vector sum of EMG magnitudes, and the index of EMG focus, a measure of the range of EMG activation recorded for each load level *(51)*. The tonic vibratory reflex is another quantifiable measure of muscle activation that is obtained when a vibrator is applied over a tendon or muscle *(3)*.

A variety of abnormal patterns of EMG activation have been described in persons with spasticity. These include inefficient muscle activation with abnormal EMG-force relationships, disturbances of spatial selection of muscles, and alterations in the time-course of EMG activation in agonist and antagonist muscles *(4)*.

Perhaps the most widely used electrophysiologic methods for evaluating spasticity is dynamic multichannel EMG, using gait-lab technology. Several variations of gait labs have been developed. They usually include multichannel EMG recording, and also simultaneously measure force and joint angles of the lower extremities during movement *(see* Fig. 4) *(52,53)*. Using video analysis, important clinical gait parameters such as cadence, velocity, and stride length are determined. Force plates record ground reaction forces. Although complex, gait-lab technology has found some clinical usefulness in planning surgery for children with cerebral palsy *(54,55)*.

The Hoffman or H-reflex is another electrophysiologic measure used to measure spasticity *(see* Fig. 5) *(1,3,56,57)*. The H-reflex is obtained by stimulating a peripheral nerve, eliciting a spinal monosynaptic reflex, and recording the resultant reflex compound muscle-action potential from a target distal muscle using an EMG electrode. A commonly measured H-reflex is obtained by stimulating the tibial nerve in popliteal fossa, eliciting a reflex response in the triceps surae muscle. The H-reflex is essentially an electrically elicited tendon jerk *(3)*. The concept is intuitively appealing, and is based on the assumption that in spastic patients, a greater percentage of the "lower motor neuron pool" can be activated reflexly by stimulating a peripheral nerve. The H-reflex is generally compared with the maximum muscle response obtained by direct supramaximal stimulation of the same nerve,

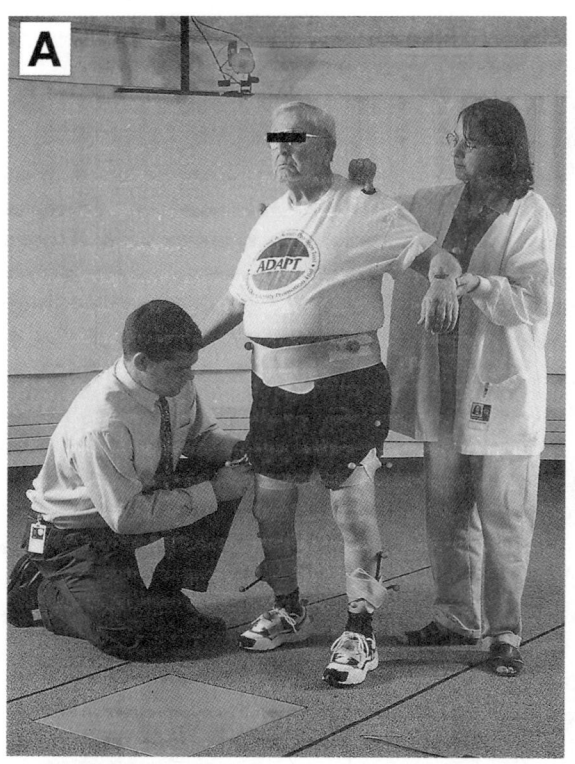

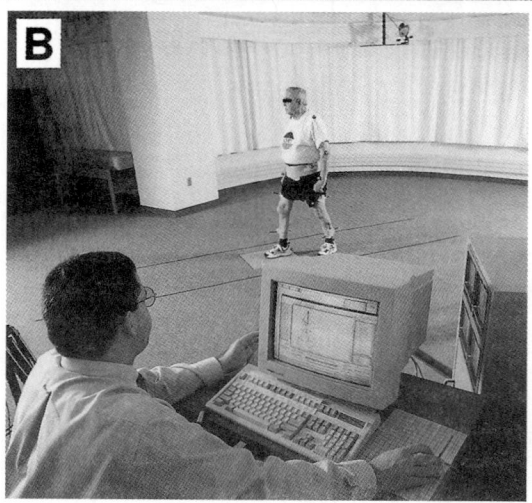

Fig. 4. (A) Markers being applied to subject in gait lab will be used to track limb and trunk position during ambulation. Note video camera and force plate on floor. **(B)** Gait analysis while subject ambulates down walkway. EMG is not being recorded on this subject.

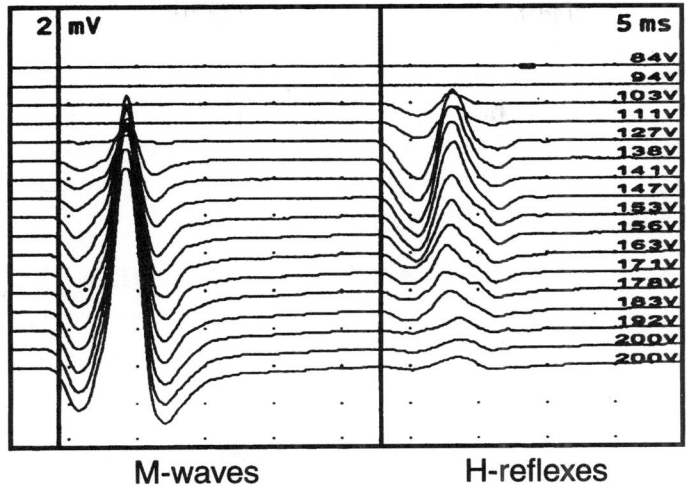

Fig. 5. Example of H-reflex recorded from a normal individual: Posterior tibial nerve H-reflexes (longer latencies responses) are recorded from the left soleus muscle using a square wave impulse of 0.2 ms during and increasing voltage stimuli. The responses are rastered from top to bottom as the voltage intensity increases. Note that the H-reflex appears at the third stimulation, increases in amplitude, and then disappears as the intensity increases further. The M-wave (shorter latency response) arises at the fifth stimulation and continues to increase in size as the stimulus intensity increases. Figure courtesy of Dr. Peter Donofrio, Department of Neurology, Wake Forest University Baptist Medical Center, Winston-Salem, NC.

recording over the same distal target muscle *(58)*. The H/M ratio is obtained by dividing the respective amplitudes. The H/M ratio tends to be higher in spastic patients with hyperactive tendon jerks *(1)*. Unfortunately, there is a wide range of normal values, and considerable overlap between the results obtained in persons with spasticity and normal individuals *(59)*. Another problem is that the H-reflex can be recorded easily only from a limited number of muscle groups *(3)*. The major usefulness of the H/M ratio is following individual patients serially over time *(60)*, especially in clinical trials evaluating the effectiveness of a specific intervention. Variations of the H reflex have been proposed *(1,56)*. For example, the H reflex is suppressed by vibration, presumably because the effect of Ia afferents is less in individuals with spasticity *(1)*. Again, this technique has been most useful in following the effects of treatment in individual subjects over time. The H reflex can also be suppressed by a "conditioning" nerve stimulus administered at 5–500 ms intervals before the H reflex stimulus *(1,3,56,61)*. In individuals with spasticity, inhibition of the H reflex by the conditioning shock is of shorter duration than in normal subjects *(1)*. This technique is referred to as the H reflex recovery curve *(1,3,56)*. As with other variations of the H reflex, calculation of the H reflex recovery curve is tedious, and is not practical for measuring spasticity in the clinical setting.

Finally, F-waves have been used to evaluate α-motoneuron excitability. This measure is not very robust, since the amplitude of the F-wave is only 1% of the amplitude of the M-wave, and multiple stimuli are required *(1,62)*.

RELEVANCE TO OTHER CLINICAL-OUTCOME MEASURES

Spasticity may certainly result in impaired function *(1,63)*. For example, spasticity can predispose to contracture, which can impede nursing care, positioning, or hygiene, or interfere with activities of daily living. In addition voluntary movements may be affected by hyperexcitable stretch reflexes or mass spasms in some patients *(64,65)*. Although these may be significant problems, the question often arises whether spasticity significantly affects overall function as reflected in commonly used measurement tools of functional abilities such as the Barthel Index (BI) or Functional Independence Measure (FIM). Although these are valid and useful measures of general functioning (particularly ADLs), they are global measures that include a wide variety of individual activities. Mild-to-moderate spasticity, although affecting specific functions, generally does not significantly influence these scales. Scales more specifically designed to measure motor abilities, for example the Fugl-Meyer scale, are more likely to correlate with increased muscle tone *(17)*. When using outcome scales to assess the effectiveness of the treatment of spasticity in individuals or groups, it is important to use a measurement tool that will be significantly affected by the components of spasticity. Quality of life can be a very abstract term that reflects a wide variety of domains. It is even less likely that spasticity would be reflected in measures of quality of life. Occasional studies have correlated changes in spasticity with quality of life, but they are relatively few *(12)*. However, quality of life is highly individualized, and the author recalls an avid golfer whose golf game deteriorated dramatically following a stroke. Although this individual was able to eventually develop a one-handed swing using his unaffected arm, he developed unwanted flexion synergy in his affected arm during his "follow-through." Local injection with botulinum toxin dramatically eliminated this problem, and the patient commented that this treatment improved his post-stroke quality of life more than any other intervention. Thus, in individual patients, treatment of spasticity can be extremely important, even when the effects of treatment can't be measured using standardized outcome assessments.

SUMMARY

The natural variability of spasticity across time and among individuals makes quantification difficult. No single measurement technique has been uniformly accepted. However, attempts at quantification are important to evaluate the efficacy of treatment in individual patients. For this purpose, a relatively simple clinical measure should suffice. The most widely used are the Modified Ashworth score, and the spasm score. For research trials, one of the many mechanical recordings of muscle torque or angular stiffness, or one of the electrophysiologic evaluation methods, such as the H reflex, can be used. For any measure of spasticity, the evaluator should be aware that increased muscle stiffness may be due to a combination of intrinsic properties of the muscle and joint as well as from increased muscle-stretch reflexes. These components are difficult to separate clinically, but treatment may differ for each. In the future, a readily available clinical tool might assist in this differentiation, but at this time there is no practical solution to this problem. Finally, the evaluation and treatment of spasticity must always be kept in the context of functional outcomes, and a specific goal of treatment should be established. Spasticity does not always need to be treated, and therefore does not always need to be measured in great detail. Again, for routine clinical purposes, simple measurement tools are best.

REFERENCES

1. Little, J. W. and Massagli, T. L. (1993) Spasticity and associated abnormalities of muscle tone, in *Rehabilitation Medicine: Principles and Practice*. 2nd ed. (Delisa, J. A., ed.), JB Lippincott Company, Philadelphia, pp. 666–680.
2. Young, R. (1994) Spasticity: a review. *Neurology* **44(Suppl. 9),** S12–S20.
3. Dimitrijevic, M. R. (1995) Evaluation and treatment of spasticity. *J. Neuro. Rehabil.* **9,** 97–110.
4. Rymer, W. Z. and Katz, R. T. (1994) Mechanisms of spastic hypertonia, in *Physical Medicine and Rehabilitation: State of the Art Reviews,* vol. 8, Hanley & Belfus, Inc., Philadelphia, pp. 441–454.
5. Ashworth, B. (1964) Preliminary trial of carisoprodol in multiple sclerosis. *Practitioner* **192,** 540–542.
6. Bohannon, R. W. and Smith, M. B. (1987) Interater reliability of a Modified Ashworth Scale of muscle spasticity. *Phys. Ther.* **67,** 206–207.
7. Lee, K.-C., Carson, L., Kinnin, E., and Patterson, V. (1989) The Ashworth Scale: A reliable and reproducible method of measuring spasticity. *J. Neuro. Rehabil.* **3,** 205–209.
8. Allison, S. C., Abraham, L. D., and Petersen, C. L. (1996) Reliability of the Modified Ashworth Scale in the assessment of plantarflexor muscle spasticity in patients with traumatic brain injury. *Int. J. Rehab. Res.* **19,** 67–78.

9. Sköld, C., Harms-Ringdal, K., Hulting, C. et al. (1998) Simultaneous Ashworth measurements and electromyographic recording in tetraplegic patients. *Arch. Phys. Med. Rehabil.* **79,** 959–965.
10. Penn, R. D. et al. (1989) Intrathecal baclofen for severe spinal spasticity. *N. Engl. J. Med.* **320,** 1517–1521.
11. Loubser, P. G. et al. (1991) Continuous infusion of intrathecal baclofen: Long-term effects on spasticity in spinal cord injury. *Paraplegia* **29,** 48–64.
12. Albright, A. L., Cervi, A., and Singletary, J. (1991) Intrathecal baclofen for spasticity in cerebral palsy. *JAMA* **265,** 1418–1422.
13. Middel, B. et al. (1997) Effect of intrathecal baclofen delivered by an implanted programmable pump on health related quality of life in patients with severe spasticity. *J. Neurol. Neurosurg. Psychiatry* **63,** 204–209.
14. Goff, B. (1976) Grading of spasticity and its effect on voluntary movement. *Physiotherapy* **62,** 358–361.
15. Das, T. K. and Park, D. M. (1989) Effect of treatment with botulinum toxin on spasticity. *Postgrad. Med. J.* **65,** 208–210.
16. Pedersen, E., Klemar, B., and Tørring, J. (1979) Counting of flexor spasms. *Acta. Neurol. Scand.* **60,** 164–169.
17. Rymer, W. Z. and Katz, R. T. (1994) Mechanical quantification of spastic hypertonia, in *Physical Medicine and Rehabilitation: State of the Art Reviews,* vol. 8, Hanley & Belfus, Inc., Philadelphia, pp. 455–463.
18. Bajd, T. and Vodovnik, L. (1984) Pendulum testing of spasticity. *J. Biomed. Eng.* **6,** 9–16.
19. Vodovnik, L., Bowman, B. R., and Bajd, T. (1984) Dynamics of spastic knee joint. *Med. Biol. Eng. Comput.* **22,** 63–69.
20. Lin, D. C. and Rymer, W. Z. (1991) A quantitative analysis of pendular motion of the lower leg in spastic human subjects. *IEEE Trans. Biomed. Eng.* **38,** 906–918.
21. Franken, H. M. et al. (1993) Identification of passive knee joint and shank dynamics in paraplegics using quadriceps stimulation. *IEEE Trans. Biomed. Eng.* **1,** 154–163.
22. Fowler, V. et al. (1998) Muscle length effect on the pendulum test. *Arch Phys. Med. Rehabil.* **79,** 169–171.
23. Kaeser, H. E. et al. (1998) Testing an antispasticity drug (Tetrazepam) with the pendulum test: a monocentric pilot study. *J. Neuro. Rehabil.* **12,** 169–177.
24. Brown, R. A. et al. (1988) Does the Wartenberg pendulum test differentiate quantitatively between spasticity and rigidity? A study in elderly stroke and Parkinsonian patients. *J. Neurol. Neurosurg. Psychiatry* **51,** 1178–1186.
25. Leslie, G. C. et al. (1992) A comparison of the assessment of spasticity by the Wartenberg pendulum test and the Ashworth grading scale in patients with multiple sclerosis. *Clin. Rehabil.* **6,** 41–48.
26. Bohannon, R. (1999) Usefulness of the pendulum test. *Neurorehab. Neural Repair* **13,** 259–260.
27. Simons, D. G. and Lamonte, R. J. (1971) Automated system for the measurement of reflex responses to patellar taps in man. *Am. J. Phys. Med.* **50,** 72–79.
28. Zhang, L.-Q. et al. (1999) System identification of tendon reflex dynamics. *IEEE Trans. Biomed. Eng.* **7,** 193–203.

29. Stam, J. and Tan, K. M. (1987) Tendon reflex variability and method of stimulation. *Electroencephalogr. Clin. Neurophysiol.* **67**, 463–467.
30. Meinders, M. et al. (1996) The stretch reflex response in the normal and spastic ankle: effect of ankle position. *Arch Phys. Med. Rehabil.* **77**, 487–492.
31. Gottlieb, G. L., Agarwal, G. C., and Penn, R. (1978) Sinusoidal oscillation of the ankle as a means of evaluating the spastic patient. *J. Neurol. Neurosurg. Psychiatry* **41**, 32–39.
32. Myklebust, B. M., Gottlieb, G. L., Penn, R. D., and Agarwal, G. C. (1982) Reciprocal excitation of antagonistic muscles as a differentiating feature in spasticity. *Ann Neurol.* **12**, 367–374.
33. Lehmann, J. F. et al. (1989) Spasticity: quantitative measurements as a basis for assessing effectiveness of therapeutic intervention. *Arch. Phys. Med. Rehabil.* **70**, 6–15.
34. Price, R. et al. (1991) Quantitative measurement of spasticity in children with cerebral palsy. *Dev. Med. Child Neurol.* **33**, 585–595.
35. Zhang, L.-Q., Rymer, W. Z. (1997) Simultaneous and nonlinear identification of mechanical and reflex properties of human elbow joint muscles. *IEEE Trans. Biomed. Eng.* **44**, 1192–1209.
36. Zhang, L.-Q. et al. (1998) *In vivo* human knee joint dynamic properties as functions of muscle contraction and joint position. *J. Biomech.* **31**, 71–76.
37. Zhang, L.-Q. et al. (1998) Reflex and intrinsic mechanical changes in spastic limbs of MS patients. Proceedings of the 20th Annual International Conference of the IEEE Engineering in Medicine and Biology Society **20**, 2321–2324.
38. Sinkjær, T. and Magnussen, I. (1994) Passive, intrinsic and reflex-mediated stiffness in the ankle extensors of hemiparetic patients. *Brain* **117**, 355–363.
39. Sinkjær, T. et al. (1988) Muscle stiffness in human ankle dorsiflexors: Intrinsic and reflex components. *J. Neurophys.* **60**, 1110–1121.
40. Sinkjær, T. et al. (1993) Non-reflex and reflex mediated ankle joint stiffness in multiple sclerosis patients with spasticity. *Muscle Nerve* **16**, 69–76.
41. Dietz, V. et al. (1993) Spastic paresis: Reflex activity and muscle tone in elbow muscles during passive and active motor tasks, in *Spasticity: Mechanisms and Management* (Thilmann, A. F., et al., eds.), Springer-Verlag, Berlin and Heidelberg, pp. 251–264.
42. Hinderer, S. R. et al. (1990) Spasticity in spinal cord injured persons: quantitative effects of baclofen and placebo treatments. *Am. J. Phys. Med. Rehabil.* **69**, 311–317.
43. Dimitrijević, M. R. and Nathan, P. W. (1971) Studies of spasticity in man 5. Dishabituation of the flexion reflex in spinal man. *Brain* **94**, 77–90.
44. Dimitrijević, M. R. and Sherwood, A. M. (1980) Spasticity: Medical and surgical treatment. *Neurology* **30**, 19–27.
45. Keenan, M.-A. E., Haider, T. T., and Stone, L. R. (1990) Dynamic electromyography to assess elbow spasticity. *J. Hand Surg.* **15A**, 607–614.
46. Fisher, M. A., Shahani, B. T., and Young, R. R. (1979) Electrophysiologic analysis of the motor system after stroke: The flexor reflex. *Arch. Phys. Med. Rehabil.* **60**, 7–11.

47. Tørring, J., Pedersen, E., and Klemar, B. (1981) Standardisation of the electrical elicitation of the human flexor reflex. *J. Neurol. Neurosurg. Psychiatry* **44,** 129–132.
48. Meinck H.-M., Küster, S., Benecke, R., and Conrad, B. (1985) The flexor reflex-influence of stimulus parameters on the reflex response. *Electroencephalogr. Clin. Neurophysiol.* **61,** 287–298.
49. Bathien, N. and Bourdarias, H. (1972) Lower limb cutaneous reflexes in hemiplegia. *Brain* **95,** 447–456.
50. Dimitrijević, M. R. and Nathan, P. W. (1968) Studies of spasticity in man. 3. Analysis of reflex activity evoked by noxious cutaneous stimulation. *Brain* **91,** 349–368.
51. Dewald J.-P. A. et al. (1995) Abnormal muscle coactivation patterns during isometric torque generation at the elbow and shoulder in hemiparetic subjects. *Brain* **118,** 495–510.
52. Conrad, B., Benecke, R., and Meinck, H.-M. (1985) Gait disturbances in paraspastic patients, in *Clinical Neurophysiology in Spasticity* (Delwaide, P. J. and Young, R. R., ed.), Elsevier Science Publishers BV, The Netherlands.
53. Fung, J. and Barbeau, H. (1989) A dynamic EMG profile index to quantify muscular activation disorder in spastic paretic gait. *Electroencephalogr. Clin. Neurophysiol.* **73,** 233–244.
54. Sutherland, D. H. (1978) Gait analysis in cerebral palsy. *Dev. Med. Child Neurol.* **20,** 807–813.
55. Shapiro, A. et al. (1990) Preoperative and postoperative gait evaluation in cerebral palsy. *Arch. Phys. Med. Rehabil.* **71,** 236–240.
56. Delwaide, P. J. (1985) Electrophysiological analysis of the mode of action of muscle relaxants in spasticity. *Ann. Neurol.* **17,** 90–95.
57. Angel, R. W. and Hofmann, W. W. (1963) The H reflex in normal, spastic, and rigid subjects. *Arch. Neurol.* **8,** 591–596.
58. Matthews, W. B. (1966) Ratio maximum H reflex to maximum M response as a measure of spasticity. *J. Neurol. Neurosurg. Psychiatry* **29,** 201–204.
59. Yanagisawa, N. et al. (1993) Methodological problems in the Hoffmann reflex study of spasticity, in *Spasticity: Mechanisms and Management* (Thilmann, A. F., et al., eds.), Springer-Verlag, Berlin-Heidelberg, pp. 273–286.
60. Little, J. W. and Halar, E. M. (1985) H-reflex changes following spinal cord injury. *Arch. Phys. Med. Rehabil.* **66,** 19–22.
61. Strassburg, H. M., Oepen, G., and Thoden, U. (1980) The late facilitation in H-reflex recovery cycles in different pyramidal lesions. *Arch. Psychiat. Nervenkr.* **228,** 197–204.
62. Eisen, A. and Odusote, K. (1979) Amplitude of the F wave: a potential means of documenting spasticity. *Neurology* **29,** 1306–1309.
63. Mayer, N. H. (1991) Functional management of spasticity after head injury. *J. Neuro. Rehabil.* **5,** S1–S4.
64. Corcos, D. M. et al. (1986) Movement deficits caused by hyperexcitable stretch reflexes in spastic humans. *Brain* **109,** 1043–1058.
65. Mizrahi, E. M. and Angel, R. W. (1979) Impairment of voluntary movement by spasticity. *Ann. Neurol.* **5,** 594–595.

II
TREATMENT MODALITIES

4
Physical and Occupational Approaches

Susan H. Pierson

INTRODUCTION

Most approaches by physical and occupational therapists are founded in neurophysiologic, neurodevelopmental, or clinical principles. Unfortunately, there is little level I evidence to support any one of these therapeutic approaches. Yet most of the enduring approaches to spasticity management by therapists persist because they are felt to be effective. These therapeutic approaches have treatment goals that include the achievement of normal motor performance, orderly developmental sequences, and functional mobility. Gillette described each of these clinical approaches as being centered about one or more clinical phenomena occurring in the neurologically injured patient. These phenomena include righting reflexes, reciprocal inhibition, synergistic patterns of movement, and sensory functions such as proprioception, vision, and temperature perception *(1)*. Physical therapy theory holds that any effective treatment program for spasticity also includes efforts aimed at enhancing normal motor control, ensuring optimal physical conditioning, and preventing deformity, skin breakdown, and other complications of spasticity. The treatment of spasticity must be cost-effective and allow for transition out of the medical model and towards resumption of daily life. Table 1 details the fundamental tenants in the management of spasticity that are central to the physical-therapeutic approach to every patient with spasticity.

PHYSICAL APPROACHES TO THE MANAGEMENT OF SPASTICITY

According to Kraft *(2)*, there are five general categories of nonpharmacologic/nonsurgical interventions available for treatment of lost motor function following neurologic injury *(see* Table 2). The point of these treatment interventions is to maximize the strength of paretic muscles, compensate for the lost local and descending inhibition, and minimize the influence of

From: *Current Clinical Neurology: Clinical Evaluation and Management of Spasticity*
Edited by: D. A. Gelber and D. R. Jeffery © Humana Press, Inc., Totowa, NJ

Table 1
Fundamental Tenants of Physical Therapy

Midline orientation and symmetry
Segmental rotation
Prevention or correction of pathologic mass reflexes and postures
Movement out of traditional planes and on the "diagonal"
Positioning of proximal segments first so that distal segments will follow
Avoidance of excessive support to the patient
Tone changes with position, time of day, and activity
Spasticity can be reduced by sustained stretch
Treatment of spasticity should enhance function
    Ease caregiving by others
    Improve hygiene
    Allow for active assisted movement
    Preserve skin integrity
    Eliminate and prevent pain
    Maintain normal tone durably and comfortably
    Allow for maximal functional interaction of the patient with the environment

Table 2
Physical Therapy Approaches for the Management of Spasticity

Facilitation (proprioceptive methods, facilitation techniques)
Conventional rehabilitation (stretching, strengthening, etc.)
Biofeedback techniques
Electrical stimulation, other physical modalities
Orthoses (splints and casts)

local hypersensitive stretch receptors. This will then result in reduction in overflow motor responses and inhibit pathologic reflexes at the brainstem and spinal levels. Within each category of treatment there are individual schools of therapeutic manipulation or physical modality, listed in Table 3. Although these methods are commonly used, none have been shown to be superior to the others, and they have not been definitively proven to be of benefit in randomized, controlled, and blinded clinical trials.

THEORETICAL BASIS OF THERAPEUTIC EXERCISE TECHNIQUES IN SPASTICITY MANAGEMENT

Any text of physical therapy will emphasize the treatment of all aspects of motor dyscontrol in the rehabilitative effort. Appropriately, the issues of the negative symptoms of the upper motor neuron syndrome, specifically

Table 3
Therapeutic Modalities Used in the Management of Spasticity

Facilitation/inhibition
   Neurodevelopmental technique
   Proprioceptive neuromuscular facilitation
   Patterning/motor learning
   Sensory integration
   Reflex inhibitory postures
   Deep pressure
   Successive induction
   Rhythmic stabilization
   Proprioceptive sensory feedback
Conventional therapies
   Reduce irritative phenomena/aversive stimuli
   Functional approach
   Positioning
   Neuromuscular reeducation
   Contract-relax-contract techniques
   Treatment of secondary orthopedic deformities/disorders
Biofeedback techniques
Physical modalities
   Cooling/heat
   Vibration
   Hydrotherapy
   Acupuncture
Electrical stimulation
   Orthotics (casting and splinting)

weakness, incoordination, and fatigability should be considered equally with the problem of hypertonia in planning treatment strategies and defining goals. Early treatment strategies were aimed at local measures when the understanding of spasticity pathophysiology was thought to be a disorder of the stretch reflex only and thought of as a local problem only. Measures such as surgery and bracing along with exercise to strengthen "weak" antagonists were employed.

Neurodevelopmental Therapy (NDT)

Bobath promulgated the expansive notion that spasticity manifests itself in patterns of hypertonus affecting not only individual muscles but involving large parts of the body in widespread patterns of posture and movement (3). She also described the influence of patterns of released or disinhibited tonic reflexes on motor behavior in children with cerebral palsy (CP). These patterns were said to prevent the execution of appropriately timed and executed postural responses in reaction to a perturbation.

The pattern of tonic reflexes is thought to be modified by the influence of compensatory or secondarily abnormal or substitution patterns of motor behavior. Additionally, structural changes that evolve over time can change the quality and character of the classic spastic-movement patterns (4). It is also well-recognized that spasticity will change according to activity, level and type of stress, and in response to different types of sensory stimuli. This concept also must be considered in the assessment of abnormal movement patterns.

Overflow patterns of spasticity have been described, as soft neurological finding on examination, which occur in response to concentrated volitional motor performance, such as the performance of stress-gait patterns or bimanual upper-extremity tasks. These overflow movements were described by Bobath as "transient shadows of patterns of lower integration when tonus increased under stress" (3). The Bobath approach (neurodevelopmental therapy; NDT) strongly emphasizes the analysis of abnormal postural reflex activity in the setting of central nervous system (CNS) insult, and treatment approaches are directed at inhibiting those pathologic reflexes and facilitating normal righting and equilibrium reactions. The phylogenetic and ontogenetic association of movement patterns stresses the evolution of the patient's motor recovery along a continuum that parallels normal motor milestones and motor development. However, more recent assessment of the neurodevelopmental technique refutes this theory and seeks to link its effectiveness to more current thinking in neural recovery (5,6).

Traditionally, NDT favors the concepts of patterns of movements, rather than specific movements of individual muscles. As illustrated in Walshe's work (7), "the cortex knows nothing of muscles, it knows only of movements." More primitive movement patterns, such as the maintenance of antigravity postures, are organized by lower level centers of integration, which are phylogenetically and ontogenetically older and more primitive. These include the cerebellum, brainstem, midbrain, and basal ganglia. It is the release of these primitive movement patterns from the descending inhibition of higher cortical centers that leads to the re-emergence of unleashed postural reflexes. These released patterns are typical and stereotyped and involve all the affected muscles of the individual's body, interfering with functional or normal movement.

The technique of managing spasticity via the neurodevelopment approach is to analyze the postural reflex activity and to normalize it to the extent possible. This is done by moving the patient, passively or by assisted active movement, through the motions of appropriate postural response. For the paretic patient this translates into appropriate positioning and facilitating the postural response by perturbations, gait training, and balance training.

In NDT training, the patients are also encouraged to bear weight on the involved extremity, as a means to enhance sensory proprioceptive feedback, encourage joint co-contraction for joint stabilization, and to reduce tone by stretching and sensory input. It is presumed that adaptation to stretch by the muscle-spindle intrafusal fibers occurs with feedback relaxation of the anterior motor neuron *(8)*. Weight bearing is also a component of the forced-use paradigm and has become a more integral part of the teachings of NDT over recent years. With this approach, the unaffected limb is restrained and the patient is "forced" to use their paretic limb. Forced use has been shown in blinded trials to enhance motor recovery *(5)*.

Proprioceptive Neuromuscular Facilitation (PNF)

The work of Knott and Voss *(9)* also emphasizes the instruction of normal patterns of movement to the spastic patient. Termed proprioceptive neuromuscular facilitation (PNF), it is based on the physiology of developing motor behavior. It assumes the recovery of motor patterns in the lesioned brain or spinal cord follows a pattern similar to that of the developing nervous system. With this technique, total movement patterns are facilitated to promote motor learning. The acquisition of normal motor patterns is thought to secondarily reduce spasticity and other abnormal movements. Movement patterns such as rolling, rising to sit, stand, and walk are taught to the patient.

The theory holds that the recapitulation of the sequence of developmental activities is valuable to the patient's recovery of normal motor control. The focus of treatment seeks to enlist less involved motor parts, to promote a balanced antagonism between reflex activity, muscle groups, and gross patterns of movement. The philosophy of PNF is that motor behavior is a series of responses to a series of sensory demands. Purposeful movements are such because they are goal-directed. Ability, strength, coordination, and endurance are developed by an active participation in the activities of daily living. Stronger or less-involved segments of the body are recruited to help stimulate and strengthen the more involved or impaired parts.

Maximal resistance is given throughout range of motion activities done on the "diagonal," using combinations of movements out of traditional planes. Motion is performed first in the strongest (usually proximal) portion of the range, progressing in a distal fashion to recruit the weaker parts of the limb (hand or foot). The movement patterns are initiated by a quick stretch to the muscle groups. This enhances the proprioceptive feedback to the muscle groups and is thought to facilitate the firing of the anterior motor neuron.

A fundamental difference between PNF and the neurodevelopment technique is that PNF will, at times, use pathologic reflexes to facilitate a desired movement. PNF thus makes use of overflow phenomena where appropriate to reach desired movement goals. In order to manage spasticity and restore upper motor neuron weakness, PNF also employs the method of rhythmic stabilization. In this technique, isometric contraction of the agonist followed by contraction of the antagonist results in enhanced response of the agonist. Another technique known as "slow reversal" uses rhythmic stabilization to alternately resist the isotonic contraction of agonist and antagonist in order to facilitate the antagonist. In managing spasticity, the antagonist is facilitated against the pull of the spastic muscle.

Facilitation of motions is begun from proximal to distal. The proximal parts are strengthened, and "normalized" prior to attending to more distal segments. It is felt that as these proximal segments improve, they provide reinforcement to distal segments of the extremities. Postural and righting reflexes are often used in an overflow technique to strengthen the head and neck, and reduce truncal spasticity. The scapula is used as proximal "pivot" on which distal upper-extremity movements are based. The premise is that the scapulae provide stability to the entire shoulder complex, which is known in both a neuromuscular and orthopedic sense. The development of a balance of power in relation to all patterns of movements and to all pivots of stabilization is deemed mandatory in this approach because it implies adequate performance of both the agonist and antagonist muscle groups.

Knott and Voss emphasize, as the ultimate therapeutic objective, the integration of these learned patterns of movement into mundane and usual activities of living. The goal is to apply these learned movements to the execution of daily living tasks, both to accomplish those tasks, and to reinforce these normalized movements. The strategy clearly emphasizes the need to select which activities, under which circumstances, are most readily learned and incorporated into daily function. There is no hard-line stand that precludes the incorporation of facilitation techniques into functional tasks, prior to the successful acquisition of the movement out of functional context. In other words, hard and fast stances on the need to master the land drill or the pre-gait skill prior to performing in context, i.e., in water or on a runway, are not emphasized by this philosophy to the degree they are by the neurodevelopmentalist.

Sensory Integration

Ayres developed an extensive evaluation tool that assesses perceptual motor function in the developmentally and neurologically disabled *(10,11)*. She developed an approach that emphasizes remediation of the underlying developmental deficit, and not one that attacks specific symptoms. This approach considers the development of so-called splinter skills to be counterproductive and favors normalization of underlying dysfunction so as to allow skills to evolve naturally as learning situations are provided. This approach went further to connect behavioral disturbances, emotional disturbances, and perceptual motor deficits in the learning-impaired child *(12)*. These techniques have also been applied to recovering lesions in adults after brain injury, but as with many of the other techniques described in this chapter, the evidence to support this treatment approach is based on open label trials or small case series.

Within the school of sensory integration, the fundamental concept is that sensory information must be organized so as to be useful to the individual. Sensory-motor integration occurs at all levels of the nervous system as an adaptive response. That adaptive response is goal-directed and purposeful and in order to achieve it the therapist both provides and controls sensory input to the patient. The theory stresses that motor learning occurs as an actual combination of sensory input-motor output and sensory feedback. Integration of this information and response is achieved at a sub-cortical level. On a neurophysiological basis, Farber and Ayre suggest that "meaningful stimuli bombarding a cell, (increases) the number of synaptic knobs" and formation of new synapses.

From a clinical standpoint, the aim of every therapeutic activity is to focus on achieving the task without heavy reliance on cortical stimulation. The approach is learning by performing the desired movement within the context of a functional task. In particular, sensory input from the muscles, joints, skin, and vestibular system are emphasized, in that input can be provided in a therapeutic manner. Impaired processing of sensory stimuli on the basis of aging, nervous-system insult, or decreased sensory stimulation may all result in abnormal motor responses. In addition, the lack of sensory stimulation is thought to result in impaired tertiary and higher-level cognitive processing and appropriate motor response.

In the case of stroke, there is thought to be a de facto case of sensory deprivation. The neurologically impaired patient is unable to utilize or respond to incoming sensory information. Controlled sensory input is thought to improve sensory processing and thereby improve motor responses in this population, and is used as a primary treatment technique by mainstream therapists. The goal of sensory integrative treatment is to direct interaction with the patients environment in such a way as to promote functional neurological change. It is founded on the premise that the CNS remains plastic throughout childhood and adult life.

As with the other approaches, there is a lack of scientific evidence to support this approach. Nonetheless, open-label studies support the theoretical basis with clinical evidence of response *(13,14)*. Deep pressure, tactile stimulation with different textures, such as spinning in a net or chair, rolling on bolsters and balls, and mobilizing on scooterboards are all used as a means of providing a sensation in order to provoke a normal motor response. This approach presumes that there will occur a transfer of training so that practice in a particular perceptual task will affect the patient's performance on similar perceptual tasks, although there is some evidence that does not support this notion of a generalization of effect *(15)*. Conversely, others have shown a generalization of effect with other forms of therapy such as constraint-induced training *(16,17)*. Recent functional magnetic resonance imaging (MRI) studies show that re-organization of the motor cortex may also occur with these treatments *(18)*.

Functionally Based Therapies

Functional approaches to the management of spasticity and the restoration of motor control make use of repetitive practice of practical tasks, such as walking and dressing. This is a handicap-driven approach aimed at alleviating the dysfunction, rather than at modifying the neurophysiology or impairment. Again, there is no level 1 evidence to support this approach, but there is a belief that it is a more pragmatic approach to rehabilitation, especially given the constraints on duration of therapy imposed by third-party payors. The forced-use paradigms and treadmill-training literature do lend conceptual support to this form of therapy being among the more efficacious because those techniques have been shown in several blinded trials to be superior to other forms of therapy *(19,20)*. On the other hand, Fetters and Kluzik found no appreciable difference between the use of rehearsal and the use of NDT techniques in developing reaching skills in children with CP. In fact, they found them to be complementary *(21)*.

In the case of the functional approach, one is training the patient to perform the same functional task over and over with rehearsal. This rehearsal of a task appears superior to other approaches that aim to train precursors of movement and function. The functional approach includes a large portion of compensation strategies, which some will interpret as learned non-use *(22)*. However, compensatory techniques are generally employed when the patient is unlikely to regain functional recovery of the limb, the side, or the visual field in a targeted time frame. Adaptation techniques supplement this compensatory approach and the patient modifies the environment or his approach to his environment so as to succeed at functional tasks he would

Physical and Occupational Approaches

not be able to perform in conventional manners; for example, the use of a wheelchair rather than abnormal gait pattern for functional mobility.

The basic tenant in each approach is that spasticity can be normalized by retraining, reproducing, patterning, or positioning normal movement. Because the resting state of the muscle or functional groupings of muscles is shortened at baseline, the muscle(s) is (are) not brought to the same amount of excursion normally seen when those muscles are used for function. The most obvious example is the state of the spastic gastroc-soleus complex at heel strike in early stance. The muscle is eccentrically contracted and the normal excursion of the muscle during active dorsiflexion is never reached. This results in impaired or no heel strike, foot-flat or toe-first stance, and an abnormally shortened stance cycle. Therapeutic interventions endeavor to return that degree of stretch without eliciting an abnormal stretch reflex and excessive contraction of the agonist.

Therapeutic Exercise Techniques/Physical Modalities

In physical and occupational therapy, a variety of "handling" techniques along with specific modalities such as heat or biofeedback are used to modulate or inhibit spasticity. All are effective to some degree as judged by a clinical response from the patient, and none produce decreases in tone that persist over hours or days. Rather they are used in concert to better achieve concurrent goals in positioning, strengthening, or function. In utilizing these techniques and modalities, spasticity is modulated by focusing on facilitating the antagonist of the spastic muscle, inhibiting the agonist spastic muscle, and by promoting generalized relaxation *(23)*. From the standpoint of neurophysiology, these techniques probably make use of reciprocal inhibition, direct fatigue of muscle, and generalized somatic and autonomic relaxation, but neurophysiologic measurement in formal studies is lacking.

Manual Pressure

Manual pressure is utilized in the sensory integrative approach as well as in some others. The maintained pressure is effective in reducing spasticity if it is applied to the tendon rather than the muscle belly. It is thought to act as a counterirritant that overwhelms sensory receptors ability to mediate other types of stimuli. H reflex testing has shown that the motor neuron is inhibited in the tendon being pressed *(24)*. Air splints, bivalve, or inhibitory casting all can provide maintained pressure via "total contact" on tendons and thereby exert an inhibitory influence on muscle tone.

Joint Cocontraction/Compression and Sustained Stretch

These techniques can be used to both facilitate or inhibit tone. When partial weight is applied across the joint as in lateral weight shifts onto the arm in sitting, stretch across the muscle is applied and this can inhibit spasticity. Co-contraction across the joint, as with weightbearing through the glenohumeral joint, is designed to achieve proximal motor control. Standing tables or tilt tables can be used to achieve weightbearing through spastic lower extremity muscles and decrease tone via sustained stretching *(25)*.

Presumably, adaptation to stretch occurs at the level of the muscle spindle as the intrafusal fibers lower their firing intensity with prolonged stretch to the extrafusal fibers *(26)*. Needle electromyography examination of spastic muscles at rest and during passive movement reveals more than one firing pattern of motor units in hypertonic muscles. In some patients the motor-unit firing is continuous and is not influenced by stretch, whereas in others continuous motor-unit activity is reduced by continuous stretch and clonus is no longer elicitable in these same muscles with quick stretch. The notion that adaptation at the level of the motor neuron in response to continuous stimuli has been suggested as the physiologic basis for this observation *(27)*.

Slow Rolling or Rocking

Activities which are slow and repetitive generally inhibit spasticity. These are passive handling techniques performed by the therapist on the patient. With this form of treatment, one body part is moved segmentally in relation to another, for example moving the hips to the right while concurrently moving the shoulders to the left. General relaxation can often be further promoted by performing tasks in an inverted position, e.g., over a "Bobath ball" or bolster. Once tone is inhibited, the patient is then asked to move actively in some functional task *(28)*.

Slow Spinning

This is a technique of Ayres by which the patient is spun slowly (less than 30 revolutions/min) in a hammock or chair *(29)*. It produces relaxation theoretically by inhibiting the anti-gravity vestibular systems such as the vestibulospinal tract, which leads to reduction in anterior horn-cell activity in the trunk and limb extensors.

Vibration

This is a facilitation technique that can be applied to the antagonist to the spastic muscle and thereby achieve relaxation of the spastic muscle via reciprocal inhibition *(30)*. Vibration is known to affect the Ia fibers and to produce a reflex contraction of the vibrated muscle, known as the TVR (tonic vibration reflex). This effect is somewhat stronger if the vibration is applied over the tendon rather than muscle *(31)*.

Heat and Cooling

Cooling the skin can reduce spasticity by decreasing Ia afferent input to the muscle spindle and decreasing the sensitivity of the spindle. Cooling also inhibits cutaneous small-fiber receptors *(32)*. In addition it is known that nerve-conduction velocities can be slower in patients with cool limbs. Cooling packs can be applied to the spastic limb for 20 min, while those muscles are placed in a sustained stretch. Active exercise or functional activity follows the cooling induced reduction in tone.

Neutral warmth achieved by wrapping the body or a limb in towels or blankets provides direct relaxation to spastic muscle and generalized relaxation via reduced sympathetic outflow *(33)*. Other methods of delivering heat to a limb include hydrotherapy, hydrocollator packs, and ultrasound. Heat may also have the effect of decreasing pain by increasing blood flow to tissue and moderating autonomic mediation of pain *(34)*.

Electrical Stimulation

Functional electrical stimulation has been extensively studied and found to be of benefit in neuromuscular re-education. In order to reduce spasticity, the antagonist to the spastic muscle is stimulated to achieve reciprocal inhibition of the agonist. In addition, directly stimulating the spastic muscle will relax it by fatiguing the muscle *(35)*. Other reasons to apply electrical stimulation in neurologically impaired patients are to improve range of motion and to facilitate voluntary muscle control. Electrical stimulation of the toe extensors has been used successfully to both improve strength of the toe extensors and reduce toe-flexor spasticity *(36)*. In one study, tonic stimulation of the sural nerve facilitated voluntary dorsiflexion in spastic patients and improved their ability to walk. It was postulated that the mechanism of recovery was owing to the activation of flexor-reflex afferents. This activation served to reset the balance between flexor and extensor tone, thus allowing active dorsiflexion with less effort than previously required in the spastic patient *(37)*. Low-intensity electrical stimulation (below motor threshold) has been shown to reduce spasticity when the stimulation is applied to the antagonist muscle. Low-intensity stimulation may also facilitate voluntary recruitment and has been reported to enhance the balance between the contraction of agonist and antagonist across the joint. This is achieved by enhancing excitation of the extensors in the wrist and biasing their strength relative to the flexors of the wrist (bias/balance therapy) *(38)*. Trancutaneous electrical nerve stimulation for muscle spasticity has also been shown to reduce tone. Initially the effect only lasted for 10 min following cessation of stimulation but with consecutive treatments over 3 mo, the duration of effect became prolonged *(39)*. Interestingly, in this study they were able to reverse the relaxation induced by stimulation with naloxone. This suggested that the effect of transcutaneous electrical nerve stimulation (TENS) in reducing spasticity may be in part mediated by endogenous opiod ligands and kappa opiate receptors in the CNS. Nonetheless, electrical stimulation remains controversial and the results showing its efficacy in reducing spasticity and in improving function are inconclusive *(40)*.

Spinal-cord stimulation has also been used to affect chronic disabling spasticity. The results have also been inconclusive. Gottlieb et al. used cervical-cord stimulation to attempt reduction in spinal spasticity and found no effect *(41)*. Sixteen patients with spinal-cord injury underwent spinal-cord stimulation. In those patients who had satisfactory electrode placement, spasticity relief was found to be substantial. Upper- and lower-extremity function was improved but follow-up revealed that nearly one-third had technical complications with their stimulating systems and that only one-third had persistence of effect at 1 yr *(42)*. This form of therapy has proven to be cumbersome, not widely available nor easily managed.

Biofeedback

Biofeedback has been used in both acute and chronic phases of motor recovery to enhance function. It is used on both agonist and antagonist muscles to decrease inappropriate co-contraction about the joint and benefits of therapy in some instances have been demonstrated to last for more than 1 yr *(43)*. Biofeedback training can take several forms. In one maneuver the patient is trained to reproduce with their paretic arm, EMG patterns produced by their normal arm during functional tasks. Biofeedback is also used to quiet EMG activity of the spastic agonist during functional tasks. Basmajian suggests that patients suppress motor-unit activity in spastic muscles by developing more control over surviving motor pathways and units *(44)*. Biofeedback data provides multimodal feedback to the patient immediately and obviously requires a patient who is cooperative and can carry over information. Auditory-signal devices have been used on head gear to encourage appropriate head position, again either by inhibiting the muscles that tonically deviate the head, or by facilitating the muscles that move opposite the undesired position. These types of devices can be effective in restoring motor control in the traumatically brain-injured population because they do not require a high degree of cortical activation or effort by the patient *(45)*. Biofeedback devices can serve to carry over therapy treatment during nontreatment times and ancillary staff and family members are readily trained to understand the principles that underlie their use.

Casting and Orthotic Devices

Both biomechanical and neurophysiologic principles underlie the treatment of upper motor neuron paresis and spasticity with splinting and casting. Within the view of neurodevelopmental therapy, static splinting is viewed to be a disadvantage because it maintains stretch at the maximal passive range of the shortened or spastic musculature. Patients then experience pain and discomfort leading to further increases in tone. Dynamic splinting is espoused as a more desirable solution. In the case of the hand and wrist, hard splint surfaces are inhibitory to the finger and wrist flexors while elastic bands over the dorsum of the forearm (orthokinetic cuff) provide increased sensory input into the antagonistic extensors, thereby facilitating them *(46)*. Although studies have not shown splints to actually reduce spasticity, as measured by resting EMG activity *(47,48)*, it is not clear if splinting might have a tone-reducing effect during physical activity or if the splints were worn for durations other than those studied; therefore, the benefit of splinting in the treatment of spasticity remains open to investigation *(49)*.

It is at least clear that contractures can be prevented by splinting. The application of prolonged, mild tension by a splint results in elongation of tendon and muscle, owing to separation of the collagen cross-links, and is more effective in contracture reduction than vigorous short-term stretching *(50)*. Case reports also support the notion of contracture reduction without worsening the underlying spasticity when dynamic splinting is used *(51)*. Inhibitory casting has also been studied but blinded controlled trials are lacking. The cost efficacy of casting vs commercially available products has been studied and the cost efficacy over traditional therapies (i.e., therapeutic exercise) appears positive *(52,53)*. Casts are applied so that the joint is positioned approx 5 degrees less than maximal endpoint of the range to avoid triggering increased spasticity. Casts are changed every 3–5 days (if the patient is otherwise tolerating them) until the deformity is maximally corrected. Casts can then be "bivalved" and transformed into a resting "clamshell" apparatus, which can be donned and doffed daily for intermittent stretch or inhibition.

The concept of total contact as experienced with serial casting or inhibitory casting is felt to play a role in spasticity reduction *(53)*. Inhibitive casts incorporate features that attempt to inhibit persistent tonic reflexes such as decerebrate extension in the lower extremities *(54)*. These might include specialized footplates that avoid pressure over the metatarsal heads and apply pressure over the calcaneus. Patients selected for casting must be appropriate, and able to tolerate it from a medical standpoint without diaphoresis, increased agitation, or skin breakdown. Some segments are less suitable for casting and pose higher risk of skin complications, such as the olecranon process, the malleoli, and the calcaneus. Some patient types, i.e., those with decorticate or decerebrate tonic reflexes and postures, are at a greater risk for contracture formation and inadequate management of spasticity and range with traditional exercise alone. They may require casting therapy more readily than some other patient types *(55)*. Persistence of the gains made with casting in terms of preserved range of motion and tone reduction have not been well-studied. Studies have not been well-controlled for patient types, or for their time-course post-injury *(56)*.

Positioning for Spasticity Reduction

In general, the term "positioning" refers to the position of the patient whether in bed or seated for mobility, i.e., in a wheelchair. There are basic principles of positioning outlined in the introduction to this chapter and should be followed whenever tone reduction or control is part of the clinical problem list. Patients should be supported to the extent they require. When support is inadequate, the patient tends to feel insecure and will likely use abnormal postural mechanisms in an attempt to maintain equilibrium. These abnormal motor responses are apt to involve overflow release of tonic postures, such as extensor thrusting, or head turning, and are unlikely to contribute in a meaningful way to the maintenance of an upright posture.

When supports are excessive, the patient is not forced to actively maintain an antigravity position and will not use trunk or neck muscles in a functional manner. Excessive gravity assisted positioning will allow the patient to be passive and utterly dependent on the device for maintenance of antigravity posture. Endurance will not be trained and environmental interaction may be limited or restricted more than is absolutely necessary, thereby further depriving the patient of meaningful stimuli. Consideration of a variety of issues must be made in approaching the patient in terms of positioning devices. These include medical stability and tolerance for upright, prone, sidelying, or other tone-inhibiting positions. Maximal environmental interaction, physical endurance, skin integrity, cost, ease of procurement/fabrication, effectiveness in reducing spasticity and facilitating active movement, and functional goals, are often factors that should be taken into account. In the case of children or young adults, consideration for growth must be given, and the issue of adaptability or customization should be addressed.

Many of the same concepts that underlie therapeutic exercise for the control and management of spasticity apply to positioning for tone. Midline orientation and symmetry are always preeminent considerations and the patients should always be seated in 90° of hip, knee, and ankle flexion. Weight should be evenly distributed over both ischial tuberosities and control of the

Physical and Occupational Approaches

trunk and upper limbs, and head should begin by proper support and positioning of the hips. If proper positing is achieved proximally, distal stabilization follows as a natural consequence. Flexible postural problems should be corrected and fixed deformities should be avoided.

A positioning system should exert a force greater than or equal to the force of gravity on the body in order to correct flexible postural deformities. Aggressive sustained stretching or applying force that is resisted by the patient in a counteractive response is unlikely to correct a deformity and likely to produce early fatigue and poor tolerance for the device. Likewise, positions or devices that cause or increase pain will also be poorly tolerated and of little lasting use. However, if the postural problem is fixed, the positioning device must be able to accommodate it, as might be the case with contoured seating systems or soft foam. Prefabricated devices are advantageous owing to low cost and should be tried and used wherever possible. They should not be expected to perform well when the problem calls for a custom solution so evaluation must extend over time and be thorough in assessing the problem, solution, and fit. The optimal position for the lower extremities is stated above: 90° at the hips, knees, and ankles, with weight distributed evenly onto both buttocks. This can be achieved through the use of pelvic straps (which open in the midline via Velcro so as to avoid restraint issues) wedges for seats; appropriate leg and foot rests, with ankle and foot straps used only as a last resort. Again, if the patient is initially positioned appropriately proximally, the more distal segments will require less attention and will fall into place on their own. Stimulating abnormal reflexes such as the tonic labyrinthine reactions should be avoided so recliner chairs that open up the hip angle or elevated leg rests should be avoided in spastic patients.

Tonic head deviation, as seen in patients with strong influence of the asymmetric tonic neck reflex, can be controlled with the use of overhead slings, headstraps, lateral outriggers, or gravity-assisted positioning (i.e., tilt in space chairs). Upper-extremity positioning is addressed last and should be maximized by allowing the shoulders to externally rotate, the scapulae to retract, and the trapezius muscles to relax. If the arms are required to actively maintain the trunk in an upright position, consideration should be given to tilt in space chairs that use gravity to assist postural control and free the arms up for functional use. Lap trays that span the entire chair will support the forearms and hands. They can control shoulder adduction/internal rotation by the use of wedges bolted to the tray, which then block excessive adduction or rotation. Lap trays need to be large enough in their cut out to accommodate the girth of the individual and must be adequately supported from below by full-length rather than desk-length arm rests. Unilateral supports may also be used and are advantageous in the hemiparetic patient in that they allow the patient to move about more freely. On the other hand, they may not allow optimal positioning of spastic but subluxed shoulders and may encourage shoulder impingement rather than relieve it. Additionally, for those patients with lateral postural bias secondary to their stroke, hemi-lap trays allow the patient to pull away from their hemiparetic side rather than weightbearing through it.

Other inhibitory positions that can effectively modulate tone are the prone and sidelying positions. Supine lying tends to allow the emergence of the tonic labyrinthine responses that facilitate head and trunk extension. Prone lying may enhance the flexion of the upper limbs. It is difficult to achieve this position for any length of time in a severely injured patient owing to the existence of respiratory compromise, and presence of, e.g., tracheostomy and feeding tubes. Prone lying may be more easily tolerated over a foam wedge, and this is a position favored by pediatric therapists when working on head control and upper-extremity weightbearing in children. Sidelying is a neutral position in relation to the influence of tonic postural reflexes and thereby avoids facilitating or inhibiting these reflexes. However, it is a difficult position to achieve in posturally disordered patients who are "pushers" and this position may be difficult to maintain. Often times large blocks of D-cell foam or moldable bean bag systems can be used to consistently position patients in sidelying, regardless of which caregiver is doing it. Sidelying will avoid the windswept or frog-legged positions commonly found in longstanding spastic quadraparetic or hemiparetic patients *(57)*.

Acupuncture

Increasingly, reports in the literature reflect the growing use of acupuncture in the management of neurologic disease. In a blinded, placebo-controlled study, acupuncture was shown to enhance recovery and motor control after stroke, but the effect on spasticity was not evaluated *(58)*. The clinical benefits of treatment lasted for 4 mo. A more recent report on the effects of acupuncture in reducing spasticity used the H reflex recovery time and curve to measure spinal motor-neuron excitability. In this study, a shorter H reflex recovery time and an abnormal recovery curve distinguished the H reflex in a spastic muscle from that in a normal limb. After treatment with acupuncture, the H reflex recovery time was found to be significantly prolonged as compared with that before acupuncture. The H recovery curve also then approximated a recovery curve from normal controls after the acupuncture had been given *(59)*.

In a subsequent study, acupuncture was combined with traditional methods of rehabilitation and compared to a control group that received only traditional rehabilitation techniques. The researchers found that not only did the acupuncture group had better outcomes as measured by objective motor and functional scales, during the 6-wk treatment period. The gains made by the acupuncture group made were still apparent throughout the year-long follow-up *(60)*.

SUMMARY

From a physical and occupational therapy perspective, the treatment of spasticity continues to use a combination of traditional forms of therapeutic exercise, casting, splinting, and positioning. Acupuncture, electrical stimulation, and other modalities are not yet widely clinically available, and are often not covered by third party payors, but research efforts are underway to better quantify and measure their effects. There is good data to support the use of forced use and repetitive treadmill training in enhancing motor recovery but neither technique is aimed specifically or solely at reducing spasticity. In fact, probably no reasonable therapeutic plan of care would direct its efforts only at spasticity management when the upper motor neuron syndrome encompasses far more than that. Clearly, the challenge in the treatment of spasticity lies not only in managing it effectively, but determining whether treating it is necessary at all.

REFERENCES

1. Gillette, H. E. (1964) Recovery of motion following cerebral insult: an appraisal of current methods of management. *Arch. Phys. Med. Rehabil.* **8,** 167–176.
2. Kraft, G. H., Fitts, S. S., and Hammond, M. C. (1992) Techniques to improve function of the hand and arm in chronic hemiplegia. *Arch. Phys. Med. Rehabil.* **73,** 220–227.
3. Bobath, B. (1985) *Abnormal Postural Reflex Activity Caused by Brain Lesions,* 3rd ed. Aspen Publications, Rockville MD.
4. Mayer, N. H., Esquenazi, A., and Wannstedt, G. Surgical planning for upper motor neuron dysfunction: the role of motor control evaluation. *J. Head Trauma Rehabil.* **11,** 37–56.
5. Keshner, E. A. (1981) Reevaluating the theoretical model underlying the neurodevelopmental theory: a literature review. *Phys. Ther.* 1035–1040.
6. Bly, L. (1991) A historical and current view of the basis of NDT. *Pedictr. Phys. Ther.* **3,** 131–135.
7. Walshe, F. M. R. (1946) *On the Contribution of Clinical Study to the Physiology of the Cerebral Cortex.* The Victor Horsley Memorial Lecture. E & S Livingstone, Edinburgh, p. 18.
8. Otis, J. C., Root, L., and Kroll, M. A. (1985) Measurement of plantar flexion spasticity during treatment with tone reducing casts. *J. Pediatr. Orthop.* **5,** 632–686.
9. Knott, M. and Voss, D. E. (1968) *Proprioceptive Neuromuscular Facilitation: Patterns and Techniques,* 2nd ed. Harper & Row, New York.

10. Ayres, J. A. (1972) *Sensor Integration and Learning Disorders.* Western Psychological Services, Los Angeles, CA.
11. Siev, E., Freishtat, B., and Zoltan, B. (1986) *Perceptual and Cognitive Dysfunction in the Adult Stroke Patient: A Manual for Evaluation and Treatment.* SLACK Inc., Thorofare, NJ.
12. Farber, S. D. and Huss, A. J. (1974) *Sensorimotor Evaluation and Treatment Procedures for Allied Health Personnel.* Indiana University Foundation, Indianapolis, IN.
13. Baker Nobles, L. and Bink, B. (1979) Sensory integration in the rehabilitation of blind adults. *Am. J. Occup. Ther.* **33,** 559–564.
14. VanBenschoten R. A Sensory integration program for blind campers. *Am. J. Occup. Ther.* **29,** 615–617.
15. Mateer C. (1997) Rehabilitation of individuals with frontal lobe impairment, in *Neuropsychological Rehabilitation: Fundamentals, Innovations, and Directions* (Leon Carrington, J., ed.), St. Lucie Press, Delray Beach, FL.
16. Wolf, S. L., LeCraw, D. E., Barton, L. A., and Jann, B. B. (1989) Forced use of hemiplegic upper extremities to reverse the effect of learned non-use among chronic stroke and head injured patients. *Exp. Neurol.* **104,** 125–132.
17. Netz, J., Lammers, T., and Homberg, V. Reorganization of motor output in the non-affected hemisphere after stroke. *Brain* **120,** 1579–1586.
18. Pritchard, J. W. and Brass, L. M. (1992) New Horizons in neurology: new anatomical and functional imaging methods. *Ann. Neurol.* **32,** 395–400.
19. Chollett, F., DiPiero, V., Wise, R. J., Brooks, D. J., and Dolan, R. J. et al. (1991) The functional anatomy of motor recovery after stroke in humans. A study with positron emission tomography. *Ann. Neurol.* **29,** 63–71.
20. Richards, C. L., Malouin, F., Wood-Dauphinee, S., Williams, J. I., Bouchard, J. P., and Brunet, D. (1993) Task specific physical therapy for optimization of gait recovery in acute stroke patients. *Arch. Phys. Med. Rehabil.* **74,** 612–620.
21. Fetters, L. and Kluzik, J. (1996) The effects of neurodevelopmental treatment versus practice on the reaching of children with spastic cerebral palsy. *Phys. Ther.* **76,** 346–358.
22. Taub, E. (1994) Overcoming learned non-use: a new approach to treatment in physical medicine, in *Clinical Applied Neurophysiology* (Carlson, J. G., Seifer, A. R., and Birnbaumer, N., eds.), Plenum, New York.
23. Giebler, K. B. (1990). Physical modalities, in *The Practical Management of Spasticity in Children and Adults* (Glenn, M. B. and Whyte, J., eds.), Lea and Febinger, Philadelphia, pp. 118–148.
24. Kukulka, C. G., Fellows, W. A., Oehlertz, J. E., and Vanderwilt, S. G. (1985) Effect of tendon pressure on alpha motor neuron excitability. *Phys. Ther.* **65,** 595–600.
25. Odeen, I. and Knuttson, E. (1981) Evaluation of the effects of muscle stretch and weight load in patients with spastic paraplegia. *Scand. J. Rehabil. Med.* **13,** 117–121.
26. Otis, J. C., Root, L., and Kroll, M. A. (1985) Measurement of plantar flexor spasticity during treatment with toner reducing casts. *J. Pediatr. Orthop.* **5,** 682–686.
27. Patajan, J. H. (1990) Spasticity: effects of physical interventions. *J. Neuro. Rehabil.* **4,** 219–225.

28. Stockmeyer, S.A. (1967) An interpretation of the approach of Rood to the treatment of neuromuscular dysfunction. *Am. J. Phys. Med.* **46,** 900–956.
29. Ayres, J. (1972) *Sensory Integration and Learning Disorders.* Western Psychological Services, Los Angeles, CA.
30. Bishop, B. (1977) Spasticity: its pathophysiology and management. Part IV: current and projected treatment procedures for spasticity. *Phys. Ther.* **57,** 396–401.
31. Griffin, J. W. (1974) Use of proprioceptive stimuli in therapeutic exercise. *Phys. Ther.* **54,** 1072–1079.
32. Knuttson, E. and Mattsson, E. (1969) Effects of local cooling on monosynaptic reflexes in man. *Scand. J. Rehabil. Med.* **1,** 126–132.
33. Stockmeyer, S.A. (1967). An interpretation of the approach of Rood to the treatment of neuromuscular dysfunction. *Am. J. Phys. Med.* **46,** 900–956.
34. Wells, H. S. (1947) Temperature equalization for the relief of pain. *Arch. Phys. Med. Rehabil.* **38,** 135–139.
35. Benton, L. S., Baker, L. L., Bowman, B. R., and Waters, R. L. (1981) *Functional Electrical Stimulation. A Practical Clinical Guide,* 2nd ed. Professional Staff Association of the Rancho Los Amigos Hospital, Downey, CA.
36. Fulbright, J. S. (1984) Electrical stimulation to reduce chronic toe flexor hypertonicity. *Phys. Ther.* **64,** 523–525.
37. Petajan, J. H. Sural Nerve stimulation and motor control of tibialis anterior muscle in spastic paresis. *Neurology* **37,** 47–52.
38. Kraft, G. H., Fitts, S. S., and Hammond, M. C. (1992) Techniques to improve function of the arm and hand in chronic hemiplegia. *Arch. Phys. Med. Rehabil.* **73,** 220–227.
39. Han, J. S., Chen, X. H., Yuan, Y., and Yan, S. C. (1994) Transcutaneous electrical nerve stimulation for treatment of spinal spasticity. *Chin. Med. J.* **107,** 6–11.
40. Barry, M. J. (1996) Physical therapy interventions for patients with movement disorders due to cerebral palsy. *J. Child. Neurol.* **(Suppl. 1)11,** S51–S60.
41. Gottlieb, G. L., Myklebust, Bm., Stefoski, D., Groth, K., Kroin, J., and Penn, R. D. (1985) Evaluation of cervical stimulation for chronic treatment of spasticity. *Neurology* **35,** 699–704.
42. Barolat, G., Myklebust, J. B., and Wenninger, W. Effects of spinal cord stimulation on spasticity and spasms secondary to myelopathy. *Appl. Neurophysiol.* **51,** 29–44.
43. Kraft, G. H. (1993) Hemiplegia: evaluation and rehabilitation of motor control disorders. *Phys. Med. Rehabil. Clin. North Am.* **4,** 687–705.
44. Basmajian, J. V. (1981) Biofeedback in rehabilitation: a review of principles and practices. *Arch. Phys. Med. Rehabil.* **62,** 469–475.
45. Rinehart, M. A. (1990) Strategies for improving motor performance, in *Rehabilitation of the Adult and Child With Traumatic Brain Injury,* 2nd ed. (Rosenthal, M., Griffith, E. R., Bond, M. R., Miller, J. D., eds.), F.A. Davis, Philadelphia, pp. 331–350.
46. Farber, S. D. and Huss, A. J. (1974) *Sensorimotor Evaluation and Treatment Procedures for Allied Health Personnel,* 2nd ed. Indiana University Foundation, Indianapolis, IN, pp. 88–97.

47. Mills, V. (1984) Electromyographic results of inhibitory splinting. *Phys. Ther.* **64,** 190–193.
48. Mathiowetz, V., Bolding, D., and Trombly, C. (1983) Immediate effects of positioning devices on the normal and spastic hand measured by electromyography. *Am. J. Occup. Ther.* **37,** 247–254.
49. McPherson, J. and Becker, A. (1985) Dynamic splint to reduce the passive component of hypertonicity. *Arch. Phys. Med. Rehabil.* **66,** 249–252.
50. Warren, C. G., Lehmann, J. F., and Koblanski, J. N. (1976) Heat and stretch procedures: an evaluation using rat tail tendon. *Arch. Phys. Med. Rehabil.* **57,** 122–126.
51. MacKay-Lyons, M. (1989) Low-load prolonged stretch in treatment of elbow flexion contractors secondary to head trauma: a case report. *Phys. Ther.* **69,** 50–54.
52. Orest, M. (1993) Casting protocol. P.T. Magazine, pp. 51–55.
53. Lehmkuhl, L. D., Thoi, L. L., Baize, C., Kelley, C. J., and Krawczyk, L., et al. (1990) Multimodality treatment of joint contractures in patients with severe brain injury: cost, effectiveness, and integration of therapies in the application of serial/inhibitive casts. *J. Head Trauma Rehabil.* **5,** 23–42.
54. Hinderer, K. A., Harris, S. R., Purdy, A. H., et al. (1988) Effects of "tone reducing" vs. standard plaster casts on gait improvement in children with cerebral palsy. *Dev. Med. Child. Neurol.* **30,** 37–77.
55. Zablotny, C., Andric, M. F., and Gowland, C. (1987) Serial casting: clinical applications for the adult head injured patient. *J. Head Trauma Rehabil.* **2,** 46–52.
56. Lehmkuhl, L. D., Thoi, L. L., Baize, C., Kelley, C. J., Krawczyk, L., et al. (1990) Multimodality treatment of joint contractures in patients with severe brain injury: cost, effectiveness, and integration of therapies in the application of serial/inhibitive casts. *J. Head Trauma Rehabil.* **5,** 23–42.
57. Hallenborg, S. C. (1990) Positioning, in *The Practical Management of Spasticity in Children and Adults* (Glenn, M. B. and Whyte, J., eds.), Lea and Febinger, Philadelphia, pp. 97–117.
58. Naeser, M. A., Alexander, M. P., Stiassny-Eder, D., Galler, V., Hobbs, J., and Bachman, D. (1993) Real versus sham acupuncture in the treatment of paralysis in acute stroke patients: a CT scan lesion study. *J. Neurol. Rehabil.* **6,** 163–173.
59. Yu, Y. H., Wang, H. C., and Wang, Z. J. (1995) The effect of acupuncture on spinal motor neuron excitability in stroke patients. *Chung Hua I Hsueh Tsa Chih* **56,** 258–263.
60. Kjendahl, A., Sallstrom, S., Osten, P. E., Stanghelle, J. K., and Borchgrevink, C. F. (1998) Acupuncture in stroke. *Tidsskr Nor Laegeforen* **118,** 1362–1366.

5
Orthotic Management

Géza F. Kogler

INTRODUCTION

Spasticity often results in biomechanical deficits that can interrupt normal neuromusculoskeletal function. A wide range of therapies, such as those detailed in other sections of this text, can be combined for the management of spasticity and its various clinical presentations. Orthoses are a fundamental component of the rehabilitation process; these can be designed to support, align, correct, or prevent a deformity and restore motion. This chapter is an overview of the basic principles and practices involved with the clinical use of orthoses for management of spasticity.

NOMENCLATURE AND CLASSIFICATION OF ORTHOSES
Description of Orthoses

An orthosis is an external force system applied to a segment of the body to control motion, and correct or prevent deformity. Orthoses are described in terms of the segment of the body they encompass and the biomechanical control parameters of their mechanical function. A device fitted for the lower leg for example is referred to as an ankle foot orthosis (AFO), whereas one for the forearm and hand is classified as a wrist hand orthosis (WHO). Accompanying the anatomical descriptor, the biomechanical function describes the intended purpose of the orthosis by indicating the mechanical controls incorporated at the joint segments. Although orthotists have adopted the use of this classification system, variations of the system have been developed by other disciplines such as physical, occupational, and hand therapists.

Based on their construction and design, orthoses are also further classified as either static or dynamic devices. Static orthoses place a body segment at rest through rigid support and possess no moving parts. Static progressive orthoses possess a variable hold feature on a joint that permits

Table 1
Symbols and Terms Used to Describe and Classify the Function of an Orthosis

Symbol	Control	Function
F	Free	Free motion permitted
A	Assist	Application of an external force to increase range, velocity, and force
R	Resist	Application of an external force to decrease range, velocity, and force
S	Stop	Elimination of undesired motion in one direction
V	Variable	An adjustable device not affecting structure
H	Hold	Elimination of all motion in one plane
L	Lock	Optional lock to eliminate motion

adjustments for joint-position change. Dynamic orthoses can permit movement of specific joints through various extrinsic mechanisms such as elastic bands, springs, and motors. These orthoses have moving parts to allow motion to be controlled in a prescribed manner. In general, the immobilization of joint segments that occurs with static orthoses is often associated with joint stiffness and muscle atrophy and should be limited to what is physiologically needed. Thus dynamic orthoses are preferred if their therapeutic benefits are equally as effective.

Functional Controls

Anatomical joints can be mechanically controlled with an orthosis through a variety of mechanisms categorized as functional controls (*see* Table 1). To improve function owing to weak musculature, for example, mechanical assists (springs, rubber bands, coils, etc.) can be incorporated into the design of a device. Restraint of motion can be achieved with a resist through the use of similar mechanisms that work to decrease the velocity and force at a joint (springs, rubber bands, coils, etc.). When motion needs to be restricted, stops strategically positioned on a mechanical joint can effectively limit the range of motion. In situations when a joint position requires adjustment during treatment the term "variable" is used to describe an adjustable feature in a functional control (i.e., variable plantar flexion stop). Hold refers to control of motion in one plane. If a joint needs to be placed in a fixed position, a lock can be used to block movement.

Orthotic Prescription

The formulation of an orthotic prescription for management of spasticity is based on a complete biomechanical assessment of the patient. The objective is to define the anatomical segments that the orthosis will encompass and to accurately describe its intended function by the biomechanical controls needed for treatment. A fundamental principle in orthotics is that an orthoses should be designed to control only those movements considered abnormal and permit free motion in anatomical segments that are not impaired. To achieve only the necessary orthotic intervention, a systematic approach to patient assessment is needed. To specify the requirements for an orthosis, a Technical Analysis Form was developed by the Committee on Prosthetics and Orthotics of the American Academy of Orthopaedic Surgeons to standardize the process of patient evaluation *(1)* *(see* Appendix). Although this Biomechanical Analysis system is time-consuming and may not be practical for all clinical situations, a focused evaluation using these guidelines is invaluable. An orthotic prescription should be based on the description of the patient impairment in functional terms and the treatment objectives. The orthotic recommendation derived from this information should indicate the anatomical joints the device will encompass and the desired control of designated function (i.e., AFO with free dorsiflexion and a variable plantar flexion stop).

Seven areas are considered in describing a patients major impairments: 1) skeletal: bone and joint; 2) neurological: sensory and motor; 3) skin condition; 4) vascular; 5) balance; 6) gait deviations; 7) other pathology. These major areas of impairments need only be grossly defined with the focused attention given to the evaluation of volitional muscle force, active and passive range of motion, hypertonicity, and proprioception. In considering muscle function, clinicians must distinguish the contributing factors associated with resistance to passive stretch and tonal response to fast and slow stretch. Patients should have both a dynamic evaluation during walking as well as a static evaluation at rest because muscle tone may vary and there is little correlation between the two *(2)*. If physical examination does not provide sufficient information of patient impairment, additional assessment through quantitative gait analysis may be warranted. Using a summary of the functional disability, treatment objectives specific to management of spasticity are categorized as: prevent/correct deformity, improve ambulation, inhibit tone, and protection of a joint body segment. These proven methods for developing an orthotic prescription will lead to an acceptable clinical recommendation. However, the dynamic nature of spasticity often requires frequent alterations to a base prescription to accommodate changes in a patients condition.

CLINICAL BASIS FOR ORTHOTIC INTERVENTION

Clinical Features Related to Orthotic Management

Orthotic intervention for the management of spasticity requires an understanding of the respective movement dysfunctions and common clinical manifestations. Lance *(3)* described four traits associated with spasticity in patients with an UMN syndrome. Enhanced stretch reflexes (spasticity) and released flexor reflexes are characterized as positive symptoms whereas loss of dexterity and weakness loss are classified as negative symptoms. The interplay of these two categories of symptoms and the related muscle stiffness and contractures owing to rheologic changes determine the functional deficit of the patient that forms the basis for the orthotic treatment plan.

Spasticity caused from an upper motor neuron (UMN) syndrome may result in motor dysfunction that limits functional abilities in walking, standing, sitting, and postural control. Clinical features of spasticity are: increased muscle tone, exaggerated tendon jerks, stretch reflex spread to the extensors, and repetitive stretch-reflex charges or clonus. The motor patterns that develop from these impairments have varied functional limitations with differing degrees of intensity. The interaction of agonist and antagonist activity determine the clinical presentation of movement dysfunction. Patients may have weakness or overactivity of agonist muscles with or without co-contractions of antagonists that result in limited movement or loss of individual muscle control. Thus weakness/overactivation of the agonists or co-activation of antagonists are important to distinguish for proper control of an extremity with an orthosis. Identification of the characteristic patterns of movement dysfunction are helpful in understanding a patient's functional impairment. Mayer et al. *(4)* described 14 common upper- and lower-extremity patterns of UMN dysfunction with seven in each respective category (*see* Table 2). Orthotic management of many of these specific motor dysfunctions are described in more detail later in this chapter.

Hypertonicity

Reduction of tone is a common orthotic treatment objective for the management of spasticity. Hypertonicity that produces movement deficits requires an understanding of how joint position and passive joint motion influences function. Knowledge of an individual's tonal patterns often gives insight to positioning and motion-control guidelines that inhibit tone. Extensor and flexor synergies are gross muscle movements over several joints that limit function and selective control of individual muscles. Positioning the affected joints opposite to the tonal response is one of the current trends of tone inhibition with orthoses. Although the mechanism for

Table 2
Common Patterns of Upper Motor Neuron Dysfunction and Muscles Contributing to Deformity

Deformity	Muscles Contributing to Deformity
	Upper extremity
Adducted/internally rotated shoulder	Pectoralis major, latissimus dorsi, teres major, subscapularis
Flexed elbow	Brachioradialis, biceps, brachialis
Pronated forearm	Pronator quadratis, pronator teres
Flexed wrist	Flexor carpi radialis and brevis, extrinsic finger flexors
Clenched fist	Various muscle slips of the flexor digitorum profundus and sublimis
Intrinsic plus hand	Dorsal interossei
Thumb-in-palm deformity	Adductor pollicis, thenar group, flexor pollicis longus
	Lower extremity
Pes equinovarus (with claw toes)	Medial gastrocnemius, lateral hamstrings, soleus tibialis
	Posterior, tibialis anterior, extensor hallucis longus, long-toe flexors, peroneus longus
Pes valgus	Peroneus longus, gastrocnemius, soleus, tibialis anterior (weak), long toe flexors (weak)
Striatal toe	Extensor hallucis longus
Extended knee	Gluteus maximus, rectus femoris, vastus lateralis, vastus
	Medialis, vastus intermedius, hamstrings, gastrocnemius, iliopsoas (weak)
Flexed knee	Medial and lateral hamstrings, quadriceps, gastrocnemius
Adducted thighs	Adductor longus and magnus, gracilis, iliopsoas (weak), pectineus (weak)
Flexed hip	Rectus femoris, iliopsoas, pectineus, adductor longus, adductor brevis (weak), gluteus maximus (weak)

Adapted with permission from ref *(4)*.

tone modification is not based on scientific study, qualitative improvements in function have encouraged clinical development in this area.

Tissue Mechanics and Orthotic Principles

Rheologic changes that occur from prolonged and chronic spasticity usually involve soft tissues such as tendon ligament and muscle. These structures have viscoelastic properties that produce stress relaxation and creep. If structures are not continually stretched, the tissue remodels without the elasticity of normal collagen and becomes stiff as it loses its elongation potential. An understanding of tissue properties is important for proper application of an orthotic-force system. These properties can be classified as: stress relaxation, creep, strain-rate dependence, elastic deformation, and plastic deformation.

Static orthoses and progressive serial casting effectively use the tissue property of "stress relaxation" to increase range of motion. Holding soft tissues in a fixed position for an extended period reduces the corrective forces over time, altering the tissue properties for gradual changes in joint position. Dynamic orthoses use the tissue attribute of creep to induce range of motion gains through continuous deformation via the constant application of a fixed load. Both creep and stress relaxation can produce plastic deformation of soft tissues, which is the permanent elongation that remains after a load is removed. Plastic deformation of soft tissue is the primary orthotic objective for gains of increased range of motion to last. Another property, elastic deformation, is the elongation that is created by loading regained after a load is removed from soft tissue. Strain-rate dependence is the reliance of tissue properties on the speed or rate a load is applied to tissue. Orthotic treatment influences strain-rate dependence by the manner in which loads are applied and through load duration wear schedules.

Chronic Spasticity and Contractures

Orthoses may be indicated for patients with chronic spasticity that often develops into soft-tissue contractures if untreated. Preventative orthotic intervention can help reduce this occurrence or resist progression of joint positioning problems and limitations in range of motion. Both static and dynamic orthoses can be used to provide prolonged stretch to prevent or correct a deformity owing to spasticity. Clinical judgment is relied on to determine the magnitude of force that can be applied to maintain joint position and stretch out a contracture. As with other therapeutic stretching techniques, slow progressive stretching is preferred over rapid forceful elongation of soft tissues. Variable position stops on a static progressive orthosis accommodate for changes in joint angulation and range as therapy progresses. Dynamic orthoses that use an assist to provide constant force often are equipped with variable control mechanisms to modulate the amount of force applied to the joint segment. Designs that incorporate variable controls tend to be more universal for management of spastic contractures because treatment usually results in frequent joint-position changes.

WRIST HAND FINGER ORTHOSES

Treatment Approaches

Orthotic management of the hypertonic hand and wrist has historically been controversial. The medical literature documents treatment protocols that both advocate the use of orthoses and oppose orthotic intervention. The use of orthoses in rehabilitation of the spastic wrist and hand developed largely from the clinical experiences of therapists, with few quantifiable measures utilized to document the efficacy of their treatment outcome (5–7). A survey of the tone-reduction orthoses for the upper limb reveals a disparity of orthotic design principles, wear schedules, functional outcome, and construction materials (8). Despite the controversies associated with orthotic management of the spastic upper limb, orthoses continue to be an adjunctive treatment procedure in many rehabilitation programs.

Two different treatment philosophies have evolved for the orthotic management of spasticity. The traditional "biomechanical approach" (9) developed from the fundamental need to control deformity and uses conventional orthotic techniques and principles to accomplish this objective. Treatment rationale for this theory suggests that prolonged stretch changes the mechanical properties of the spastic muscle, which permits increased range of motion and a reduction of tone (10,11). An alternative rationale, referred to as the "neurophysiologic approach," is based on movement and positioning techniques to inhibit spasticity. Spastic-muscle inhibition may occur through prolonged stretch in a muscles maximum range. Proponents of the neurophysiologic rationale theorize two mechanisms may be activated: stimulation of the neurotendinous spindle and the release of Ia receptors of the intrafusal muscle fiber (6,12–14).

Types of Orthoses

Numerous types of orthoses have been developed for flexor-tone reduction in the upper limb. Because the majority of tone-reduction orthoses are based on subjective clinical observations and case studies, the rationale for certain design criteria is often not well-documented. Basic design features such as the dorsal vs volar approach for the management of the hypertonic wrist and hand have been assessed with varied conclusions of their performance capabilities. Chariat *(5)* studied dorsal and volar orthoses in hemiplegia and concluded the dorsal design was more effective at reducing tone than the palmar devices. This concurs with the works of Kaplan *(6)* and Snook *(15)*, who made similar observations. In contrast, there have also been reports that show volar orthoses produce a decrease in flexor tone *(16–18)*. One study comparing dorsal and volar resting hand orthoses deemed both designs effective at reducing flexor tone *(19)*. The disparity in the literature on this topic is owing in part to the diversity of research methodology making comparisons between studies difficult. Studies using similar quantifiable measures and methods will be useful in future investigations.

The primary objectives for management of the spastic hand are flexor-tone reduction, increased passive range of motion, and the prevention of palm maceration. Positioning of the upper limb and hand is fundamental to the functional outcome and may require changes throughout the treatment process. Trombly *(20)* suggests that both the wrist and hand be included for orthoses intended for spasticity reduction because extension of one joint segment often results in a flexion contracture if both are not orthotically controlled.

Some of the more common tone-reduction wrist hand finger orthoses (WHFO) are the: Snook splint *(15)*, cone splint, Bobath splint, Becker splint, finger-abduction splint, and serial casting. The upper limb can be controlled using dorsal, volar, and circumferential designs dependent on the treatment philosophies and individual needs of the patient. Although the orthotic objective may be similar for tone-reduction devices, the treatment approach and philosophies may be notably different.

The reflex-inhibitive pattern suggested by Bobath is the basis for positioning with the Snook splint *(15,18)*. The orthosis aims to position the wrist in 30° of hyperextension, the metatarsal phalangeal (MP) joints in 45°, interphalangeal (IP) joint extension, finger abduction, thumb abduction, and extension. For spasticity isolated to the hand, reflex-inhibition through finger abduction is recommended by Bobath *(21)*. This can be accomplished with varying orthotic designs ranging from a simple foam block with an array of holes for the fingers and thumb (*see* Fig. 1) to thermoplastic devices with finger troughs and holes (*see* Fig. 2). For inhibition of finger-flexion tone, a cone-type device held in the hand is another common orthotic technique. The finger-hand cone control has also been incorporated into WHOs *(22)* (*see* Fig. 3A,B) and slings *(13)* designed to reduce flexor tone.

Orthotic therapy that provides deep pressure and warmth combined with movement therapy has also been proposed for management of wrist-hand spasticity *(23)*. An inflatable wrist-hand immobilization orthosis commonly used in emergency situations has been adopted for spasticity inhibition. The

Orthotic Management

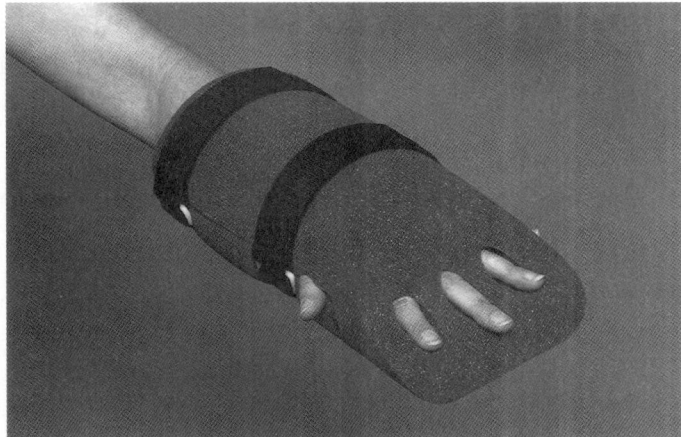

Fig. 1. A bi-valved prefabricated foam block type wrist hand finger orthosis for a left hand. Troughs located on the dorsal and volar halves maintain the fingers in abduction when they are pressed together via the Velcro® closures. (Sammons™ Preston, Bolingbrook, IL)

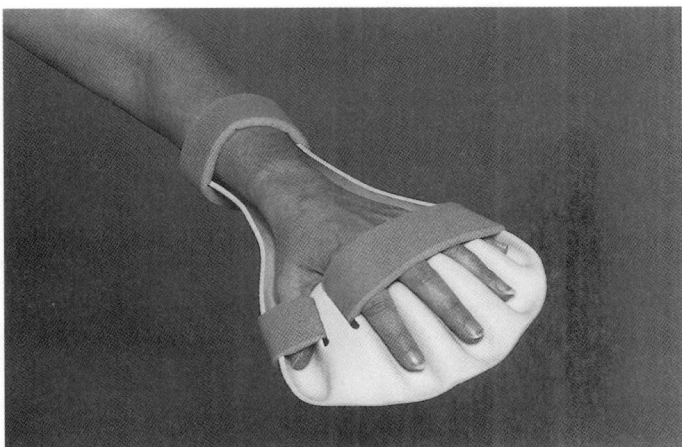

Fig. 2. A prefabricated thermoplastic wrist hand finger orthosis designed to maintain the wrist in neutral and the fingers and thumb in abduction. (Sammons™ Preston, Bolingbrook, IL)

affected joints are stabilized through mild air-pressure compression with orthotic cuffs that encompass the limb segment. The orthosis is worn for 20 min prior to therapeutic exercise and stretching continuing through the

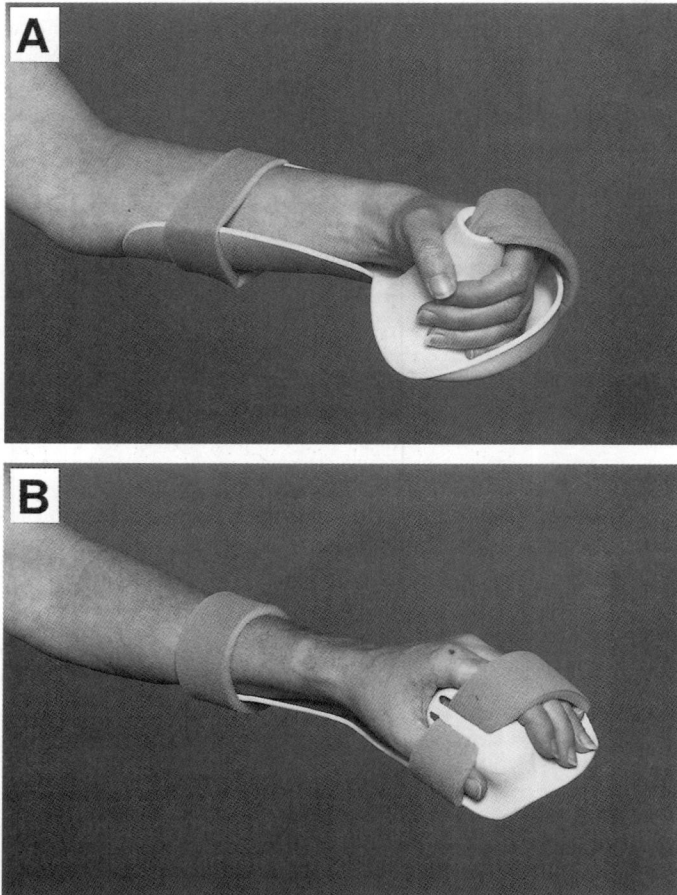

Fig. 3. Prefabricated thermoplastic wrist hand finger orthoses designed to reduce flexor tone in spasticity and prevent palm maceration. (**A**) A cone-type orthosis with the wrist positioned at neutral and the fingers accommodated in slight flexion. (**B**) A volar-design orthosis with the wrist positioned in 20 degrees of extension with the thumb posted in slight extension (Sammons™ Preston, Bolingbrook, IL)

therapy session *(24)*. The orthosis maintains joint position and provides sensory stimulation during therapeutic exercises that simulate weight-bearing *(23)*.

Prolonged immobilization through serial casting is a method that has been used effectively for management of spasticity in brain-injured and stroke patients *(18,25)*. The biomechanical approach for spasticity inhibition is the basis for this type of orthotic-treatment therapy. Proponents of serial casting state therapeutic benefits including decreased spasticity, increased range of motion, and stimulation of antagonist muscle tone in certain regions *(18,25)*. The technique consists of the application of plaster bandage or fiber resin tape with the affected limb segments positioned in full stretch. The casts can be bi-valved to permit access to the limb for additional therapeutic stretching and periodic bathing. Casts are changed according to a patients progress based on range of movement increases for up to 3 mo. To avert complications of skin irritation and pain associated with serial casting patients must be monitored closely. Skill in the application of casts is also a necessity if problems are to be avoided. Custom and prefabricated orthoses that can be progressively adjusted as a patient's situation changes have also been introduced. The time and cost saved with these systems are an alternative to conventional casting methods.

ELBOW ORTHOSES

Spasticity affecting the elbow usually presents as increased flexion tone with extensor tone being rare. In moderate to severe cases, the flexion attitude can lead to skin breakdown, hygiene problems, and malodor *(4)*. Both custom and prefabricated elbow orthoses have been developed for treatment of increased elbow flexor tone with various orthotic approaches used to increase range of motion and reduce the occurrence of contractures. The application of an increased amount of force for a short duration or a decreased amount of force for a short duration are the two basic approaches used to improve range of motion caused from spasticity. In most cases orthotic management is an adjunct to stretching and other forms of physical therapy.

Types of Orthoses

To improve range of motion with an elbow flexion contracture or decrease flexor tone, a static progressive orthosis is effective. A static progressive orthosis provides static incremental changes in elbow positioning, which can reduce secondary inflammation associated with therapeutic stretching. The basic design consists of thermoplastic forearm and humeral cuffs with an adjoining mechanical joint and a turnbuckle rod (Fig. 4). The trimlines of the humeral cuff extend to the axilla and the forearm cuff terminates at the radial styloid. The cuffs are situated anteriorly with Velcro® closures encompassing the open posterior segments of the cuffs. The turnbuckle component of the elbow orthosis provides the progressive joint angular changes in the device. The posterior Velcro straps nearest the elbow joint and the distal segments of the anterior cuffs provide the corrective forces to reduce the flexion contracture. Although the success of the turnbuckle mechanism for management of flexor tone has not been reported,

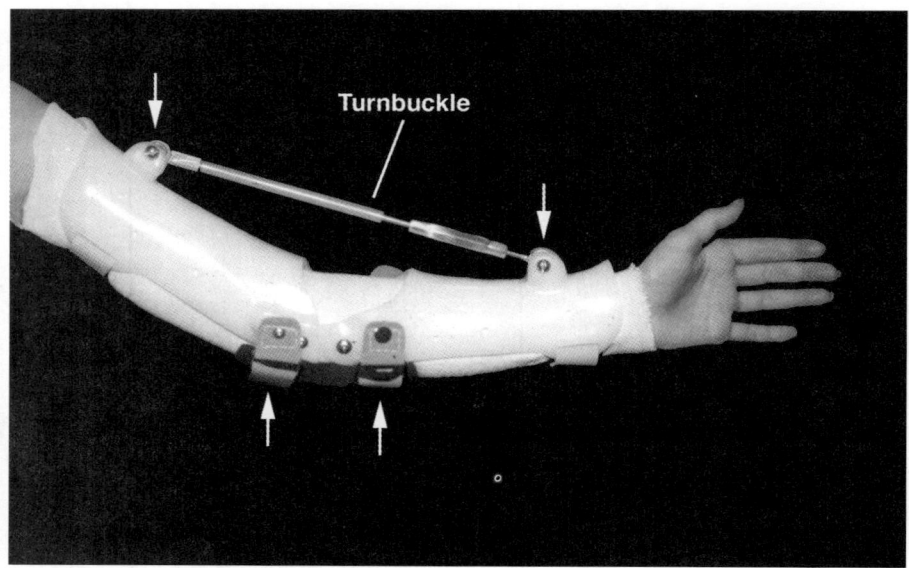

Fig. 4. An adjustable custom elbow orthosis with a turnbuckle attachment for managing elbow-flexion contractures. Posterior straps positioned close to the elbow joint form one common force-application point and the anterior humeral and forearm components apply two opposing force application points, resulting in a simple three point-force system (arrows) to the extremity to resist flexion of the elbow.

Green and McCoy *(26)* reported contractures owing to acute injuries produced an average increase in range of motion of 43 degrees and an average deformity reduction of 37 degrees. An adjustable extension joint possessing an internal locking mechanism is another means of control for an elbow orthosis.

A dynamic orthosis is indicated in patients that have mild-to-moderate spasticity at the elbow where nominal corrective forces are needed to resolve undesirable joint posture. The dynamic assist has the advantage of applying continued corrective forces to the contracted or spastic muscles but still allow full range of motion of the elbow. Although the constant force may be beneficial for mild contractures, in some instances the active stretch can also trigger increase tone for some forms of spasticity. The orthosis consists of forearm and humeral cuff segments with Velcro closures and a mechanical joint with an assist mechanism. The dynamic assist can be in the form of an elastic band, spring, or spring coil. Joints and their accompanying assist mechanism should have design features that allow for diverse adjustment of the force application. Several prefabricated dynamic elbow joints and orthoses are available that can provide control comparable to custom devices (Fig. 5).

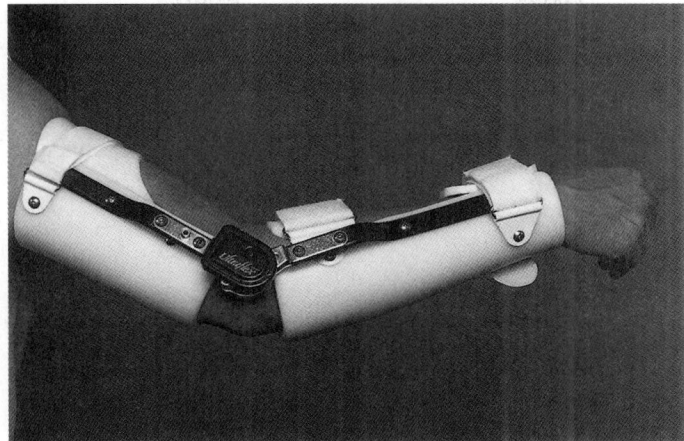

Fig. 5. A custom elbow orthosis equipped with an extension-assist joint uses a coiled-spring mechanism to apply the external force to the extremity via thermoplastic cuffs and Velcro straps. (UltraFlex® Systems Inc., Malvern, PA).

Overall, elbow orthoses are most effective for the management of mild-to-moderate spasticity. The short lever arms and the magnitude of the corrective forces required to control severe tone at the elbow are usually not sufficient enough to treat severe tonal problems at the elbow. Serial progressive casting may be considered for severe spasticity if an orthotic therapy is preferred over other treatment regimens.

ANKLE FOOT ORTHOSES

Types of Orthoses

AFOs may be used in the management of spasticity to inhibit tone, increase range of motion, prevent contracture, and enhance function. Because clinical problems associated with spasticity vary greatly among patients, the orthotic goals may also differ. In some instances two different types of orthoses may be needed for treatment. For example, orthotic management may include one orthosis for static positioning to maintain range of motion for night-time use and another orthosis to provide a dynamic stretch to a joint segment. Therefore, careful consideration should be given to each issue so that orthotic intervention can be maximized. In the lower extremities, movement dysfunction owing to spasticity can have a dehabilitating effect that limits joint movements and impairs selective control of certain muscles. A primary concern for treatment with orthoses is identifying the compensatory muscle activity that results from the hypertonicity. Subtle design changes in an AFO can have a profound effect on functional potential and should be carefully scrutinized. This section describes the orthotic rationale for management of the most common problems related to spasticity in the lower extremity.

The AFO can be effective in the rehabilitation of patients with mild-to-moderate spasticity of the lower leg. The use of thermoplastic AFOs over conventional metal double-upright designs is the current trend in the management of spasticity, because patients prefer their light-weight, total-contact interface and greater aesthetic appeal. These orthoses are durable, highly adjustable, and easily maintained. A diversity of orthoses can be prescribed for treatment of hypertonicity, however, maximum success is based on critical assessment of the individual goals and needs of the patient. Once the orthotic treatment objectives are established, the desired biomechanical controls built into the orthosis determine functional outcome. Material selection and design play a secondary role to these basic requirements in developing the optimal orthotic system for the patient.

Several clinical features that may accompany spasticity and influence orthotic recommendations are: loss of sensation, type of spasticity, and stretch response. Loss of sensation puts a patient at increased risk of developing pressure sores from the orthosis. Attention to fit of the orthosis and the manner in which corrective forces are applied to the limb are critical to avert skin-related problems. The stretch response, whether slow or fast with passive or active dorsiflexion of the foot, may be an indicator whether dorsiflexion motion from midstance to terminal stance of walking will provoke spasticity and increase tone. Therefore, clinical evaluation of a patient's response to a brisk and slow stretch of the triceps surae is an important determinant for considering functional controls such as free dorsiflexion, and dorsiflexion assists on AFOs. A slow stretch response usually will not trigger increased tone in AFO when walking at an average speed. However if a brisk stretch reflex induces tone, patients will likely experience an increase in tone during the later portion of stance with an AFO that has a dorsiflexion assist or permits free dorsiflexion. Thus considerable clinical judgment is needed to determine the appropriate orthotic functional controls for an AFO in patients with certain types of stretch responses.

Basic treatment approaches for patients that walk with an ankle equinus (drop foot) from increased tone, require the control of plantar flexion. The orthotic goal is to maintain the ankle foot in a plantargrade position (90°) for stability during standing and to achieve toe clearance at swing phase. This can be accomplished with an AFO through several different motion-control mechanisms. A solid-ankle AFO achieves the maximum orthotic control by restricting the movements of both plantar flexion and dorsiflexion. With a thermoformed plastic AFO, the motion control is achieved through a combination of its structural shell shape, the mechanical properties of the material, special reinforcements at the ankle region and the orientation of the trimlines. Plantar flexion within an AFO is restricted through an anterior-control strap at the ankle and partially by the shoe closure (i.e., laces, Velcro). The control strap maintains the heel within the foot-piece section of the orthosis and limits the motion between the foot and orthosis. The solid ankle AFO can provide swing-phase clearance for the toe and reduces hyperextension of the knee during stance phase of walking, both problems associated with increased tone in the lower extremity. AFO systems using an ankle joint to control motion have the added advantage of being adjustable if changes in tone are likely to occur.

Although a solid ankle AFO or an AFO with a plantar-flexion stop may achieve the desired toe clearance during the swing-phase portion of gait, consideration must be given to the compromises borne during stance phase with the restriction of plantar flexion. During normal walking the foot plantar flexes just after heel strike (deceleration) to provide a stable base at foot flat as the limb accepts the load of body weight and advances over the foot. Although, the concession for a plantar-flexion stop appears to be costly in gait, careful shoe selection and small changes in step length can minimize the effects on walking. To emulate the eccentric contraction of the dorsiflexors that are not active with a plantar-flexion stop during heel strike, a shoe with a cushioned heel will permit a smoother transition to foot flat and reduce the knee flexion moment during the heel contact portion of gait. A properly selected running or walking-type shoe may provide the additional shock absorption necessary to normalize walking during the initial phase of stance. Shoes can also be converted to a cushioned heel if the desired hardness (durometer) of the heel is not acceptable. If the heel is too soft, patients with a tendency towards knee hyperextension may not have adequate knee control. The importance of the shoe is often overlooked and should be assessed with the same care and attention as the AFO in the overall performance evaluation of the patient.

Free dorsiflexion may be an important feature to maintain in an AFO in some patients. The hinged or articulated AFO provides a plantar-flexion stop for swing-phase toe clearance but permits dorsiflexion from midstance to terminal stance. This yields a normal step length on the opposite side as the body's weight line moves anterior to the axis of rotation of the ankle, which is restricted with rigid solid-ankle designs. The additional therapeutic gain of passive stretch of the gastroc soleus muscles is also possible with free dorsiflexion in an articulated ankle AFO *(27)*. One must be cautious with permitting passive stretch of the plantar flexors as it may induce a stretch-reflex pattern that induces plantar flexion in some patients. In general, a dorsiflexion assist/plantar-flexion resist AFO is limited in its use in the management of hypertonicity, because the assists are usually not powerful enough to overcome the increased tone and have also been known to trigger a plantar-flexion response. They are usually reserved for inadequate dorsiflexion rather than treatment of spasticity.

Preventing deformities because of contractures is an important consideration in orthotic management of spasticity. In the non-ambulatory patient where increased plantar flexion tone is present the rehabilitation goal may be to improve sitting posture and prevent the development of permanent ankle deformities. For sitting balance and comfort in wheelchairs the ankle should be situated at 90°. A rigid, solid ankle AFO with an ankle control strap can maintain adequate ankle foot position and resist progression of the deformity. An articulated AFO is indicated only if the ankle equinus cannot be reduced to neutral and progressive correction of the deformity is a treatment goal.

Inhibitive and progressive serial casting have influenced current orthotic-treatment approaches *(28–30)*. These concepts are now integrated into the design of tone-reducing ankle foot orthoses (TRAFOs) that inhibit the extensor synergy patterns through dorsiflexion of the toes in patients with a hyperactive flexor-grasp reflex *(31)*. Additional modifications to the AFO foot plate theorized to inhibit tone include: metatarsal pads, interphalangeal joint support (sulcus pad), toe-extension plates, heel and forefoot wedges, metatarsal head and calcaneal reliefs. Although these orthotic techniques have demonstrated clinical success in some patients, the mechanisms responsible for the tone inhibition are not well-understood. The tone inhibiting response is not reliable in all situations, making patient selection criteria for tone inhibiting AFOs difficult.

The idea of progressive stretching for management of spasticity with serial casts can also be achieved with an AFO. For moderate to severe spasticity, progressive stretch with an adjustable hinged AFO can reduce the magnitude of deformity and prevent progression. These orthoses have been used in the management of closed-head injuries and other upper motor neuron injuries that can produce an equinus foot position owing to increased plantar-flexion tone. A thermoplastic custom AFO is usually required to manage this type of problem. An anterior posterior clamshell design with an adjustable plantar-flexion stop can provide infinite adjustments for sagittal plane foot-ankle positioning (*see* Fig. 6). Corrective forces are applied at the proximal posterior calf section, the plantar distal foot piece, and by a padded anterior ankle strap or anterior shell. Because patients are at risk of developing skin ulceration, relief zones and padding are often incorporated to avoid pressure

Orthotic Management

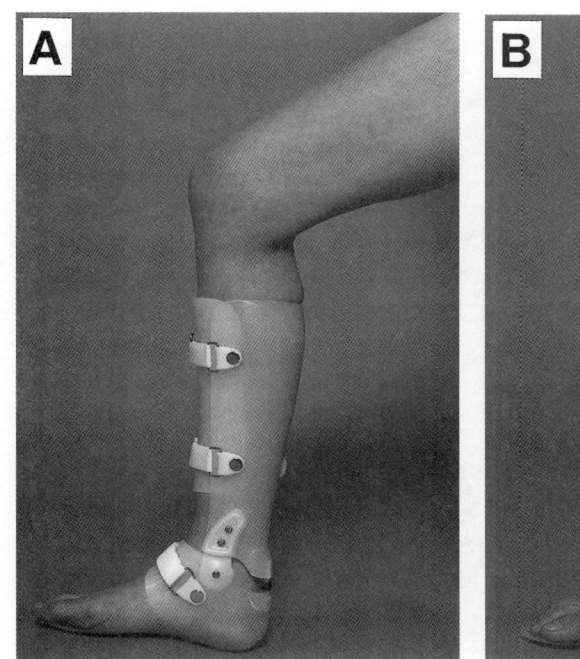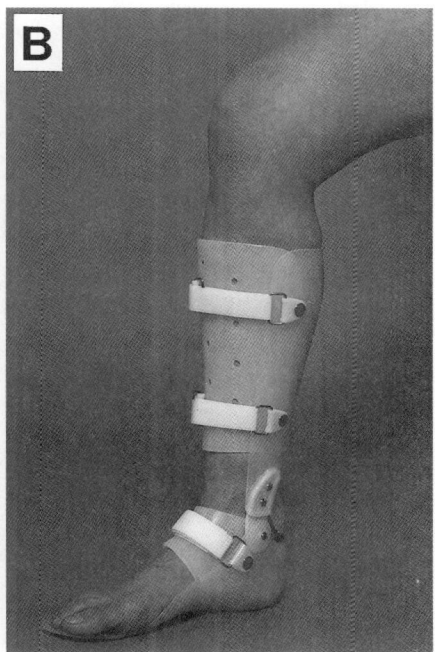

Fig. 6. A custom AFO designed to reduce plantar-flexion contractures. The orthosis has an anterior posterior clamshell closure with an adjustable plantar-flexion stop that provides adjustment for foot-ankle positioning in the sagittal plane. **(A)** Oblique view showing the design of anterior foot and tibial shells that apply the posterior-directed forces for controlling plantar flexion. **(B)** Sagittal view showing the posterior adjustable stop (arrow).

problems over bony prominences (i.e., posterior heel, malleoli). Special coiled springs that provide constant corrective forces are an example of a dynamic AFO design for management of spasticity and contractures (*see* Fig. 7). Progressive correction with an AFO must be accompanied with a regular stretching program through physical therapy. Patients should be monitored regularly to assure pressure sores (decubitus ulcers) do not develop.

An extensor synergy is characterized by increased tone in the plantar flexors, which causes an ankle equinus and restricts weight-bearing to the ball of the foot *(32)*. The plantar-flexed ankle creates an artificial leg length difference that is further complicated by inadequate knee flexion. Patients have difficulty with toe clearance and compensate by circumducting the hip and with exaggerated trunk shifts. If plantar flexion can be successfully controlled with an AFO, a 1-cm sole lift on the unaffected side can assist in full swing-phase clearance.

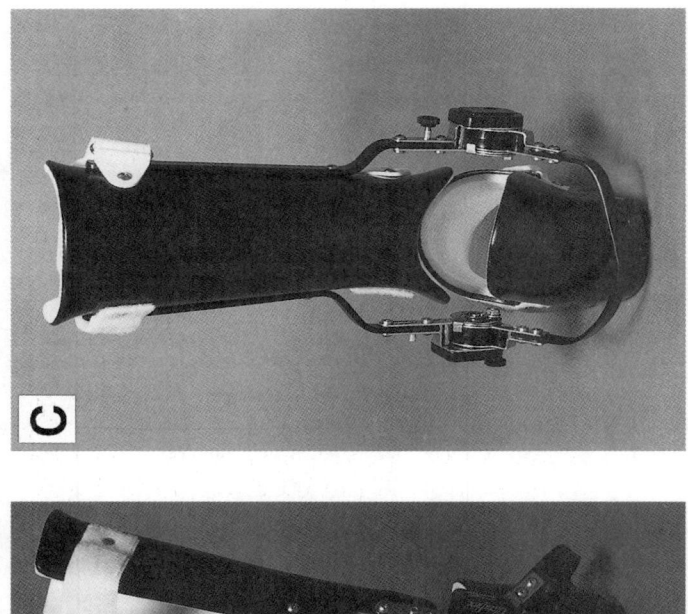
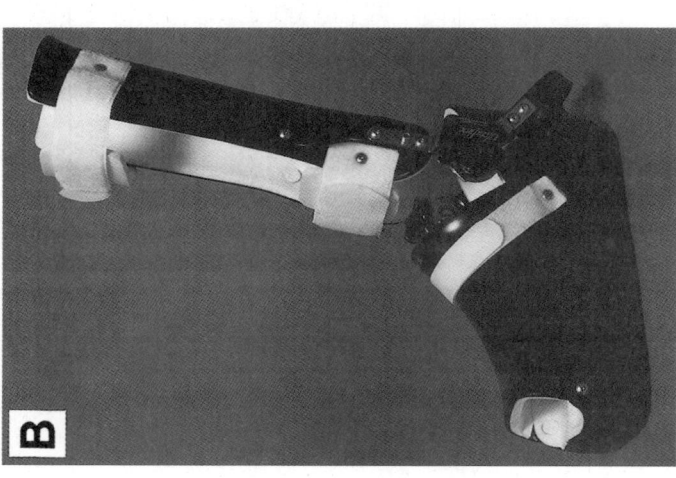

Fig. 7. A prefabricated AFO designed to reduce contractures at the talocrural and subtalar joint with a coiled-spring ankle-joint mechanism. (**A**) The AFO shown with the anterior-foot shell held open to accept the limb. (**B**) The AFO with the anterior-foot shell in the closed position. (**C**) Posterior view of the AFO showing the components that permit positioning adjustments in the coronal plane. (UltraFlex® Systems Inc., Malvern, PA).

Clinical problems related to hypertonicity acting on the knee can often be controlled with an AFO. To control knee hyperextension caused by equinus position at the ankle, a solid-ankle AFO positioned in 5–10° of dorsiflexion can adequately reduce this knee posture. From early stance to midstance the AFO applies a flexion force at the knee resisting knee extension. The range of dorsiflexion and quadriceps strength are determinant factors in the amount of dorsiflexion the AFO is set in. If the achilles tendon is tight the amount of ankle dorsiflexion will be limited. Knee instability may occur with quadricep weakness if the ankle position of the AFO is situated in excessive dorsiflexion.

Flexor synergies of the lower extremity are more difficult to treat orthotically than extensor synergies. Persistent hip flexion and knee flexion and ankle dorsiflexion produce a "crouch-like" gait pattern commonly seen with some forms of cerebral palsy (CP). Moderate spasticity that produces excessive knee flexion can be treated with several types of AFOs. A custom plastic solid-ankle AFO with an anterior clamshell with the ankle foot positioned at 90° can adequately control knee-flexion spasticity. A hinged clamshell closure AFO with a dorsiflexion stop and free plantar flexion is an alternative design. The floor-reaction AFO and variations of this design are very effective at encouraging knee extension for patients with knee-flexion hypertonicity (*see* Fig. 8).

Prefabricated Orthoses

With the economics of rehabilitation medical care a growing concern, the consideration to use "off-the-shelf" stock orthoses has increased in recent years. Numerous prefabricated orthoses are available as an alternative or adjunct treatment option to custom fabricated devices. With proper fit and selection, some problems related to the orthotic management of spasticity can be effectively treated with stock orthoses.

Prefabricated AFOs used for positioning the foot and ankle during the early stages of spasticity may be one of the most appropriate places to use stock orthoses. In nonambulatory patients with mild spasticity, several prefabricated AFO systems have been devised to prevent contractures, improve ankle positioning, and reduce the risk of skin breakdown. Appropriate design considerations include: relief for the posterior aspect of the heel, control for internal and external rotation, padded anterior ankle-control strap, adjustability for alignment, durability of materials, and features to aid in hygiene.

Prefabricated orthoses are designed to fit the general population with minimal accommodations for specific individual variations. Orthotic systems usually have a limited selection of sizes (i.e., small, medium, large)

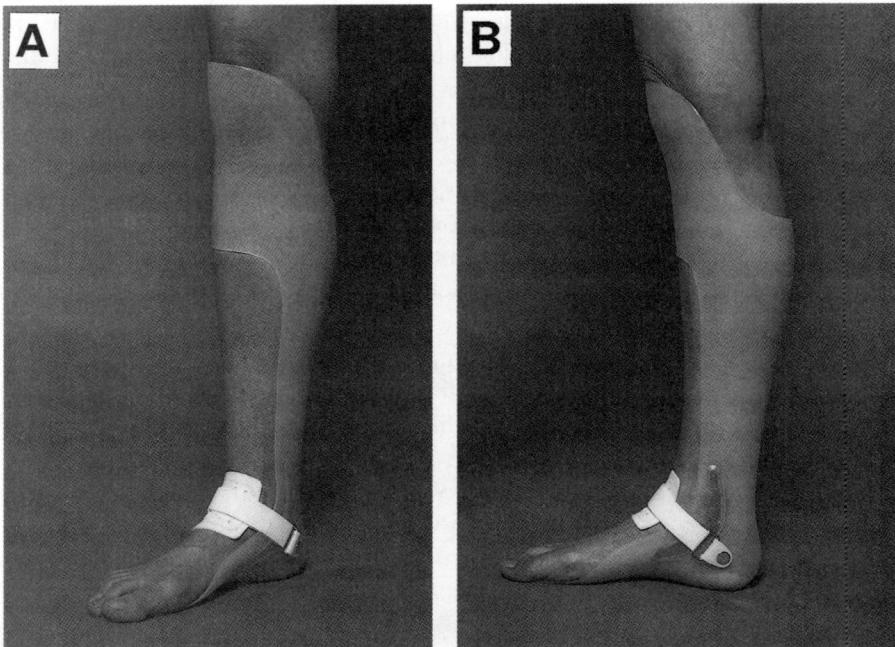

Fig. 8. The floor-reaction AFO designed to control knee flexion. **(A)** Oblique view showing anterior proximal trimlines around the knee. **(B)** Sagittal view of the AFO showing carbon reinforcement at the ankle to resist deflection of the plastic during the stance portion of the gait cycle.

determined by a few measurements of the patient. Problems associated with prefabricated AFOs usually relate to inadequate fit, decreased efficiency in maintaining foot-ankle position, skin breakdown, and general discomfort. Contraindications for the use of prefabricated AFOs include: excessive deformity, moderate to severe spasticity, and patients at risk of skin problems. Although some commercial systems are appropriate for temporary use during physical therapy sessions, patients should be fit with custom orthoses for definitive treatment.

KNEE ORTHOSES

The use of knee orthoses (KOs) for management of spasticity is limited owing to mechanical limitations of their design. The primary mechanical disadvantage with knee orthoses is that the proximal and distal lever arms tend to be too short for the efficient application of forces. KOs designed to maintain the knee in extension apply corrective forces posteriorly over soft tissue that usually is not sufficient enough to resist the deforming forces comfortably in patients with spastic paresis.

In nonambulatory patients with increased knee-flexion tone a knee ankle foot orthosis (KAFO) with a variable stop at the knee joint will provide the necessary knee control and reduce the risk of skin-pressure problems. A KAFO redistributes corrective forces over a larger area compared to the KO. Patients that have mild to moderate tone are best-suited for management with a KAFO. For more difficult cases, some patients may require a long leg cast to prevent deformity and control knee position.

In general, a knee orthosis is not recommended for increased flexion tone at the knee in the ambulatory patient. Instead, an AFO positioned in slight plantar flexion with a rigid ankle is usually beneficial via an extension moment produced at the knee during stance while providing free knee flexion in swing.

For control of knee hyperextension owing to increased extensor tone during stance, a knee orthosis with an extension stop and free knee flexion (Swedish Knee Cage) is of benefit for gait-training purposes in therapy (*see* Fig. 9). The short lever arms on the Swedish knee orthosis usually prevent it from being used as definitive knee hyperextension-control device. The orthosis is commonly used in conjunction with an AFO to encourage knee flexion during stance. The orthosis is most commonly used for management of pes equinus in hemiplegia patients to control knee hyperextension *(33,34)*.

KNEE ANKLE FOOT ORTHOSES

With the exception of some forms of CP in children and young adults, KAFOs are usually contraindicated for the management of spastic paresis in the ambulatory patient. If the extent of functional impairment is severe enough to warrant the use of a KAFO, loss of selective control and increased energy expenditure will prevent improvement in functional ambulation. Only in instances where knee stability may aid in transfers is a KAFO indicated for management of increased tone.

A KAFO can be used effectively to manage the nonambulatory patient that has a knee-flexion contracture or chronic flexor tone with mild-to-moderate spasticity. If the magnitude of the deformity is not severe, the use of KAFOs for night-time use may be all that is needed to maintain joint position and alignment. Although most need to be custom fabricated, some commercial systems may be beneficial if use is only temporary and they are carefully fitted.

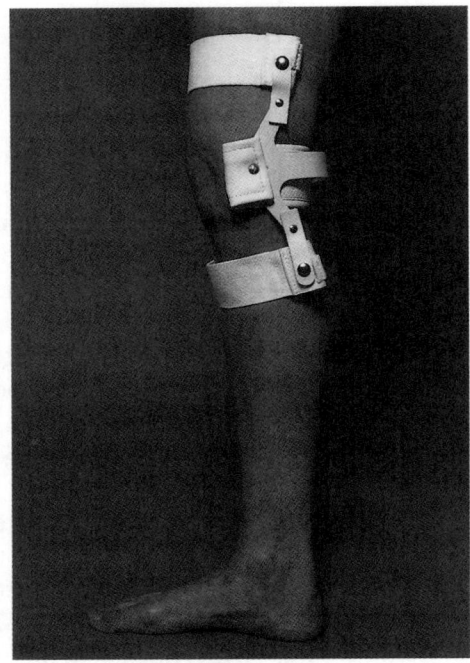

Fig. 9. Knee orthosis (Swedish knee cage) designed to resist knee hyperextension while permitting free knee flexion (United States Manufacturing Company, Pasadena, CA).

HIP ORTHOSES

The typical patterns of spasticity afflicting the hip are flexion, adduction, and internal rotation. Although orthoses have been used to manage all of these deformities, adduction and internal rotation are the most common for orthotic intervention and preventative care. Adduction of the thighs can lead to difficulties with dressing, standing, transfers, walking, sitting, and perineal hygiene. To prevent deformity and maintain desirable hip posture, hip-abduction orthosis are used. With the clinical goal to prevent scissoring of the thighs owing to hypertonicity of the adductors, an orthosis must resist or stop the medial progression of the thighs. For nonambulatory patients, V-shaped foam blocks with Velcro closures are very effective at preventing contractures and ideal for acute, early orthotic intervention. For the seated patient, thigh cuffs with an adjustable spreader bar positioned just proximal to the knee can be used to maintain the thighs in abduction. Proper fit of a hip orthosis should ensure that femoral pelvic symmetry is attained at both hips. Rotation control owing to hypertonicity usually requires orthotic positioning at the feet. As increased tone at the hip is often accompanied by spasticity in the lower legs, positioning devices to control rotation are commonly attached to AFOs. Hip-abduction and rotation-control orthoses for standing and ambulation have been developed. However, these orthoses have been designed for management of spasticity in CP and are not widely used for adult motor dysfunctions.

SUMMARY

So diverse is the use of orthoses in the management of spasticity that this chapter constitutes only a brief introduction to the subject. The formulation of an orthotic prescription requires a thorough assessment of functional impairments and selection of appropriate treatment objectives. Although orthotic intervention can be implemented as the primary treatment, it is usually an adjunct to other therapeutic approaches. Any treatment plan should be flexible enough to accommodate for the frequent changes associated with the management of hypertonicity. Periodic reassessment of the patient is helpful to monitor whether treatment goals are being met and to address any changes needed in orthotic control.

REFERENCES

1. McCollough, N. C., III. (1985) Biomechanical analysis systems for orthotic prescription, in American Academy of Orthopaedic Surgeons *Atlas of Orthotics: Biomechanical Principles and Application,* 2nd ed. CV Mosby, St. Louis, pp. 35–75.
2. Gage, J. R. (1991) Gait analysis in cerebral palsy. MacKeith Press, London.
3. Lance, J. W. (1980) Symposium synopsis, in *Spasticity, Disordered Motor Control* (Feldman, R. G., Young, R. R., and Koella, W. P., eds.), Year Book Medical Publishers, Chicago.
4. Mayer, N. H., Esquenazi, A., and Childers, M. K. (1997) Common patterns of clinical motor dysfunction. *Muscle Nerve* **(Suppl. 6),** S21–S35.
5. Charait, S. E. (1968) A comparison of volar and dorsal splinting of the hemiplegic hand. *Am. J. Occup. Ther.* **22,** 319–321.
6. Kaplan, N. (1962) Effects of splinting on reflex inhibition and sensorimotor stimulation in treatment of spasticity. *Arch. Phys. Med.* **43,** 565–569.
7. Rosenada, J. P. and Ellwood, P. M. (1961) Review of physiology, measurement and management of spasticity. *Arch. Phys. Med.* **42,** 167–174.
8. Neuhaus, B. E., Ascher, E. R., Coullon, B. A., Donohue, M. V., Einbond, A., Glover, J. M., et al. (1981) A survey of rationales for and against hand splinting in hemiplegia. *Am. J. Occup. Ther.* **35,** 83–90.
9. Ogden, R. (1918) Systematic therapeutic exercise in the management of the paralysis in hemiplegia. *J. Am. Med. Assoc.* **70,** 828–833.
10. Kottke, F. J., Pauley, D. L., and Ptak, R. A. (1966) Rationale for prolonged stretching for correction shortening of connective tissue. *Arch. Phys. Med. Rehabil.* **47,** 345–352.

11. Tabary, J. C., Tabary, C., Tardieu, C., Tardieu, G., and Goldspink, G. (1972) Physiologic and structural changes in cat's soleus muscle due to immobilization at different lengths by plaster casts. *J. Physiol.* (Lond.) **224,** 231–244.
12. McPherson, J. J., Becker, A. H., and Franszczak, N. (1985) Dynamic splint to reduce the passive component of hypertonicity. *Arch. Phys. Med. Rehabil.* **66,** 249–252.
13. Farber, S. D. and Huss, A. J., (eds.). (1974) *Sensorimotor Evaluation and Treatment Procedures for Allied Health Personnel,* 2nd ed. Indiana University Foundation, Indianapolis, IN.
14. Harris, F. A., Spelman, F. A., and Hymer, J. W. (1974) Electronic sensory aids as treatment for cerebral-palsied children: inapproprioception: part II. *Phys. Ther.* **54,** 345–365.
15. Snook, J. H. Spasticity reduction splint. *Am. J. Occup. Ther.* **33,** 648–651.
16. Zislis, J. M. (1964) Splinting of the hand in the spastic hemiplegia patient. *Arch. Phys. Med. Rehabil.* **45,** 41–43.
17. Long, C. (1966) Upper extremity limb bracing, in Orthotics, Etcetera (Licht, S., ed.), Elizabeth Licht Publisher, New Haven, CT.
18. Brennan, J. (1959) Response to stretch of hypertonic muscle groups in hemiplegia. *BMJ* **1,** 1504–1507.
19. McPherson, J. J., Kreimeyer, D., Aalderks, M., and Gallager, T. (1982) A comparison of dorsal and volar resting hand splints in the reduction of hyper tonus. *Am. J. Occup. Ther.* **36,** 664–670.
20. Trombly, C. A. (1989) *Occupational Therapy for Physical Dysfunction,* 3rd ed. Williams and Wilkins, Baltimore, MD, pp. 329–355.
21. Bobath, B. (1978) *Adult Hemiplegia: Evaluation and Treatment,* 2nd ed. Heinemann Medical Books, London.
22. Kiel, J. L. (1974) Making the dynamic orthokinetic wrist splint for flexor spasticity in hand and wrist, in *Sensorimotor Evaluation and Treatment Procedures for Allied Health Personnel,* 2nd ed., (Farber, S. D. and Huss, A. J., eds.), Indiana University Foundation, Indianapolis.
23. Johnstone, M. (1983) *Restoration of Motor Function in the Stroke Patient,* 2nd ed. Churchill Livingstone, London.
24. Johnstone, M. (1975) Inflatable splint for the hemiplegic arm. *Physiotherapy* **61(12),** 377–379.
25. King, T. I. (1982) Plaster splinting as a means of reducing elbow flexor spasticity: a case study *Am. J. Occup. Ther.* **36,** 671–673.
26. Green, D. P. and McCoy, H. (1979) Turnbuckle orthotic correction of elbow flexion contractures after acute injuries. *J. Bone Joint Surg.* **61A,** 1092–1095.
27. Middleton, E. A., Hurley, G. R. B., and McIlwain, J. S. (1988) The role of rigid and hinged polypropylene ankle-foot orthoses in the management of cerebral palsy: a case study. *Prosthet. Orthot. Int.* **12,** 129–135.
28. Ada, L. and Scott, D. (1980) Use of inhibitory weight bearing plasters to increase movement in the presence of spasticity. *Aust. J. Physiother.* **26,** 57–61.
29. Hayes, N. K. and Burns, Y. R. (1970) Discussion on the use of weight bearing plasters in the reduction of hypertonicity. *Aust. J. Physiother.* **16,** 108–112.

30. Sussman, M. D. and Cusick, B. (1975) Preliminary report: the role of short-leg, tone-reducing casts as an adjunct to physical therapy of patients with cerebral palsy. *John Hopkins Med. J.* **145,** 112–114.
31. Ford, C., Grotz, R. C., and Shamp, J. K. (1986) The neurophysiologic ankle-foot orthosis. *Clin. Prosth. Orthot.* **10,** 15–23.
32. Winters, T. F., Gage, J. R., and Hicks, R. (1987) Gait patterns in spastic hemiplegia in children and young adults. *J. Bone Joint Surg.* [Am] **69,** 437–441.
33. Lehneis, H. R. (1968) The swedish knee cage. *Artif. Limbs* **12,** 54–57.
34. Farncombe, P. M. (1980) The swedish knee cage: management of the hyperextended hemiplegic knee. *Physiotherapy* **66,** 33–34.

6
Electrical Stimulation

Peter W. Rossi

INTRODUCTION

Spasticity is one of the most common problems faced by rehabilitation physicians. It represents a disorder of upper motor neuron pathways and is often a permanent clinical accompaniment of a variety of illnesses including stroke, traumatic brain injury, multiple sclerosis (MS), spinal-cord injury, and cerebral palsy (CP). It is estimated that spasticity affects approx 6 million people each year *(1)*. Spasticity may disrupt activities of daily living, produce disabling and debilitating pain, and limit the efficacy of physical therapy.

Spasticity has been defined as "a motor disorder characterized by a velocity dependent increase in tonic stretch reflexes (muscle tone) with exaggerated tendon jerks resulting from the hyperexcitabilty of the stretch reflex, as one component of the upper motor neuron syndrome" *(2)*. The treatment of spasticity typically begins with appropriate general nursing management, reduction in painful stimuli, and a regular program of physiotherapy. The treatment of spasticity may be further supplemented by pharmacologic treatment, nerve blocks, motor blocks, or surgical treatment.

Electrical stimulation represents an experimental and controversial treatment for spasticity. Although there are proponents of its use, there is little agreement as to the appropriate stimulation sites or parameters to be used *(3)*. Additionally, there have been no well-defined studies that quantify the appropriate amount of electrical stimulation or duration of use *(4,5)*. Although there are a few studies that suggest that long term treatment with electrical stimulation may reduce muscle tone *(4,5)*, there are conflicting series that demonstrate worsening spasticity following electrotherapy *(6,7)*. Although therapists in rehabilitation centers often employ electrical stimulation in their treatment programs for spasticity because of central nervous

From: *Current Clinical Neurology: Clinical Evaluation and Management of Spasticity*
Edited by: D. A. Gelber and D. R. Jeffery © Humana Press, Inc., Totowa, NJ

system (CNS) disorders, it is not considered a well-established or conventional treatment modality at this time.

HISTORY

The first use of electrical stimulation for treatment of a spastic limb was recorded by Duchenne in 1871, when he applied electrical currents to the antagonist of a spastic muscle *(7)*. Many years later, in 1950, Lee et al. noted up to 14 h of spasticity reduction following the application of cutaneous electrical stimulation to the spastic muscles of 27 spinal cord-injured patients *(8)*. In 1952, Levine et al. used tetanizing current applied to the antagonistic muscle of a spastic muscle, which resulted in a reduction in spasticity *(9)*. Subsequent studies by Alfieri *(10)*, and Bajd and Vodovnik *(11)* demonstrated the effect of cutaneous electrical stimulation on the reduction of muscle tone.

Chronic cerebellar stimulation was evaluated by Cooper in 1972 after animal experiments in spastic cats and monkeys demonstrated a reduction in motor tone when the anterior cerebellum was stimulated electrically *(12)*. Subsequent studies, however, demonstrated that cerebellar stimulation produced only a modest reduction in spasticity and gain in function *(13,14)*. At present, cerebellar stimulation for spasticity remains investigational at best, and limited to only specialized centers. Complications of this therapy include headache, hydrocephalus, death from intracranial hemorrhage, and the necessity for re-exploration and revision of electrical leads in implantable units.

Since the early 1970s, electrical stimulation of the spinal cord has been used to treat spasticity. Most commonly, electrodes are placed in the epidural space in the cervical or thoracic region over the posterior columns. Electrode stimulation is then performed percutaneously or through the use of a radio-frequency transmitter to an implanted receiver.

There are many issues facing the investigator and clinician who wish to use electrical stimulation for the treatment of spasticity. Published reports document a variety of sites of stimulation and there is no clear consensus as to which site is most efficacious. Methodologies include: 1) transcutaneous or percutaneous electrical stimulation of muscles or nerves *(15,16)*; 2) electrical stimulation of skin below muscle threshold or above muscle threshold *(17)*; and 3) transcutaneous spinal-cord stimulation *(18)*, epidural spinal-cord stimulation *(19)*, repetitive magnetic stimulation, and therapeutic electrical stimulation, defined as low-intensity stimulation below motor threshold in sleep.

Further issues that remain unresolved in the treatment of spasticity by electrical stimulation include appropriate stimulation parameters, duration of electrical stimulation programs, duration of effective electrical stimulation, and diagnostic groupings for which the use of electrical stimulation is most efficacious. There is little information that allows the clinician to predict which patients are most appropriate for the use of electrical stimulation as treatment for their spasticity.

The goals of the treatment of spasticity with electrical stimulation are similar to those with other modalities and include: 1) increase in functional abilities; 2) reduction in pain; and 3) improvement in positioning, cosmesis, and avoidance of orthopedic complications.

TREATMENT OF HEMIPLEGIA

There are numerous reports documenting the effectiveness of electrical stimulation on spastic hemiplegia. Most commonly, electrical stimulation has been applied trans- or percutaneously, although transcutaneous spinal-cord stimulation has also been tested. In addition, electrical stimulation has been combined with other treatment modalities including the use of botulinum toxin.

Baker et al. reported in 1979 that cyclical electrical stimulation applied during a 4-wk treatment program to the wrist and finger extensors of 16 hemiplegia patients produced only a general trend in decreasing spasticity. Despite this, they noted increase in range of motion in the wrist and fingers following a treatment program that consisted of three half-hour periods a day 7 d/wk for 4 wk. Contractures were prevented at the wrist, metacarpophalangeal, and proximal interphalangeal joints and a statistically significant increase in wrist extension was observed (20).

Alfieri reported a dramatic reduction in spasticity when cutaneous electrical stimulation was applied to "weak muscles" rather than the antagonistic spastic muscles. Ninety-six patients were treated with cutaneous electrical stimulation to the flexors of the wrist and fingers, plantar flexors, and supinators of the foot, or pectoralis major. Treatment sessions lasted 10 min and from 5–16 treatments were performed daily. Ninety percent of patients demonstrated a reduction in spasticity immediately following the application of electrical stimulation in spastic antagonistic muscles. This effect lasted from 10–15 min up to a maximum of 2 or 3 h with an average duration of approx 1 h. The 10% failures were patients who had severe spasticity. It was theorized that the mechanism of action was the activation of alpha-motoneurons in the stimulated agonist muscles and reciprocal inhibition and Golgi organ activation of the antagonistic spastic muscles (10).

Vodovnik et al. applied cyclical electrical stimulation to 10 hemiparetic patients with clinical signs of knee-joint spasticity. None of the patients were on medications to reduce spasticity. Thirty minutes of stimulation were applied to the hamstrings followed by another 30 min of stimulation to the hamstrings and quadriceps. Although some researchers had feared providing electrical stimulation to an "overstimulated" muscle, no increased spasticity was noted. Five patients gained at least some slight improvement in selective knee flexion and three patients reported improved gait patterns, although the reduction in spasticity varied markedly between patients. It was not determined whether stimulation of the antagonist muscle was preferable to stimulation of the spastic muscle.

Subsequently, Levin and Hui-Chan have reported on the effects of long-term repetitive transcutaneous electrical nerve stimulation (TENS) on spastic hemiplegia. Their previous studies had demonstrated that a single 45-min application of TENS prolonged soleus-H and stretch-reflex latencies (electrophysiologic measures of spasticity) in hemiparetic subjects. They subsequently studied the effects of 15 daily 60-min TENS treatments over a 3-wk period applied to the peroneal nerve of the affected leg. They were able to demonstrate that repeated applications of TENS increased vibratory inhibition of the soleus H reflex, produced decreased clinical spasticity, and a marked improvement in voluntary dorsiflexion of the foot. They theorized that the mechanism of action was owing to an enhancement in presynaptic inhibition of the spastic plantar flexors and possibly to disinhibition of descending voluntary commands to the paretic dorsiflexor motor neurons *(21)*.

Hummelsheim et al. investigated the effects of super-threshold electrical stimulation of the extensor and flexor carpal radialis muscles in 12 patients with hemiplegia secondary to middle cerebral-artery stroke. Following 20 min of electrical stimulation twice daily for 2 wk, they were able to demonstrate a decrease in muscle tone in the hand and finger flexors as assessed by means by the modified Ashworth scale. However they were unable to demonstrate improved functional use of the paretic hand or arm *(15)*.

Dewald and Given studied nine hemiparetic stroke subjects with application of electrical stimulation of the biceps muscles for a period of 10 min at an intensity level below motor threshold but above sensory threshold. They were able to demonstrate reduced spasticity for at least 30 min following stimulation *(22)*.

Hesse et al. investigated a combined approach of botulinum toxin type A and electrical stimulation in six upper-limb spastic flexor muscles following stroke. Muscle tone was evaluated by the modified Ashworth score. They demonstrated that the most significant reduction in spasticity was observed in patients who received both botulinum toxin and electrical stimulation relative to either placebo or the injection of botulinum toxin alone. However, no significant difference was found between the combined approach of botulinum toxin type A and electrical stimulation when compared with the electrical stimulation alone *(17)*.

Wang et al. investigated a novel approach of transcutaneous spinal cord stimulation applied at the twelfth thoracic and first lumbar vertebrae in an effort to decrease lower-extremity spasticity following stroke. Ten patients with hemiparesis received electrical stimulation for 45 min for five treatment sessions. Stimulation intensity was adjusted so that each patient perceived a sensory stimulation. Significant reduction in the Ashworth score was noted in the affected calf muscle following treatment *(18)*.

In summary, the use of cutaneous electrical stimulation to reduce spasticity following stroke remains empirical at best. There is ample evidence that electrical stimulation can reduce spastic tone for short periods following its application. However, there is little evidence that long-term benefits of electrical stimulation are achieved for spastic hemiparesis or that significant changes in functional abilities are achieved in a rehabilitation setting.

TREATMENT OF SPINAL-CORD INJURY

Spasticity resulting from spinal-cord injury represents a difficult rehabilitation problem. Painful flexor spasms and spastic posturing can significantly impact the quality of life for persons living with spinal-cord injury. Most of the initial studies focused on the effect of TENS, however, more recent series have evaluated the effect of epidural spinal-cord stimulation. The latter represents a more invasive approach, accompanied by both increased risk and cost.

In 1985, Bajd et al. studied the effect of TENS applied to dermatomes belonging to the same spinal-cord level as the selected spastic-muscle group. Of six spinal cord-injured patients evaluated, only three demonstrated a noticeable decrease in spasticity. The benefit lasted no longer than 2 h *(23)*.

In contrast, a study by Franek et al. studied 44 patients with traumatic damage to the spinal cord. They applied TENS to the upper hips, the anterior aspects of the thigh, and the central area of the buttocks. Thirty-five nonelectrically stimulated spinal cord-injured patients were used as a control. In the treated group, 22 patients (50%) demonstrated a temporary reduction in spasticity lasting a few hours to a few days, whereas the other 22 treated patients reported a "permanent" reduction in their spasticity. It was suggested that the effectiveness of electrical stimulation depends on the electrical parameters as well as the points of application *(24)*.

Seib et al. evaluated five traumatically brain-injured and five spinal cord-injured subjects using cutaneous electrotherapy over spastic tibialis anterior musculature. Following 20 min of stimulation, 9 of 10 subjects demonstrated decreased spasticity and 8 of the 9 demonstrated decreased spasticity for up to 24 h poststimulation. A stimulation parameter was used that mimicked normal timing of the gait cycle on the tibialis anterior muscle. It was felt that the presence of clonus pre-treatment could be used as a clinical indicator of the spinal cord-injured patients most likely to benefit from this treatment *(3)*.

Goulet et al. also demonstrated that there were short-term beneficial effects on spasticity by the use of TENS for 14 spinal cord-injured patients. The reduction in spasticity was measured by the modified Ashworth score and could be demonstrated up to 30 min after the application of TENS in lower extremity muscles including the gastrocnemius, vastus medialis, and tibialis anterior *(25)*.

Epidural spinal-cord stimulation has been reported to reduce spasticity in patients with spinal-cord injury *(26)* as well as extrapyramidal motor disorders, spasmodic torticollis, and MS. The mechanism of action is unclear. It has been suggested that spinal-cord stimulation inhibits spinal circuits that are hyperexcitable owing to a loss of inhibition from higher neurologic centers *(27)*. Overall, epidural spinal stimulation has been demonstrated to produce both immediate and short-term relief of spasticity. Recently, Midha and Schmitt investigated the long-term efficacy of epidural spinal-cord spasticity. They conducted a retrospective study of 17 patients who had undergone implantation of an epidural spinal stimulator following spinal-cord injury. In only one of the patients did the epidural stimulator produce symptomatic relief. Among the possible reasons for failure included dislodgment of the electrode and tachyphylaxis to electrical stimulation. The total cost of the procedures for this series was over $500,000. In view of the high cost and low efficacy, it was suggested that epidural stimulation be considered only when more conventional measures have clearly failed *(19)*.

In summary, the use of electrical stimulation for the treatment of spasticity following spinal-cord injury has had mixed results. In part, this may be attributed to differences in the site of stimulation and stimulation parameters. The use of epidural spinal-cord stimulation is associated with the risk of complications attendant with an invasive procedure and is also costly.

Although immediate and short-term relief from spasticity is often obtained, significant long-term benefits have not been demonstrated.

TREATMENT OF MS

One of the earliest reports that chronic dorsal-column stimulation produced a reduction in spasticity and spasms of MS was reported by Cook and Weinstein in 1973 *(28)*. Subsequently, Berg et al. reported on 11 patients,

10 with definite MS and 1 with probable MS who underwent epidural spinal-cord stimulation using techniques similar to those described by Cook and Weinstein. The most striking result was a subjective improvement in bladder function. Of the nine patients with bladder dysfunction, seven reported long-lasting improvement. Five patients felt that they had improved their ambulatory and motor skills. No improvement was noted in the Kurtzke scale. None of the patients reported side effects from spinal-cord stimulation *(29)*.

A recent study reported the effects of repetitive magnetic stimulation in a double-blind, placebo-controlled study in the treatment of spasticity associated with MS. Repetitive magnetic stimulation was administered twice daily at the mid-thoracic level for seven consecutive days. Improvement was noted in the clinical spasticity score, and the stretch-reflex threshold suggesting that repetitive magnetic stimulation has an anti-spastic effect on MS *(30)*.

In summary, a review of the literature reveals relatively few studies that have addressed the issue of electrical stimulation for the treatment of spasticity associated with MS. No definite conclusions may be reached at this time regarding the efficacy of electrical stimulation for this patient population.

TREATMENT OF CP

The use of electrical stimulation for the treatment of spasticity in CP has not been extensively studied. An anecdotal report in 1993 demonstrated significant improvement in "local motor efficiency" following the use of neuromuscular electrical stimulation to the lower extremities of three children with hemiplegia owing to CP *(31)*.

An additional study was reported in 1997 by Steinbok et al. They performed a randomized controlled trial to determine the efficacy of therapeutic electrical stimulation in improving the functional abilities of children with spastic CP who had undergone selective posterior lumbosacral rhizotomy more than a year previously. Therapeutic electrostimulation was delivered using a muscle stimulator to the abdominal and most proximal lower-limb muscles demonstrating weakness for 8–12 h per night at a low amplitude barely noticeable by the patient. Treatment was continued for at least 6 nights/wk and was continued for 12 mo. A control group did not receive electrical stimulation. Therapeutic electrical stimulation was found to be simple to use without adverse complications and was well-accepted by the children. A significant change in motor function was noted but no change was noted in the Ashworth scale among those subjects who received therapeutic electrical stimulation. It was suggested that although the mechanism by which low-level electrical stimulation was to produce a beneficial effect was not known, it might possibly increase blood flow and metabolic activity of muscle and increase muscle bulk and contractility *(32)*.

Overall, given the paucity of studies, no definitive recommendations can be made regarding the use of electrical stimulation for children with CP.

SUMMARY

A review of the current medical literature reveals that the efficacy of electrical stimulation for the treatment of spasticity is unresolved. The mechanism of action of electrical stimulation is unclear and it is difficult to demonstrate long-term effects. Most commonly transcutaneous electrical nerve or muscle stimulation has been used and has relatively few side effects. Short-term reductions in spasticity have been demonstrated in hemiplegia and spinal-cord injury. Epidural spinal-cord stimulation is expensive, has potential complications, and has not been convincingly shown to produce long-term improvement. Cerebellar stimulation to reduce spasticity remains investigational.

REFERENCES

1. Bishop, B. (1977) Spasticity: its physiology and management: part II. Neurophysiology of spasticity: current concepts. *Phys. Ther.* **57,** 377–383.
2. Lance, J. W. (1980) Spasticity and disordered motor control (Feldman, R. G. and Young, R. R., eds.), Yearbook, Chicago, pp. 485–494.
3. Seib, T. P., Price, R., Reyes, M. R., and Lehmann, J. F. The quantitative measurement of spasticity: effective cutaneous stimulation. *Arch. Phys. Med. Rehabil.* **75,** 746–750.
4. Weingerden, H. P., Zeilig, G., Heruti, R., Shemesh, Y., Ohry, A., Dar, A., et al. (1998) Hybrid functional electrical stimulation orthosis system for the upper limb: effects on spasticity in chronic stable hemiplegia. *Am. J. Phys. Med. Rehabil.* **77,** 276–280.
5. Walker, J. B. (1982) Modulation of spasticity: prolonged suppression of spinal reflex by electrical stimulation. *Science* **216,** 203–204.
6. Dimitrijevic, M., Illis, L., Nakajima, K., Sharkey, P., and Sherwood, A. (1986) Spinal cord stimulation for the control of spasticity in patients with chronic spinal cord injury: II neurophysiologic observations. *CNS Trauma* **3,** 145–152.
7. Robinson, C., Kett, N., and Bolam, J. (1988) Spasticity in spinal cord injured patients: initial measures and long term effects of surface electrical stimulation. *Arch. Phys. Med. Rehabil.* **69,** 862–868.
8. Vodovnik, L. (1981) Therapeutic affects of functional electrical stimulation. *Med. Biol. Eng. Comput.* **19,** 470–478.
9. Levine, M., Knott, M., and Kabat, H. (1952) Relaxation of spasticity by electrical stimulation of the antagonist muscles. *Arch. Phys. Med. Rehabil.* **33,** 668–673.

10. Alfieri, V. (1982) Electrical treatment of spasticity. *Scand. J. Rehabil. Med.* **14**, 177–182.
11. Bajd, D. T., Kralj, A., Turkh, H., Benko, H., and Sega, J. (1989) Use of functional electrical stimulation in the rehabilitation of patients with incomplete spinal cord injuries. *J. Biomed. Eng.* **11**, 96–102.
12. Cooper, I. S. (1973) Effect of stimulation of posterior cerebellum on neurological disease (Letter). *Lancet* **1**, 1321.
13. Cooper, I. S., Riklan, M., Amin, I., Waltz, J. M., and Cullihan, M. (1976) Chronic cerebrallar stimulation in cerebral palsy. *Neurology* **16**, 744–753.
14. Cooper, I. S., Riklan, M., Tabaddor, K., Cullihan, T., Amin, I., and Walkins, E. S. (1978) Cerebellar stimulation in man. (Cooper, I. S., ed.), Raven Press, New York, NY, pp. 59–99.
15. Hummelsheim, H., Maier-Loth, M., and Eickhof, C. (1997) Functional value of electrical muscle stimulation for the rehabilitation of the hand in stroke patients. *Scand. J. Rehabil. Med.* **29**, 3–10.
16. Goulet, C., Arsenault, A. B., Bourbonnais, D., Laramee, M. T., and Lapage, Y. (1996) Effects of transcutaneous electrical nerve stimulation on the H-reflex on spinal spasticity. *Scand. J. Rehabil. Med.* **28**, 169–176.
17. Hesse, S., Reiter, F., Konrad, M., and Jahnke, M. T. (1998) Botulinum toxin type A in short term electrical stimulation in the treatment of upper limb flexor spasticity after stroke: a randomized, double blind, placebo controlled trial. *Clin. Rehabil.* **12**, 381–388.
18. Wang, R. Y., Tsai, M. W., and Chan, R. C. (1998) Effects of surface spinal cord stimulation on spasticity and quantitative assessment of muscle tone in hemiplegic patients. *Am. J. Phys. Med. Rehabil.* **77**, 283–287.
19. Midha, M. and Schmitt, J. K. (1998) Epidural spinal cord stimulation for the control of spasticity in spinal cord injured patients lacks long term efficacy and is not cost effective. *Spinal Cord.* **36**, 190–192.
20. Baker, L., Yeh, H. C., Wilson, D., and Waters, R. L. (1979) Electrical stimulation of wrist and fingers for hemiplegic patients. *Phys. Ther.* **5912**, 1495–1499.
21. Levin, M. F. and Hui-Chan, C. W. Y. (1992) Relief of hemiparetic spasticity by TENS is associated with importance in reflex and voluntary motor functions. *Electroencephalogr. Clin. Neurophysiol.* **85**, 131–142.
22. Dewald, J. P., Given, J. D., and Rymer, W. Z. (1996) Long lasting reductions of spasticity induced by skin electrical stimulation. *IEEE Trans. Rehabil. R. Eng.* **4**, 231–242.
23. Bajd, T., Gregoric, M., Vodovnik, L., and Benko, H. (1985) Electrical stimulation in treating spasticity resulting from spinal cord injury. *Arch. Phys. Med. Rehabil.* **66**, 515–517.
24. Franek, A., Turczynski, B., and Opara, J. (1988) Treatment of spinal spasticity by electrical stimulation. *J. Biomed. Eng.* **10**, 266–270.
25. Goulet, C., Arsenault, A. B., Bourbonnais, D., Laramee, M. T., and Lapage, Y. (1996) Effects of transcutaneous electrical nerve stimulation on H-reflex and spinal spasticity. *Scand. J. Rehabil. Med.* **28**, 169–176.
26. Barolat-Romana, G., Myklebust, J. B., Hemmy, D. C., Myklebust, B., and Wenninger, W. (1985) Immediate effects of spinal cord stimulation in spinal spasticity. *J. Neuro. Surg.* **62**, 558–562.

27. Gildenberg, P. L. (1978) Treatment of spasmodic torticollis by dorsal column stimulation. *Appl. Neurophysiol.* **31,** 113–121.
28. Cook, A. W. and Weinstein, S. P. (1973) Chronic dorsal column stimulation in multiple sclerosis. Preliminary report. *NY State J. Med.* **73,** 286–287.
29. Berg, V., Bergmann, S., Hovdal, H., Hunstad, N., Johnsen, H. L., Levin, L., and Sjaastad, O. (1982) The value of dorsal column stimulation in multiple sclerosis. *Scand. J. Rehabil. Med.* **14,** 183–191.
30. Nielsen, J. F., Sinkjaer, T., and Jakoben, J. (1996) Treatment of spasticity with repetitive magnetic stimulation; a double-blind placebo-controlled study. *Mult. Scler.* **2,** 227–232.
31. Carmick, J. (1993) Clinical use of neuromuscular electrical stimulation with cerebral palsy, Part I: Lower extremity. *Phys. Ther.* **73,** 505–513.
32. Steinbok, P., Reiner, A., and Kestle, J. R. W. (1997) Therapeutic electrical stimulation following selective posterior rhizotomy in children with spastic diplegic cerebral palsy: a randomized clinical trial. *Dev. Med. Child. Neurol.* **39,** 515–520.

7
Baclofen

Eric P. Bastings and Amelito Malapira

INTRODUCTION

In spastic patients, suprasegmental lesions interfere with descending control of interneuronal systems in the spinal cord. A better understanding of neurotransmitters and neuromodulators active in these interneuronal circuits has been the basis for pharmacological manipulation of spasticity (*see* Chapter 2 for further details). One of the most powerful drugs and certainly the most widely used in the past 30 years has been baclofen. Baclofen (4-amino-3-[p-chlorophenyl]-GABA) was initially developed as an antiepileptic medication. It did not prove to be very effective in this indication, and later studies actually suggested a possible procomitial action *(1,2)*. However, during its clinical evaluation, baclofen was noted to reduce spasticity. Numerous clinical-efficacy studies were conducted in the 1970s, and after that the interest became mostly oriented towards a comparison with the newly available tizanidine in the 1980s. At the same time, several studies addressed the mechanisms of action of baclofen, both at the cellular and spinal-tissue levels. In this chapter, we will first review the chemistry and cellular mechanisms of action, the physiologic effect at the spinal-cord level, and the pharmacokinetics of baclofen. We will thereafter consider the clinical effects on spastic patients, and summarize a systematic review of published studies of patients with a variety of neurological disorders since the drug became available in 1966. We will also describe the possible side and toxic effects of baclofen, and finally present a recommended schedule of administration in different patient populations. Intrathecal baclofen (ITB) is discussed in Chapter 15.

CHEMISTRY

Baclofen has the structure of 4-amino-3-[p-chlorophenyl]-ganuna aminobutyric acid (Fig. 1).

From: *Current Clinical Neurology: Clinical Evaluation and Management of Spasticity*
Edited by: D. A. Gelber and D. R. Jeffery © Humana Press, Inc., Totowa, NJ

GABA

cl

Baclofen

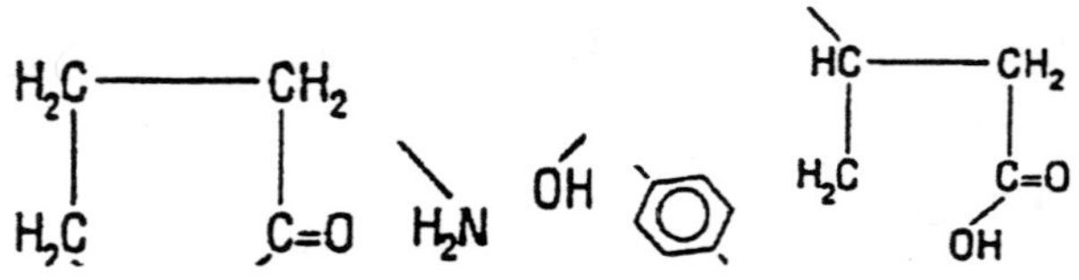

Fig. 1. Comparative structure of GABA and baclofen.

CELLULAR LEVEL MECHANISM OF ACTION

There has been much speculation about the exact mechanism of action of baclofen. Although earlier hypotheses suggested a binding to the classical gamma-amino butyric acid ($GABA_A$) receptor, later reports supported the hypothesis that baclofen acts upon bicuculline-insensitive $GABA_B$ receptors, both at the spinal-cord level and more rostrally (3,4). $GABA_B$ receptors are primarily located pre-synaptically, on afferent neurons and GABAergic interneurons. The activation of the pre-synaptic $GABA_B$ receptor decreases the calcium conductance, leading to a reduced release of excitatory neurotransmitters glutamate and aspartate.

Some $GABA_B$ receptors are also located post-synaptically on the la sensory afferent terminal. The binding of baclofen at these receptors leads to an increase of W conductance producing slow inhibitory postsynaptic potentials and hyperpolarization of the motoneuron. Baclofen, therefore, leads to a reduction of neuronal excitability by its activity on both pre-synaptic and postsynaptic $GABA_B$ receptors (5,6). In addition, $GABA_B$ autoreceptors potentially depressing the release of GABA have been isolated but their activity in vivo is uncertain (7). Furthermore, baclofen, at higher concentrations, has been shown to have a direct inhibitory effect on anterior horn cells, producing muscle weakness.

CENTRAL NERVOUS SYSTEM
LEVEL MECHANISM OF ACTION

Baclofen is a powerful and widely acting neuronal depressant. Baclofen reduces the symptoms of spasticity in patients with complete spinal transsections as well as in patients with incomplete lesions, suggesting that its major site of action is in the spinal cord (8). This concept is well-supported by animal studies. The effect on spinal reflexes is the same in intact, decerebrate, and spinal-transacted cats *(8)*.

The monosynaptic H-reflex used to investigate the Ia-afferent input upon the alpha-motoneuron is depressed earlier and more strongly than the F-waves which assess alpha-motoneuron activity, suggesting that baclofen inhibits neuronal transmission more effectively by blocking pre-synaptic $GABA_B$ receptors than decreasing the alpha-motoneurons excitability *(5)*. It is not clear then if the reduction of the alpha-motoneurons excitability is a primary effect of baclofen or secondary to reduced transmission of excitatory influence from Ia-afferents, interneurons, or alteration of some other segmental mechanisms. A variety of other effects have been ascribed to baclofen, including an augmentation of Renshaw-cell activity and depression of fusimotor activity, but their importance in the therapeutic manifestations of the drug is currently unknown *(8)*.

PHARMACOKINETICS

Absorption

Oral baclofen is readily absorbed from the gastrointestinal tract *(9)*. It also appears that the ingestion of food does not affect the bioavailability of baclofen *(10)*. After oral administration, baclofen appears in the blood within half an hour *(11)* with peak concentrations after about 2 h. As the serum half-life is 3–4 h *(12)*, split daily doses are necessary. The plasma kinetics of baclofen in spastic patients receiving long-term treatment with daily oral doses between 30 and 90 mg is similar to that observed after a single dose *(9)*.

Distribution

Animal studies suggests that baclofen is fairly evenly distributed in most organs and body tissues, although concentrations in the brain remain low up to 30 min after intravenous administration. Blood levels are high initially and then decline rapidly, whereas concentrations in the brain and nerve tissues are initially lower, but decrease much more slowly. This may be because of a relatively slow passage of baclofen through the blood-brain barrier (BBB) in both directions. As only about 30% of baclofen is bound to human serum protein at wide concentration range, displacement from binding sites by other drugs is unlikely *(9,12)*.

Metabolism and Elimination

After oral administration of baclofen, about 85% is excreted unchanged in the urine and feces and the remainder is oxidatively dearninated in the liver to produce beta-(p-chlorophenyl)-gamma-hydroxybutyric acid as a major metabolite. Quantitative measurement in the urine reveals that this metabolite is less than 10% of the radiolabeled baclofen. Complete excretion after oral administration is noted within 72 h, whereas 80% of the drug is excreted within 24 h *(9,12)*.

A slight active secretion in addition to the dominant transport mechanism of glomerular filtration may be present, but passive tubular reabsorption is not significant *(13)*. These findings are important for elderly patients with lower creatinine clearance as they are more prone to toxic/adverse effects even at relatively low doses.

Baclofen shows no evidence of hepatic enzyme induction and no significant change in half-life even with long-term administration. In animal studies, plasma-to-brain baclofen ratio was estimated at about 10. In the human, plasma-to-cerebrospinal fluid (CSF) baclofen ratio is more variable, with no simple correlation between therapeutic efficacy and concentrations *(9,14)*.

Clinical Effects

The evaluation of drug effects in patients suffering from muscle spasticity is difficult and takes into account many different parameters. For example, environmental temperature variations and emotion can affect the degree of spasticity in many patients. There is often in this population with chronic disability a very high suggestibility in both patients and families *(15)*. Ideally, objective measurements should be used. Surface electromyography has proven valuable, but no mechanical aid entirely replaces accurate clinical evaluation. Also, spasticity may in some cases be beneficial. For example, the patient who uses his spasticity in the lower extremities "as a crutch" to enable him to walk may well lose this ability if his spasticity is overtreated.

Overall, baclofen remains the most established oral agent for the treatment of spasticity. However, baclofen is not effective in all types of spasticity, nor is it effective against all symptoms of spasticity. Baclofen has proven to be most effective in patients with lesions of the spinal cord, the most common of which are multiple sclerosis (MS) or traumatic lesions. Baclofen reduces slow passive-stretch responses *(11)*, increased muscle tone, and ankle clonus *(16)*. The effect on deep tendon reflexes is controversial, with some authors suggesting a reduction *(17)*, whereas others report no changes of deep tendon reflexes *(18)*. One of the most appreciated effects of baclofen is the reduction of the number and severity of painful flexor and/or extensor spasms, which often awaken patients at night, or render voluntary movements more difficult *(18–20)*. Baclofen can also diminish tonic flexor and adductor contractions in the lower extremities, thereby permitting the resumption of more normal posture, making much easier the patient's hygiene and nursing care, permitting the use of orthotic devices, and facilitating transfers *(21)*. Another controversial effect is a possible benefit on bladder and bowel control in patients with spinal lesions. If present, this benefit is certainly less dramatic than the effect on flexor spasms. Despite these positive effects, a clear demonstration of a functional benefit from baclofen treatment is lacking. For example, baclofen does not improve the spastic stiff gait that many patients have, nor does it increase manual dexterity *(22)*. It may even worsen ambulation in patients with spastic paraparesis. A possible reason for that lack of functional improvement was suggested by McLellan *(11)*. By recording surface electromyographic (EMG) activity from the quadriceps and hamstring muscles of 11 patients with lower-limb spasticity during a cyclic flexion and extension of the knee, he demonstrated that the effect of voluntary effort on the magnitude of the stretch reflex differs according to the degree of spasticity. Voluntary effort in mild spasticity tends to abolish the stretch reflex, whereas it enhances the reflex if the spasticity is severe. By measuring the amount of co-contraction in antagonist muscles during a passive movement, he showed that baclofen has no effect on the amount of contraction during the active exercise, whereas during passive movement it was reduced by up to 30%.

Given the difficulty of objective assessment of spasticity and the subjectivity of spastic patients, placebo-controlled studies of anti-spastic medications must be preferred. However, as the nature of the effects and side effects of effective agents may enable patients and investigators to distinguish active from inactive medication, much of the necessary therapeutic information and evidence of efficacy has been obtained from open trials *(12)*. Table 1 summarizes the results of all clinical studies of baclofen efficacy published in a peer reviewed journal in the English language and listed in the MEDLINE database in the past 30 yr. These results for different types of neurological conditions in which baclofen has been tried will be analyzed here.

Multiple Sclerosis

Baclofen has emerged as a first-line medication in the treatment of spasticity in MS. Hudgson and Weightman published one of the first studies (double-blind, placebo-controlled) in 1971. Based on clinical assessment in 18 MS patients, they found a statistically significant improvement in spasticity with both the placebo and the active preparation, but the improvement was significantly higher with baclofen *(23)*.

In a double-blind crossover paradigm, Cartlidge et al. (1974) compared baclofen and diazepam in the treatment of spasticity in 40 patients (34 of which had MS in remission). They used clinical assessment (Ashworth scale) for scoring. They recorded the observer and patient's impressions of

Table 1
Summary of Clinical Studies of Baclofen in Spasticity

Investigator/ Reference	Year	Diagnosis	Study type	Duration	Dosage (mg)	Tone improvement	Flexor spasms improvement	Results	Comments
Jones et al. J Neurol Neurosurg Psych 33:464	1970	SCI (n=6)	Double-blind vs placebo	2 wk	15–60	83%	50%	Baclofen> placebo	Electromyographic assessment of spasticity.
Pedersen et al. Acta Neurol Scand 46:257–266	1970	(n=15)	Double-blind vs placebo	2 wk	75	73%	NA	Baclofen> placebo	Continued in an open study in 69 patients for 3 yr: improvement of tone in 66% and of spasms in 43%.
Hudgson and Weightman. BMJ 4:15–17	1971	MS (n=18) SCL (n=5)	Double-blind vs placebo	10 d	30	NA	NA	Baclofen> placebo	Average improvement considered only.
Pinto et al. Postgrad Med J 48 (Suppl.5): 18–25	1972	(n=616)	Open trial meta-analysis	Up to 2 yr	30–225	>70%	>70%	Reports improvement in ability to walk in >70%	Validity of data questionable.

Study	Year	Patients	Design	Duration	Dose (mg)	Serum level	Outcome	Comments
Rigby. Postgrad Med J 48 (Suppl.) 28–29	1972	MS (n=8)	Open trial	2 wk	30	NA	NA	Anecdotal report of beneficial effect in 77%	Validity of data questionable.
Hudgson et al. Postgrad Med J 48 (Suppl.5): 37–40	1972	MS (n=18) SCL (n=5)	Double-blind against placebo	20 d	30	NA	NA	Baclofen > placebo	Limited study.
Cartlidge et al. J Neurol Sci 23:17–24	1974	MS (n=34)	Double-blind Other (n = 6)	8 wk vs placebo	30–60	NA	NA	Baclofen diazepam > placebo	
Basmajian Am J Phys Med 54:175–177	1975	MS (n=14)	Double-blind	9 wk vs placebo	NA	NA	NA	Baclofen > placebo	No statistical analysis.
Hedley et al. Postgrad Med J 51:615–618	1975	MS (n=36)	Open study		ND	15–60	44%	61%	No functional improvement.

MS, multiple sclerosis; SCL, spinal cord lesion; NA, not available; CP, cerebral palsy; ALS, amyotrophic lateral sclerosis; SM, spondylotic myelopathy; SCI, spinal cord injury.

the effects of the drug. Both baclofen and diazepam proved to be highly effective spinal spasmolytic agents. There was no significant difference between the two drugs, either in high or low dosage *(24)*.

In 1978, Feldman et al. published another report including an initial double-blind crossover study of baclofen vs placebo, followed by a 3-yr open-label study. Patient receiving baclofen showed a significant decrease in frequency of spasms and severity of knee and ankle clonus. Fifteen of the 23 patients showed improvement in performance of range of motion exercises with baclofen, while 4/23 patients also improved on placebo. Ten of the 16 patients with painful spasms of the legs showed a significant reduction in frequency of spasms during the double-blind trial. Of these 10 patients with spasms, 9 were on baclofen and only 1 on placebo. Twelve of 15 patients with either induced or spontaneous clonus reported reduction of clonus on baclofen. All patients maintained the benefit throughout 3 yr of open-label study *(19)*. These results were confirmed in several other studies comparing baclofen against placebo, diazepam, and tizanidine (*See* Table 1). Baclofen was consistently found superior to placebo and equal to the other antispastic agents in term of efficacy.

Spinal-Cord Injury

The second most extensively studied condition in baclofen treatment trials has been spinal-cord injury. Jones et al. published one of the largest studies in 1977. They reported their experience in the management of spasticity and muscle spasms in 113 patients (104 spinal cord injuries and 9 cerebral lesions) treated for up to 6 yr with baclofen. Baclofen was found to be of little help in the 9 patients with spasticity of cerebral origin, but was effective in reducing spasticity of spinal origin in 70% of patients. It also reduced the number and severity of spasms in 87% of patients who presented with that complaint. Side effects necessitating reduction of dosage were experienced by 20% of patients *(20)*.

Duncan et al. conducted a double-blind, crossover study vs placebo in patients with spinal lesions (mixed population of MS, trauma, and degenerative lesions). No improvement was noticed for muscular strength in comparison with pre-treatment level. There was no unmasking of residual voluntary movement that had been prevented by spasticity. Transfer activities were generally improved because of the reduction of flexor spasms induced by the cutaneous stimulation during movement and the greater ease in passive manipulation of the limbs. Flexor spasms and resistance to passive movements were the two symptoms most improved by baclofen. Weakness, clonus, and tendon reflexes were not significantly modified. Gait was not improved in these patients, despite the considerable reduction in resistance to passive stretch of leg muscles. This again exemplifies the lack of clear functional improvement provided by baclofen *(18)*.

Baclofen was also found superior to placebo and equal to clonazepam in a spinal cord-injured population *(25)*, equal to diazepam *(26)*, and to clonidine and cyprohetadine *(27)*.

Stroke

Sporadic reports have suggested that baclofen can be useful in the treatment of patients with stroke. These claims have never been confirmed in a large double-blind study. In addition, stroke patients are much more subject to side effects from baclofen than are patients with lesions limited to the spinal cord. This may be more evident in elderly patients, who are prone to these adverse effects and in whom drug metabolism and clearance may be impaired because of reduced renal and hepatic function. Nevertheless, baclofen continues to be used by many clinicians on empirical grounds with various success. Alternative approaches such as botulinum toxin are probably more effective and appropriate in selected stroke patients.

Amyotrophic Lateral Sclerosis

Baclofen is also used in amyotrophic lateral sclerosis (ALS), despite any supportive study. Norris published the only trial investigating its efficacy in ALS in 1979. Twenty patients completed a 5-wk double-blind trial (9 receiving baclofen and 11 receiving a placebo). Several patients in the baclofen-treated group noted reduction of spasticity and diminution of painful cramps, but such benefits also occurred in the placebo-treated patients. There was no statistically significant difference between the groups *(28)*.

Cerebral Palsy

Although oral baclofen is not as effective for cerebral spasticity as it is for spinal spasticity, it is nevertheless one of the most commonly used medications to treat cerebral spasticity in children. Mills reported the only double-blind study in 20 children suffering from cerebral palsy (CP) *(15)*. Baclofen performed significantly better than placebo in reducing spasticity and in allowing both active and passive movements to be carried out. Side effects were minimal and responded promptly to dose reduction. Notable improvement was also seen with scissoring. Fourteen patients improved on baclofen, whereas only two patients improved on placebo. Improvements in manual dexterity, working ability, and scissoring were reported in some cases *(15)*.

Comparison with Other Antispastic Agents

Two double-blind trials have compared baclofen to diazepam *(26,29)*. In both trials a dosage of 15–30 mg of diazepam was compared to 30–60 mg of baclofen. There was no significant difference in the therapeutic efficacy, but baclofen was better-tolerated. The advantage of baclofen over diazepam becomes more apparent with the higher dosage levels required to control spasticity and muscle spasms in traumatic paraplegia and quadriplegia. In these patients, an effective dose of baclofen can usually be achieved without the sedation.

A clinical trial of clonazepam vs baclofen was carried out in a group of 63 MS patients. No significant difference in therapeutic efficacy was reported between the two drugs. However, there was a trend for clonazepam to be more beneficial in patients with spasticity of cerebral origin, whereas patients with spinal spasticity benefited rather from baclofen treatment. There was also a suggestion that a combination of the two drugs may be more effective in some patients than clonazepam or baclofen alone *(29)*. Since 1980, baclofen has been extensively studied against tizanidine, more recently introduced as an alternative oral treatment *(30–34)*. Overall, the efficacy was found equal for both agents, but some authors reported a trend for tizanidine to be more beneficial in improving the activities of daily living and bladder function *(31)*.

Baclofen was found equally effective as cyproheptadine and clonidine in a recent study *(27)*, using a video-pendulum test to evaluate spasticity. Oral baclofen has not been compared to dantrolene in rigorously controlled studies.

ADVERSE EFFECTS

In general, side effects with baclofen are quite common, with a reported incidence of 30–75% *(35)*, most disappearing within a few days of initiating therapy. The side-effect profile of baclofen shows similarities among different studies. However, variation of frequency exists along with unusual adverse effects. Among the most frequently reported, depressant side effects of baclofen include sedation, somnolence, and less commonly ataxia and respiratory depression. A variety of other side effects have been reported; these include headache, insomnia, paresthesia, muscle pain, tinnitus, coordination disorders, tremor, rigidity, dystonia, ataxia, bluffed vision, nystagmus, strabismus, diplopia, dysarthria, hallucinations, and seizures (*see* Table 2).

In studies involving spasticity of cerebral origin *(22)*, neuropsychiatric side effects such as confusion, hallucination, and drowsiness may be more common even at lower dosage. These more pronounced effects maybe secondary to age and more extensive cerebral damage *(36)*. Weakness is often reported by patients. Subjective reports of weakness do not appear to be related to alterations of the physiological properties of contraction, and probably are a subjective interpretation that less stiffness is weakness because of less resistance to muscle contraction *(37)*.

There has also been a report suggesting that baclofen can alleviate neuroleptic-induced tardive dyskinesia but can increase extrapyramidal symptoms. Dyskinesia as a side effect has also been reported, mostly at the initiation of the treatment. A baclofen-induced frontal-lobe syndrome was described with prominent perseverative behavior after treatment with low-dose baclofen. The clinical symptoms cleared up in 72 h after the medication was discontinued *(38)*. Although the pathogenesis of the baclofen-induced frontal-lobe syndrome is unknown, it is possible that the inhibitory effect of baclofen of the GABA receptors-rich frontal lobes may have caused the frontal-lobe symptoms. Baclofen should therefore be started with a smaller dose in the elderly to allow for physiological accommodation to the drug *(38)*. Baclofen-induced psychotic depression and pseudo-psychosis have also been reported *(39,40)*.

Most of the studies show that baclofen has no significant effect on the bone marrow, kidney, liver, and gastrointestinal tract. Less than 1% of patients on baclofen in phase III trials had transaminase elevations. Transient elevations in transaminases, alkaline phosphatase, and blood sugar may occur in some patients *(41)*. A case in which elevated transaminases was reduced by half within 2 d of baclofen dose reduction has also been reported *(42)*.

TOXICITY

Previous studies show that despite a wide variability in optimal dosage and corresponding serum levels between individuals, there is some correlation between baclofen serum levels and clinical control of spasticity *(43)*. The therapeutic blood level for baclofen is considered to be 80–400 ng/ml *(22)*. As previously discussed, reduced renal function may predispose the patient to baclofen toxicity in elderly patients. In a spinal cord-injured population, a reduction in glomerular filtration that may be related to recurrent urinary-tract infection and reflux has been reported *(20)*. Toxic effects related to high serum levels of baclofen are detailed in Table 3.

At a dose of 20–80 mg, baclofen is active primarily at the spinal-cord level but at more rostral level, it exerts central effects by virtue of its being lipophilic through its parachlorophenyl ring, acting upon the $GABA_A$

Table 2
Side Effects of Baclofen

Investigator/ Reference	Year	Diagnosis	Study type	Duration	Dosage (mg)	Tone improvement	Flexor spasms improvement	Results	Comments
From and Heltberg (29)	1975	MS (n=17)	Double blind crossover vs.	8 wk	30–120	NA	58%	Baclofen = Diazepam	No effect on bladder dysfunction.
Duncan et al. Neurology 26:441	1976	SCL (n=25)	Double blind crossover vs. Placebo	9 wk	Up to 100	55%	72%	Baclofen > placebo	
Jones et al. Arch Neur 34:422–428	1977	MS (n=113)	Open study	1–6 yr	30–200	81%	88%	NA	Poor efficacy in spasticity of cerebral origin.
Sachais et al. Arch Neurol 34:422–428	1977	MS (n=106)	Double blind	5 wk vs placebo	70–80	NA	42%	Baclofen > placebo	Baclofen effective on flexor spasms, tone, pain, and stiffness.
Mills and Jackson J Intl Med Kos 5:398–404	1977	CP (n=20)	Double blind crossover vs. placebo	8 wk	30–60	70%	NA	Baclofen > placebo	
Cendrowski and Sobczyck Eur Neurol 16:257–262	1977	MS (n=63) SCL (n=5)	Baclofen vs. clonazepam vs. placebo	8–16 wk	30–90	60%	NA	Baclofen = clonazepam > placebo	Combination of clonazepam + baclofen might be more effective in some patients.

Study	Year	Population	Design	Duration	Dose (mg)	% Improved (active)	% Improved (placebo)	Result	Notes
Feldman et al. Neurology 28:1094–1098	1978	MS (n=33)	Double blind crossover vs. placebo	10 wk	80	65%	56%	Baclofen > placebo	Prolonged in an open study placebo for 3 yr in 12. Clinical benefit maintained in 100% of patients.
Sawa and Paty J Can Neurol Sci 6:351–354	1979	MS (n=21)	Double blind crossover vs. placebo	7 wk	60	72%	NA	Baclofen > placebo	Prolonged in an open study for 6 in 11 patients, up to 200 mg/d. Clinical benefit maintained in 64%.
Norris et al. Arch Neurol 36:715–716	1979	ALS (n=20)	Double blind vs. placebo	5 wk	80	NA	NA	Baclofen = placebo	Prolonged in an open study: 4 patients reported to benefit from baclofen.
Smolenski et al. Curr Med Res Opin 7:374–383	1981	MS (n=11)	Double blind vs. tizanidine	6 wk	10–80	81%	27%	Baclofen = tizanidine (spasticity)	Trend for tizanidine > baclofen for activities of daily living and bladder function improvement.

Table 3
Toxic Effects of Baclofen

Investigator/Reference	Year	Diagnosis	Study type	Duration	Dosage (mg)	Tone improvement	Flexor spasms improvement	Results	Comments
Newman et al. Eur J Clin Pharmacol 23:31–35	1982	MS (n=32) SM (n=4)	Double blind crossover vs tizanidine	13 wk	40	30%	NA	Baclofen = tizanidine	
Roussan et al. Pharmatherapy 4:278–284	1985	MS (n=7) TM (n=1) SCI (n=5)	Double blind crossover vs. diazepam	19 wk	25–60	NA	NA	Baclofen = diazepam	Rebound of spasticity noted in 7/13 patients after discontinuing baclofen.
Roussan et al. Pharmatherapy 4:278–284	1985	(n=18)	Open study	4 yr	25–60	NA	NA	No evidence of drug tolerance	83% of patients had worsening of spasticity after discontinuing baclofen.
Stien et al. Acta Neurol Scand 75:190–194	1987	MS (n=40)	Double blind vs. tizanidine	6 wk	20–90	65%	65%	Baclofen = tizanidine	No improvement of functional status with either drug.

Reference	Year	Population	Study design	Duration	Dose			Result	Comments
Bass et al. Can J Neurol Sci 15:15–19	1988	MS (n=66)	Double blind crossover vs. tizanidine	8 wk	80	68%	NA	Baclofen = tizanidine	
Eysette et al. Curr Med Res Opin 10:699–708	1988	MS (n=100)	Double blind vs tizanidine	8 wk	15–60	100%	48.5%	Baclofen = tizanidine	Clinical assessment of locomotion, spasms, clonus strength, tone.
Hinderer et al. Am J Phys Med Rehab 69:311–317	1990	SCI (n=5)	Double-blind vs. placebo	2.5–4.5 weeks	40–80	NA	NA	Baclofen = placebo	Objective measurement of ankle stiffness using an original device.
Smith et al. Neurology 41:1829–1831	1991	MS (n=112)	Retrospective study.	43.7 mo	40–80 or more	NA	NA	15% of patients identified received dose >80 mg/d	No evaluation of efficacy.
Nance PW J Am Paraplegia Soc 17:150–156	1994	SCI (n=25)	Double-blind vs. cyproheptadine vs clonidine	3 wk	80	NA	NA	Baclofen = cyproheptadine = clonidine > placebo	Video-pendulum test found equal to Ashworth scale in evaluation of spasticity.

receptors; this may explain some of the findings in toxicity. The adult cases resulting in baclofen toxicity had doses ranging from 420–2500 mg and a single pediatric case reported ingestion of 120 mg. Most of the patients, however, recovered full neurologic function with supportive care *(44)*.

ADVERSE EFFECTS SECONDARY TO WITHDRAWAL

Although drug withdrawal-rebound phenomena are thought as being associated with withdrawal of narcotics, barbiturates, and some cardiovascular agents, a number of clinical investigators have described a phenomenon of rebound spasticity in baclofen withdrawal. Cumming *(45)* reported that rebound spasticity occurred within 48 h after discontinuing baclofen and that rebound had ameliorated after another 48 h. Such a time-course was noted not only in the seven baclofen cases but in three cases of diazepam therapy. The most comprehensive evaluation of the rebound phenomenon following abrupt discontinuation of baclofen therapy was reported by Knuttson et al. by using EMG recordings and graphs of resistance to passive movement of the knee joint *(17)*. This study showed that the rebound phenomenon was maximum on the second day after the abrupt withdrawal of baclofen therapy and that by the sixth day, muscle activity returned to the baseline level. As with long-term diazepam therapy, when given chronically, baclofen should be discontinued gradually to avoid the painful spastic-rebound phenomenon and a more serious hallucinosis-seizure complication *(46)*. Abrupt withdrawal after long-term use can lead to central nervous system (CNS) excitation, inducing psychosis with hallucinations, dyskinesias, hyperthermia, or seizures *(47,48)*. Baclofen withdrawal appears to be a problem only after many months of therapy and has not been noted after only 1 or 2 mo of therapy *(14)*. Major reduction in dose or discontinuation after long-term use should be done with caution. These withdrawal symptoms are usually noted between 12–96 h after the last dose. The mechanism underlying the clinical findings is uncertain and may reflect a rebound phenomenon after the removal of inhibitory influences of the GABA agonist *(49)* and may also involve supersensitivity of dopamine receptors *(48)*.

DOSAGE

Like that of any medication, the dosage should be the lowest that produces an optimal therapeutic response without major side effects. Treatment should be continued only if benefits are derived. It is often difficult to evaluate subjective impressions of improvement with baclofen. Although the recommended adult dose is 40–80 mg/d, with 70–80 mg being adequate for most patients *(50)*, dosage should be individualized according to the pa-

Table 4
Side Effects of Baclofen

Side effects	%
Neuropsychiatric	
Somnolence/ drowsiness	7–70
Hallucinations	5.3–10
Insomnia	3.3–10
Euphoria	1.7–10
Confusion	5.2
Depression	1.7–4.5
Anxiety	0.9
Psychotic depression	Rare
Neurological	
Paresthesia	21.7
Vertigo	17.5
Dizziness/lightheadedness	3.8–27
Weakness	0.9–22
Imbalance	10
Bluffed vision	1.7–8.7
Headache	1.7–4.5
Jerking tremor	1.7
Perioral numbness	0.9
Diplopia	0.9
Dyskinesia	Rare
Frontal-lobe syndrome	Rare
Gastro-intestinal	
Nausea/vomiting	1.7–27
Diarrhea	5
Abdominal pain	10
Dry mouth	3.3–21.7
Anorexia	8.3
Sore mouth	4.6
Cardiovascular	
Hypotension	4.5
Chest pain, dyspnea, syncope	Rare
Genito-urinary	
Urinary frequency	12.5
Erectile dysfunction	7.6
Enuresis, retention, dysuria	Rare
Miscellaneous	
Weight gain	2.7–5
Leg edema	4.5–7.6
Sweating	0.9
Rash, pruritus, nasal congestion	Rare

tient's need, response, and concomitant medical problems. Some patients require less while others may require more, even up to 225 mg/d *(20,51,52)*. Some clinicians will prescribe beyond the recommended maximum when a satisfactory effect does not occur within the usual range. Smith et al. *(51)* reviewed a random sample of charts from an outpatient clinic for MS to determine the frequency with which baclofen was prescribed for spasticity above 80 mg/d *(51)*. About 20% of patients had taken high-dose baclofen, which was well-tolerated in most cases.

It is recommended to start at 5 mg three times a day and increase by 15 mg at 3-d intervals, until an optimum effect is achieved. In some patients, a four times a day dosing provides a smoother control of spasticity. Patients with co-existing brain damage or psychiatric disorder appear to be more prone to psychological side effects. These may be minimized by starting at a lower dose or by titrating more slowly every 7 d *(41)*.

Although the safety of oral baclofen for the pediatric population under age 12 has not been established, it has been used in management of spasticity from CP. It has been suggested that the starting dose for children between 2–7 yr should be 5–10 mg daily, increasing gradually to a maximum daily dose of 30–40 mg over a period of 2 wk. For children over 8 yr, a starting dose of 10 mg is recommended with the 2-wk incremental period used to titrate for the optimum therapeutic dose *(29)*. Finally, it is occasionally advantageous to withdraw the drug periodically to determine whether spasticity worsens *(3)*.

CONCLUSIONS AND FUTURE DIRECTIONS

Baclofen has been widely accepted as an effective oral antispastic agent in patients with spasticity of spinal origin. Its efficacy in patients with spasticity of hemispheric origin is more controversial and certainly not as robust. It remains a good first-line oral agent in most spastic patients, although in selective cases alternative approaches such as other medications or botulinum toxin injections may be considered first.

Side effects are frequent but usually subside after a few days. Care must be taken in initiating the treatment progressively, and also in withdrawing it progressively, especially if the treatment was administered during several months prior to withdrawal. A combination with other modalities (physical therapy, etc.) or drugs (benzodiazepine, tizanidine) may be beneficial in some patients. Finally, the use of the isolated L-enantiomer of baclofen instead of the racemic mixture constituting the commercially available baclofen may be another way to improve its efficacy. Some studies indicate that oral L-baclofen is approx five times as effective as a racemic mixture

Table 5
Toxic Effects of Baclofen

Toxic effects	%
Hyporeflexia	100
Coma	100
Respiratory depression	100
Hypotonia	100
Bradycardia	50
Generalized epilepsy	42
Myoclonic jerking	42
Hypotension	33
Tachycardia	33
Hypertension	25
Cardiac conduction abnormalities	8

into treating trigeminal neuralgia. The D-enantiomer may even partially antagonize the response to the L-enantiomer. It is possible that L-baclofen would be more dose-effective and have fewer CNS side effects than the racemic mixture. Studies to evaluate that possibility are underway *(53)*.

REFERENCES

1. Rush, J. M. and Gibberd, F. B. (1990) Baclofen-induced epilepsy. *J. R. Soc. Med.* **83,** 115–116.
2. Zak, R., Solomon, G., Petito, F., and Labar, D. (1994) Baclofen-induced generalized nonconvulsive status epilepticus. *Ann. Neurol.* **36,** 113–114.
3. Rice, G. P. A. (1987) Pharmacotherapy of spasticity: some theoretical and practical considerations. *Can. J. Neurol. Sci.* **14,** 510–512.
4. Bowery, N. (1989) GABA-B receptors and their significance in mammalian pharmacology. *Trends Pharmacol. Sci.* **10,** 401–407.
5. Dressnandt, J., Carola, A., and Conrad, B. (1995) Influence of baclofen upon the alpha-motoneuron in spasticity by means of F-wave analysis. *Muscle Nerve* **18,** 103–107.
6. Young, R. R. et al. (1997) Current issues in spasticity. *Neurology* **3,** 261–275.
7. Fromm, G. H. (1994) Baclofen as an adjuvant analgesic. *J. Pain. Symptom. Manag.* **9,** 500–509.
8. Davidoff, R. A. (1985) Antispasticity drugs: mechanisms of action. *Neurology* **17,** 107–116.
9. Faigle, J. W., Keberle, H., and Degen, P. H. (1980) Chemistry and pharmacokinetics of baclofen, in *Spasticity: Disordered Motor Control* (Feldman, R. G., Young, R. R., and Koella, W. P., eds.), Yearbook Medical, Chicago, pp. 94–100.

10. Peterson, G. M., McLean, S., and Millingen, K. S. (1985) Food does not affect the bioavailability of baclofen. *Med. J. Aust.* **42,** 689–690.
11. McEllan, D. L. (1977) Co-contraction and stretch reflexes in spasticity during treatment with baclofen. *J. Neurol. Neurosurg. Psych.* **40,** 30–38.
12. Brogden, R. N., Speight, T. M., and Avery, G. S. (1974) Baclofen: a preliminary report of its pharmacological properties and therapeutic efficacy in spasticity. *Drugs* **8,** 1–14.
13. Wuis, E. W., Dirks, M. J. M., Termond, E. F. S, Vree, T. B., and Van der Kleijn, E. (1989) Plasma and urinary excretion kinetics of oral baclofen in healthy subjects. *Eur. J. Clin. Pharmacol.* **37,** 181–184.
14. Terrence, C. F. and Fromm, G. H. (1981) Complications of baclofen withdrawal. *Arch. Neurol.* **38,** 588–589.
15. Mills, P. J. and Jackson, A. D. M. (1977) A controlled trial of baclofen in children with cerebral palsy. *J Intl. Med Res.* **5,** 398–404.
16. Milanov, I. G. (1992) Mechanisms of baclofen action on spasticity. *Acta Neurol. Scand.* **85,** 305–310.
17. Knutsson, E., Lindblom, U., and Martensson, A. (1973) Differences in effects in gamma and alpha spasticity induced by the GABA derivative baclofen (Lioresal). *Brain* **96,** 29–46.
18. Duncan, G. W., Shamani, B. T., and Young, R. R. (1976) An evaluation of baclofen treatment for certain symptoms in patients with spinal cord lesions. *Neurology* **26,** 441.
19. Feldman, R. G., Kelly-Hayes, M., Conomy, J. P., and Foley, M. G. (1978) Baclofen for spasticity in multiple sclerosis: double-blind crossover and three-year study. *Neurology* **28,** 1094–1098.
20. Jones, R. F. and Lance, J. W. (1976) Baclofen in the long term management of spasticity. *Med. J. Aust.* **1,** 654–656.
21. Young, R. R. (1987) Physiologic and pharmacologic approaches to spasticity. *Neurol. Clin.* **5,** 529–539.
22. Young, R. R. and Delwaide, P. J. (1981) Drug therapy: spasticity (second of two parts). *N. Engl. J. Med.* **304(2),** 96–99.
23. Hudgson, P. and Weightman, D. (1971) Baclofen in the treatment of spasticity. *BMJ* **4,** 15–17.
24. Cartlidge, N. E. F., Hudgson, P., and Weightman, D. (1974) A comparison of baclofen and diazepam in the treatment of spasticity. *J. Neurol. Sci.* **23,** 17–24.
25. Cendrowski, W. and Sobczyk, W. (1977) Clonazepam, baclofen and placebo in the treatment of spasticity. *Eur. Neurol.* **16,** 257–262.
26. Roussan, C., Terrence, G., and Fromm, G. H. (1985) Baclofen versus diazepam for the treatment of spasticity and long-term follow-up of baclofen therapy. *Pharmatherapy* **4,** 278–284.
27. Nance, P. W. (1994) A comparison of clonidine, cyproheptadine, and baclofen in spastic spinal cord injured patients. *J. Am. Paraplegia Soc.* **17,** 150–156.
28. Norris, H., Sang, K., Sachais, B., and Carey, M. (1979) Trial of baclofen in arnyotrophic lateral sclerosis. *Arch. Neurol.* **36,** 715–716.
29. From, A. and Heltberg, A. (1975) A double-blind trial with baclofen and diazepam in spasticity due to multiple sclerosis. *Acta Neurol. Scand.* **51,** 158–166.

30. Eysette, M., Rohmer, F., Serratrice, G., Warter, J. M., and Boisson, D. (1988) Multi-center, double-blind trial of a novel antispastic agent, tizanidine, in spasticity associated with multiple sclerosis. *Curr. Med. Res. Opin.* **10,** 699–708.
31. Smolenski, C., Muff, S., and Smolenski-Kautz, S. (1981) A double-blind comparative trial of a new muscle relaxant, tizanidine, and baclofen in the treatment of chronic spasticity in multiple sclerosis. *Curr. Med. Res. Opin.* **7,** 374–383.
32. Newman, P. M., Nogues, M., Newman, P. K., Weightman, D., and Hudgson, P. (1982) Tizanidine in the treatment of spasticity. *Eur. J. Clin. Pharmacol.* **23,** 31–35.
33. Stien, R., Nordal, H. J., Oftedal, S. I., and Slettebo, M. (1987) The treatment of spasticity in multiple sclerosis: a doubleblind clinical trial of a new antispastic drug tizanidine compared with baclofen. *Acta Neurol. Scand.* **75,** 190–194.
34. Bass, B., Weinshenker, B., Rice, G. P. A, Noseworthy, J. H., Cameron, M. G. P., Hader, W., Bouchard, S., and Ebers, G. C. (1988) Tizanidine versus baclofen in the treatment of spasticity in patients with multiple sclerosis. *Can. J. Neurol. Sci.* **15,** 15–19.
35. Jamous, A., Kenedy, P., and Grey, N. (1994) Psychological and emotional effects of the use of oral baclofen: a preliminary study. *Paraplegia* **32,** 349–353.
36. Hulme, A., MacLennan, W. J., Ritchie, R. T., John, V. A., and Shotton, P. A. (1985) Baclofen in the elderly stroke patient: its side effects and pharmacokinetics. *Eur. J. Clin. Pharmacol.* **29,** 467–469.
37. Smith, M. B., Bar, S. P., Nelson, L. M., and Franklin, G. M. (1992) Baclofen effect on quadriceps strength in multiple sclerosis. *Arch. Phys. Med. Rehabil.* **73,** 237–240.
38. Liu, H., Tsai, S., Liu, T., and Chi, C. (1991) Baclofen-induced frontal lobe syndrome: case report. *Paraplegia* **29,** 554–556.
39. Sommer, B. R. and Petrides, G. (1992) Cases of baclofen-induced psychotic depression. *J Clin. Psych.* **53,** 211–212.
40. Roy, C. W. and Wakefield, I. R. (1986) Baclofen pseudopsychosis: a case report. *Paraplegia* **24,** 318–321.
41. Merritt, J. L. (1981) Management of spasticity in spinal cord injury. *Mayo Clin. Proc.* **56,** 614–622.
42. Chui, L. K. and Pelot, D. (1984) Hepatic enzyme elevations associated with baclofen. *Clin. Pharm.* **3,** 196–197.
43. Aisen, M. L., Dietz, M., McDowell, F., and Kutt, H. (1994) Baclofen toxicity in a patient with subclinical renal insufficiency. *Arch. Phys. Med. Rehabil.* **75,** 109–111.
44. Nugent, S., Katz, M. D., and Little, T. E. (1986) Baclofen overdose with cardiac conduction abnormalities: case report and review of the literature. *Clin. Toxicol.* **24(4),** 321–328.
45. Cumming, R. (1972) Multiple sclerosis in the Shetlands, with an evaluation of Lioresal. *Postgrad. Med. J.* **Oct. (Suppl.),** 34–37.
46. Harrison, S. A. and Wood, C. A. (1985) Hallucinations after preoperative baclofen discontinuation in spinal cord injury patients. *Drug. Intell. Clin. Pharmacol.* **19,** 747–749.
47. Mandac, B. R., Hurvitz, E. A., and Nelson, V. S. (1993) Hyperthermia asso-

ciated with baclofen withdrawal and increased spasticity. *Arch. Phys. Med. Rehabil.* **74,** 96–97.
48. Rivas, D. A., Chancellor, M. B., Hill, K., and Freedman, M. K. (1993) Neurological manifestations of baclofen withdrawal. *J. Urol.* **150,** 1903–1905.
49. Garabedian-Ruffalo, S. M. and Ruffalo, R. (1985) Adverse effects secondary to baclofen withdrawal. *Drug Intell. Clin. Pharm.* **19,** 304–306.
50. Sachais, B. A., Logue, J. N., and Carey, M. S. (1977) Baclofen, A new antispastic drug. *Arch. Neurol.* **34,** 422–428.
51. Smith, C. R., LaRocca, N. G., Giesser, B. S., and Scheinberg, L. C. (1991) High-dose oral baclofen: experience in patients with multiple sclerosis. *Neurology* **41,** 1829–1831.
52. Pinto, O. S., Polikar, M., and Debono, G. (1972) Results of international clinical trials with Lioresal. *Postgrad. Med. J.* **Oct. (Suppl.),** 18–23.
53. Albright, A. L. (1996) Baclofen in the treatment of cerebral palsy. *I Child Neurol.* **11,** 77–83.

8
Tizanidine

David A. Gelber

INTRODUCTION

Spasticity develops as a consequence of central nervous system (CNS) lesions that affect descending tracts in the brain and spinal cord that normally inhibit spinal-reflex pathways *(1)*. This results in a velocity-dependent increase in muscle tone (spasticity) and is often accompanied by an increase in muscle-stretch reflexes, abnormal cutaneous and autonomic reflexes, muscle weakness, poor dexterity, painful spasms, and co-contraction of agonist and antagonist muscles *(2,3)*. Treatment of spasticity is generally considered when it results in pain, or interferes with functional activities, such as ambulation, transfers, posture, and hygiene *(4,5)*. Medications, such as tizanidine, are often used to manage spasticity, when more conservative interventions, such as nursing cares, physical therapy, splints, and orthoses have been ineffective *(6)*.

Tizanidine is the newest of medications approved in the United States for the treatment of spasticity and has become a first-line pharmacologic agent for spasticity management. It has been shown to be effective in reducing muscle tone and lessening painful spasms in patients with multiple sclerosis (MS), spinal-cord injury, stroke, and other CNS disorders. Its side-effect profile is favorable in comparison to other antispasticity medications. The following review will focus on the pharmacology and mechanisms of action of tizanidine, and will highlight clinical studies involving the drug.

PHARMACOLOGY

Tizanidine is a imidazoline derivative; it acts primarily as an alpha$_2$ receptor agonist and has noradrenergic activity in the spinal cord and brain *(8)*. It has been shown that tizanidine decreases alpha-motor neuron excitability by reducing the release of excitatory neurotransmitters in the spinal cord (by enhancing presynaptic inhibition) *(8,9)*, and decreasing the

From: *Current Clinical Neurology: Clinical Evaluation and Management of Spasticity*
Edited by: D. A. Gelber and D. R. Jeffery © Humana Press, Inc., Totowa, NJ

action of excitatory neurotransmitters at their receptors (via Ia reciprocal and IIb nonreciprocal postsynaptic inhibition) *(10,11)*. At high doses, tizanidine has antinocieptive properties through its activity at adrenergic receptors in the dorsal horn; it inhibits releases of substance P from small sensory afferent-nerve fibers *(3,12)*. Tizanidine has also been shown to slow the firing of the locus ceruleus, which normally facilitates spinal-cord reflexes through descending ceruleospinal pathways *(13–16)*. In addition, tizanidine is active at imidazoline receptors in the spinal cord. Although the physiologic function of these receptors are unknown, they are thought to be involved in the modulation of the noradrenergic pathways discussed *(17)*.

Through these actions tizanidine reduces spasticity preferentially by decreasing spinal-cord polysynaptic reflexes. This is in contrast to baclofen, which primarily reduces monosynaptic reflexes *(11,18)*. Tizanidine also weakly depresses monosynaptic reflexes and suppresses acetylcholine-induced excitation of Renshaw cells *(11)*. Flexor and extensor muscle tone as well as painful spasms are reduced *(19)*.

PHARMACOKINETICS

Tizanidine hydrochloride is most commonly administered as a 4 mg (immediate-release) tablet. Fifty-three to sixty-six percent is absorbed from the gut *(11)*. Only 30% is bound to plasma proteins. Tizanidine is absorbed rapidly, reaching a peak concentration in the blood in 1–2 h; efficacy is noted as early as 30 min and persists for 3–4 h *(7,20)*. The effect correlates directly with plasma level and the pharmacokinetics are linear *(21,22)*.

Tizanidine is metabolized extensively by hepatic metabolism (oxidation and conjugation) to inactive compounds *(7)*. Less than 3% of the drug is excreted unchanged *(23)*. Approximately 30% is excreted in the feces, 70% in the urine. The elimination half-life is 2–4 h, but increases up to 13 h in patients with renal disease (creatinine clearance < 25 mL/min) *(11)*.

Available in Europe, and currently under investigation in the US, is a modified-release formulation of tizanidine. The bioavailability is the same as for the immediate-release form. The half-life for the 6 and 12 mg capsules is 12.6 and 14.7 h, respectively *(24)*.

EFFICACY STUDIES

There have been three major phase III multicenter, double-blind, randomized, placebo-controlled trials of tizanidine in the treatment of spasticity and painful spasms in patients with MS and spinal-cord injuries *(25–27)*. All of the trials had a similar study design. Other antispasticity medications were withdrawn during a washout period. Patients were treated with either placebo or tizanidine, begun at 2 or 4 mg and titrated upwards to the highest tolerated dose or 36 mg split three times a day over a 3-wk period and then maintained at that dose for 4–9 wk. The primary outcome measure was the Ashworth score *(28)*, measured in the upper and lower extremities in the MS studies and the lower extremities in the spinal cord-injury study. Two of the studies evaluated changes in spasms and clonus *(25,26)*. All three studies evaluated muscle strength by the British Medical Research Council Scale (BMRC) *(29)*.

A combined data analysis has been done for these three studies, yielding a total of 525 patients *(30)*. A significant improvement in Ashworth score, spasm counts, and clonus was found for patients treated with tizanidine at the conclusion of the maintenance phase of the study compared to patients given placebo. More severely spastic patients showed a better response to tizanidine. There was no difference in response based on gender, age, or race. Despite an improvement in muscle tone, tizanidine was not shown to cause any muscle weakness *(30)*.

A recently completed multicenter trial demonstrated the efficacy of tizanidine in the treatment of spasticity associated with chronic stroke *(31)*. Forty-seven patients with stroke at least 6 mo prior and who had at least moderate spasticity were treated for 16 wk in an open-label nonrandomized format, beginning at doses of 2 mg daily and titrating upwards to a maximum of 36 mg/d. The primary outcome measure was the change from baseline to follow-up examination in the total Modified Ashworth Scale score *(28)*. Secondary efficacy variables included changes from baseline to follow-up of a pain score, and strength, as measured by the BMRC Scale *(29)*. A significant reduction in muscle tone was found after 16 wk of treatment with tizanidine. Although not statistically significant, there was actually an increase in strength noted on both the affected and nonaffected sides as measured by the BMRC and grip dynamometry. As well, there was trend towards improvement in functional abilities as measured by the Barthel Index *(32)*, and in spasticity-associated pain.

In addition, there have been 20 short-term studies (performed during the development stages of tizanidine, 1977–1987) that have compared the efficacy of tizanidine to other antispasticity medications in patients with MS, stroke, cerebral palsy (CP), traumatic brain injury, and amyotrophic lateral sclerosis (ALS). Many of the studies used a similar design with patients randomized in a double-blind fashion to receive either tizanidine or an active control (baclofen or diazepam) for 4–8 wk. Tizanidine was administered at a starting dose of 2 or 4 mg/d and was increased in 2–6 mg increments every fourth day until optimal clinical effect or side effects developed (maximum dosage of 36 mg/d). In 11 of these studies, the protocols and evaluation methods were similar *(33–43)*, allowing for a combined analysis *(44)*. This included a total of 288 patients, 144 treated with tizanidine, 106 with baclofen, and 38 with diazepam.

In these studies tizanidine reduced muscle tone significantly in 30% of patients by the third week; this was felt to be clinically relevant *(44)*. A similar improvement was noted for clonus and muscle spasms. Muscle strength actually improved with tizanidine; this, as well, was statistically significant after 3 wk of treatment.

In comparison to baclofen and diazepam, tizanidine had a similar effect on tone reduction; however, tizanidine was found to be more effective than the other drugs in reducing clonus. In addition, while patients treated with tizanidine generally showed an improvement in muscle strength, treatment with baclofen often caused muscle weakness; this, in fact, led to a discontinuation of the baclofen in over 10% of the patients studied *(44)*. When combining data from the 20 comparative trials, fewer patients discontinued tizanidine than those on other medications *(44)*. In addition, when the physicians in these studies were asked to assess medication tolerability, they generally rated tizanidine better than baclofen or diazepam; the difference was statistically significant *(44)*.

There have been several studies that have evaluated the efficacy of tizanidine in children with CP. In one series, 11 children, age 4 mo to 13 yr, were treated with tizanidine at doses 0.75–6 mg/d for 3–16 wk. A reduction in spasticity was found for 55% of patients, while 27% showed improvement in their ability to perform activities of daily living *(45)*. In another study, 18 children with CP were treated with tizanidine for 8–32 wk at doses beginning at 0.5 mg and titrated upwards by 1 mg increments. Improvement in muscle tone and activities of daily living were seen in 67 and 44%, respectively *(46)*.

In summary, a number of open-label and placebo-controlled studies have clearly demonstrated the efficacy of tizanidine in treating spasticity, painful spasms, and clonus associated with disorders of the brain and spinal cord, including MS, spinal-cord injury, traumatic brain injury, stroke, and CP. The drug has been shown to benefit both children and adults with these disorders. Studies have found tizanidine to be at least as effective as baclofen and benzodiazepines and better-tolerated when compared to these drugs. Most importantly, in contast to baclofen, tizanidine has not been found to cause muscle weakness.

SIDE EFFECTS

In the placebo-controlled trials, the most common side effects of tizanidine were dry mouth (49%), somnolence (48%), asthenia (41%), and dizziness (16%) *(30)* (*see* Table 1). These symptoms were generally dose-related

Table 1
Side Effects of Tizanidine
(From Placebo-Controlled Trials)

Side effect	Tizanidine	Placebo
Dry mouth	49%	10%
Somnolence	48%	10%
Asthenia	41%	16%
Dizziness	16%	4%
Headache	12%	13%
Insomnia	8%	8%
Nausea	7%	7%

Adapted from ref. *30*.

and were minimized by slow titration of dose. Of 284 patients treated with tizanidine in these studies, 3 reported hallucinations. In all of the cases the hallucinations were visual and recognized by the patient as being unreal. The hallucinations typically occurred with the first 5 wk of treatment and were temporary. In only one case was the tizanidine discontinued because of this *(30)*. Two patients developed significant elevations in alanine aminotransferase values (defined as 3 times the upper limit of normal or 2 times baseline values if elevated pre-treatment). In animal and human studies the liver-enzyme values generally have returned to normal when tizanidine was discontinued or the dose decreased *(30)*. More patients treated with tizanidine (35%) developed a drop in blood pressure compared to those on placebo (24%) *(30)*. With tizanidine the hypotension appears to be dose-related and peaks 2–3 h after administration; the drop in blood pressure is similar to that of another alpha$_2$-adrenergic agonist, clonidine, but shorter in duration *(48)*.

Prolongation of the QT interval and bradycardia were found in studies of dogs treated with doses of tizanidine equivalent to the maximum human dose *(47)*. However, in human studies there is only one report of a tizanidine-treated patient developing bradycardia and ventricular premature beats; this patient also had severe hypokalemia, which may have been responsible for the cardiac abnormalities noted. There is a case report of sinus bradycardia and heart block that occurred in a patient with a tizanidine overdose *(49)*.

In animal studies with tizanidine 10% of rats developed corneal opacities. However, there were no ophthalmologic side effects in studies of dogs and, to date, none have been seen in human studies *(47)*. There has been no documented carcinogenic effects of tizanidine in animal or human studies *(47)*.

Table 2
Pediatric Dosing of Tizanidine

	Body weight			
	10kg	20kg	30kg	40kg
Day	Total daily dose (mg)			
1	0.5	0.5	0.5	0.5
2–4	1	1	1	1
5–7	1	1	1	1
8–9	1.5	1.5	1.5	2
10–11	1.5	1.5	1.5	3
12–13	1.5	2	2	4
14–15	2	2	2	5
16–17	2	2.5	2.5	6
18–19	2.5	3	3	7
20–21	2.5	3.5	4	8
22–24	3	4	5	9
25–26	3	4.5	6	10
27–28	3	5	7	11
Maintenance	3	7	11	12

ADMINISTRATION

In the United States, tizanidine is available only as a 4-mg immediate-release formulation. A 2-mg immediate-release preparation is currently being evaluated. The usual starting dosage is either a half or one 4-mg tablet administered at bedtime. As noted previously, beginning at a low dose at night and titrating upwards slowly may help minimize the sedative and hypotensive side effects of the medication. The dose is then increased by a half of a tablet (2 mg) every 3–7 d to a maximum of 36 mg divided 3 or 4 times a day. Dosing flexibility is recommended because the severity of spasticity and spasms may fluctuate throughout the day. For children, tizanidine is generally dosed based on body weight (*see* Table 2).

Available in Europe are a 6 and 12 mg modified-release formulation. These are generally administered twice a day. These preparations are currently under investigation in the United States.

PRECAUTIONS AND DRUG INTERACTIONS

Tizanidine should be used cautiously in patients with impairment in renal function. For patients with a creatinine clearance of < 25 mL/min, tizanidine clearance is reduced by more than 50%. For these individuals the dosage should be reduced and the drug administered only once or twice a day, with careful attention paid to the development of side effects *(47)*. Similarly, a dose reduction may be necessary in women taking oral contraceptives; in these individuals the clearance of tizanidine is reduced by approx 50% *(47)*.

Because of the potential of hepatotoxicity, tizanidine should be avoided or used cautiously in patients with impaired liver function *(50)*. It is recommended that transaminase levels be monitored during treatment, at baseline, 1, 3, and 6 mo, and periodically thereafter *(47)*. The drug should be discontinued or dosage decreased if the transaminase values rise to greater than three times the upper limit of normal values.

Because of the hypotensive side effects of tizanidine, it should be used cautiously in patients already taking antihypertensive medications; the dosage of the latter may need to be decreased in these individuals. It is recommended that tizanidine not be given to patients taking other alpha$_2$-adrenergic agonists, such as clonidine *(47)*.

Tizanidine is considered a category C drug as it has not been formally studied in pregnant women. It is not known whether tizanidine is excreted in breast milk *(47)*.

OTHER CLINICAL USES OF TIZANIDINE

In patients with spinal-cord lesions, bladder-sphincter dyssynergia often develops. In this condition the urinary sphincters contract simultaneously with the bladder, leading to development of increased bladder pressures, injury to upper urinary-tract structures, and urinary retention. Treatment is, in part, directed at decreasing the overactivity of the external urinary sphincter, which is composed of skeletal muscle. Baclofen, dantrolene, and botulinum toxin have been previously shown to be effective in this regard *(52–54)*. Studies of tizanidine in the treatment of bladder-sphincter dyssynergia are currently underway.

Tizanidine has been evaluated for the treatment of various pain conditions. In a study of 105 patients with acute low-back pain, the combination of tizanidine (4 mg three times daily) plus ibuprofen (400 mg three times daily) was more effective in reducing pain than ibuprofen plus placebo *(55)*. In a study of 30 patients with acute neck, shoulder, or back pain treated in an open-label fashion with either 1, 2, or 4 mg administered three times daily, there was a significant decrease in pain and muscle spasms seen with all three dosage regimens *(56)*. In another series, tizanidine given 4 mg three times daily was found to be more effective than placebo in treating pain and following prolapsed disc surgery *(57)*. In several comparative studies of patients with neck and back pain, tizanidine was found to be at least as effective and faster-acting than diazepam and traditional muscle relaxants in reducing pain and muscle spasms *(58–61)*.

Tizanidine has also been shown to be effective in the treatment of tension headaches. In a randomized, double-blind, crossover comparison trial of 37 women with tension headache, patients were treated for 6 wk with either tizanidine or placebo, and then crossed over to the other treatment after a 2-wk washout period *(62)*. Tizanidine was started at 2 mg three times daily and titrated to a maximum of 6 mg three times daily. A significant percentage of patients (90%) considered their headache to be milder when treated with tizanidine compared to those treated with placebo (60%). As well, there was significantly less analgesic use during the tizanidine phase of treatment. Several open-label studies have also reported benefit of tizanidine in the treatment of tension headache *(63,64)*. Further studies evaluating the efficacy of tizanidine in the treatment of acute and chronic painful conditions are being planned or are currently underway.

SUMMARY AND CONCLUSIONS

Tizanidine should be considered a first-line agent for the management of spasticity and painful spasms resulting from brain and spinal-cord diseases, including MS, stroke, traumatic brain injury, spinal-cord injury, and CP. Studies have shown it to be at least as effective as other available medications, including baclofen. Overall, it is tolerated reasonably well, especially when started at a low dose and titrated slowly. The greatest advantage of tizanidine is that in contrast to baclofen and dantrolene, tizanidine has not been shown to cause muscle weakness. Therefore, tizanidine may be the preferred treatment for spasticity and spasms in patients with marginal strength. Tizanidine is currently being evaluated for a variety of other disorders, including chronic-pain syndromes and bladder-sphincter dyssynergia.

REFERENCES

1. Gelber, D. A. and Jozefczyk, P. B. (1999) Therapeutics in the management of spasticity. *Neurorehabil. Neural Repair* **13,** 5–14.
2. Young, R. R. (1987) Physiologic and phamacological approaches to spasticity. *Neurolog. Clin.* **5,** 529–39.
3. Young, R. R. (1994) Spasticity: a review. *Neurology* **44(Suppl. 9),** S12–S20.
4. Young, R. R. (1995) Spastic paresis, in *Diagnosis and Management of Disorders of the Spinal Cord* (Young, R. R. and Woolsey, R. M., eds.), Saunders, Philadelphia, pp. 363–376.
5. Little, J. W. and Massagli, T. L. (1993) Spasticity and associated abnormalities of muscle tone, in *Rehabilitation Medicine: Principles and Practice,* 2nd ed. (DeLisa, J. A., ed.), Lippincott, Philadelphia, pp. 666–680.

6. Gelber, D. A. and Jozefczyk, P. B. (1999) Management of spasticity in multiple sclerosis. *Intl. J. MS Care* **1**, 16–21.
7. Nance, P. W. (1997) Tizanidine: an alpha$_2$ agonist imidazoline with antispasticity effects. *Today's Therapeut. Trends* **15**, 11–25.
8. Coward, D. M. (1989) Pharmacology and mechanisms of action of tizanidine (Sirdalud), in *Spasticity: The Current Status of Research and Treatment.* (Emre, M. and Benecke, R., eds.), Parthenon, Carnforth, UK, pp. 131–140.
9. Davies, J. and Johnston, S. E. (1983) Inhibition by DS 103-282 of D-(3-H)-aspartate release from spinal cord slices. *Br. J. Pharmacol.* **78**, 2P.
10. Curtis, D. R., Leah, J. D., and Peet, M. J. (1983) Spinal interneuron depression by DS-103-282. *Br. J. Pharmacol.* **79**, 9–11.
11. Wagstaff, A. J. and Bryson, H. M. (1997) Tizanidine: a review of its pharmacology, clinical efficacy and tolerability in the management of spasticity associated with cerebral and spinal disorders. *Drugs* **53**, 435–452.
12. Davies, J., Johnston, S. E., Hill, D. R., and Quinlan, J. E. (1984) Tizanidine (DS 103-282), a centrally acting muscle relaxant, selectively depresses excitation of feline dorsal horn neurons to noxious peripheral stimuli by an action at alpha$_2$-adrenoreceptors. *Neurosci. Lett.* **48**, 197–202.
13. Foote, S. L., Bloom, F. E., and Aston-Jones, G. (1983) Nucleus locus coeruleus: a new evidence of anatomical and physiological specificity. *Physiol. Rev.* **63**, 844–914.
14. Strahlendorf, J. C., Strahlendorf, H. K., and Kinglsey, R. E., et al. (1980) Facilitation of the lumbar monosynaptic reflexes by locus coeruleus stimulation. *Neuropharmacology* **19**, 225–230.
15. Chen, D. F., Bianchetti, M., and Wiesendanger, M. (1987) The adrenergic agonist tizanidine has differential effects on flexor reflexes of intact and spinalized rats. *Neuroscience* **23**, 641–647.
16. Maramatsu, I. and Kigoshi, S. (1992) Tizanidine may discriminate between imidazoline-receptors and alpha-2 adrenoreceptors. *Jpn. J. Pharmacol.* **59**, 457–459.
17. Li, G., Regunathan, S., and Barrow, C. J., et al. (1994) Agmatine: an endogenous clonidine-displacing substance in the brain. *Science* **263**, 966–969.
18. Davies, J. (1982) Selective depression of synaptic transmission of spinal neurones in the cat by a new, centrally acting muscle relaxant, 5-chloro-4-(2-imidazolin-2yl-amino)-2,1,3-benzothiadiazole (DS-103-282). *Br. J. Pharmacol.* **76**, 473–481.
19. Hassan, N. and McLellan, D. L. (1980) Double-blind comparison of single doses of DS103-282, baclofen, and placebo for suppression of spasticity. *J. Neurol. Neurosurg. Psychiatry* **43**, 1132–1136.
20. Mathias, C. J., Luckitt, J., Desai, P., Baker, H., El Masri, W., and Frankel, H. L. (1989) Pharmacodynamics and pharmacokinetics of the oral antispastic agent tizanidine in patients with spinal cord injury. *J. Rehabil. Res. Dev.* **26**, 9–16.
21. Emre, M., Leslie, G. C., Muir, C., Part, N. J., Pokorny, R., and Roberts, R. C. (1994) Correlations between dose, plasma concentrations, and antispastic action of tizanidine (Siralud®). *J. Neurol. Neurosurg. Psychiatry* **57**, 1355–1359.

22. Nance, P. W., Sheremata, W. A., Lynch, S. G., Vollmer, T., Hudson, S., Francis, G. S., and O'Conner, P., et al. (1997) Relationship of the antispasticity effect of tizanidine to the plasma concentration in patients with multiple sclerosis. *Arch. Neurol.* **54,** 731–736.
23. Heazlewood, V., Symoniw, P., Maruff, P., and Eadie, M. J. (1983) Tizanidine-initial pharmacokinetic studies in patients with spasticity. *Eur. J. Clin. Pharmacol.* **25,** 65–67.
24. Hutchinson, D. R. (1989) Modified release tizanidine: a review. *J. Intl. Med. Res.* **17,** 565–573.
25. Smith, C., Birnbaum, G., Carter, J. L., Greenstein, J., Lublin, F. D., and the US Tizanidine Study Group. (1994) Tizanidine treatment of spasticity caused by multiple sclerosis: results of a double-blind, placebo controlled trial. *Neurology* **44(Suppl .9),** S34–S43.
26. Nance, P. W., Bugaresti, J., Shellenberger, K., Sheremata, W., Martinez-Arizala, A., and the North American Tizanidine Study Group. (1994) Efficacy and safety of tizanidine in the treatment of spasticity in patients with spinal cord injury. *Neurology* **44(Suppl. 9),** S44–S52.
27. The United Kingdom Tizanidine Trial Group. (1994) A double-blind, placebo-controlled trial of tizanidine in the treatment of spasticity caused by multiple sclerosis. *Neurology* **44(Suppl. 9),** S70–S78.
28. Ashworth, B. (1964) Preliminary trial of carisoprodel in multiple sclerosis. *Practitioner* **192,** 540–542.
29. Medical Research Council. (1976) Aids to the Examination of the Peripheral Nervous System: Her Majesty's Stationary Office, London, 1976.
30. Wallace, J. D. (1994) Summary of combined clinical analysis of controlled clinical trials with tizanidine. *Neurology* **44 (Suppl 9),** S60–S69.
31. Gelber, D. A., Dromerick, A., Richardson, M., and Good, D. An open-label dose titration safety and efficacy study of Zanaflex (Tizanidine HCl) in the treatment of spasticity associated with chronic stroke. *Stroke.* In press.
32. Mahoney, F. I. and Barthel, D. W. (1965) Functional evaluation: The Barthel Index. *MD Med. J.* **14,** 61–65.
33. Eysette, M., Rohmer, F., and Serratrice, G., et al. (1988) Multicentre double-blind trial of a novel antispastic, tizanidine, in spasticity associated with multiple sclerosis. *Curr. Med. Res. Opin.* **10,** 699–708.
34. Chrzanowski, C. (1980) A new muscle relaxant, DS 103-282, vs baclofen in the treatment of chronic spasticity (abstract), in Proceedings of the 8th International Congress of Physical Medicine and Rehabilitation, vol. 45, (Pedersen, E., ed.), Print MINAB, Stockholm.
35. Newman, P. M., Nogues, M., and Newman, P. K., et al. (1982) Tizanidine in the treatment of spasticity. *Eur. J. Clin. Pharmacol.* **23,** 31–35.
36. Rinne, U. K. (1980) Tizanidine treatment of spasticity in multiple sclerosis and chronic myelopathy. *Curr. Ther. Res.* **28,** 827–836.
37. Smolenski, C., Muff, S., and Smolenski-Kautz, S. (1981) A double-blind comparative trial of a new muscle relaxant, tizanidine, and baclofen in the treatment of chronic spasticity in multiple sclerosis. *Curr. Med. Res. Opin.* **7,** 374–383.

38. Stien, R., Nordal, H. J., and Oftedal, S. I., et al. (1987) The treatment of spasticity in multiple sclerosis: a double-blind clinical trial of a new antispastic drug tizanidine compared with baclofen. *Acta. Neurol. Scand.* **75,** 190–194.
39. Van Ouwenaller, C. and Chantraine, A. (1985) A new myorelaxant in neurological affectations. *J. Neurol.* **235 (Suppl.),** 305.
40. Hoogstraten, M. C., van der Ploeg, R. J., Vreeling, A., van Marle, S., and Minderhoud, J. M. (1988) Tizanidine vs baclofen in the treatment of spasticity in multiple sclerosis patients. *Acta. Neurol. Scand.* **77,** 224–230.
41. Jellinger, K. (1984) Zur Behandlung der Spastizitat bei multipler Sklerose-Ergebnisse einer Doppelblindstudie mit Tizanidin und Diazepham, in Die klinische Wertung der Spastizitat. (Conrad, B., Benecke, R., and Bauer, H. J., eds.), Schattauer, Stuttgart, pp. 171–185.
42. Bes, A., Eyssette, M., and Pierrot-Deseilligny, E., et al. (1988) A multicentre double-blind trial of a new antispastic agent tizanidine, in spasticity associated with hemiplegia. *Curr. Med. Res. Opin.* **10,** 709–718.
43. Bass, B., Weinshenhenker, B., Rice, G. P., Noseworthy, J. H., Cameron, M. G., Hader, W., Bouchard, S., and Ebers, G. C.. (1988) Tizanidine vs baclofen in the treatment of spasticity in patients with multiple sclerosis. *Can. J. Neurol. Sci.* **15,** 15–19.
44. Lataste, X., Emre, M., Davis, C., and Groves, L. (1994) Comparative profile of tizanidine in the management of spasticity. *Neurology* **44 (Suppl. 9),** S53–S59.
45. Mizue, H. (1985) Clinical experience with tizanidine on infantile spastic paralysis. *Jpn. J. Pediatr.* **39,** 701–708.
46. Imamura, S., Sakuma, K., Hirano, S., and Satou, N. (1985) Tizanidine treatment of hypertonus in cerebral palsied children. *Jpn. J. Clin. Pediatr.* **33,** 325–331.
47. Kastrup, E. K. (ed.) (1999) *Drug Facts and Comparisons.* Wolters Kluwer Co, St. Louis.
48. Miettinen, T. J., Kanto, J. H., Salonen, M. A., and Scheinin, M. (1996) The sedative and sympatholytic effects of oral tizanidine in healthy volunteers. *Anesth. Analg.* **82,** 817–820.
49. Luciani, A., Brugioni, L., Serra, L., and Grazilna, A. (1995) Sino-atrial and atrio-ventricular node dysfunction in a case of tizanidine overdose. *Vet. Human. Toxicol.* **37,** 556–557.
50. de Graaf, E. M., Oosterveld, M., Tjabbes, T., and Stricker, B. H. (1996) A case of tizanidine-induced hepatic injury. *J. Hepatol.* **25,** 772–773.
51. Gelber, D. A. (1997) Neurogenic bowel and bladder, in Neurorehabilitation (Lazar, R. B., ed.), McGraw-Hill Inc., New York, pp. 289–307.
52. Leyon, J. F., Martin, B. F., and Sporer, A. (1980) Baclofen in the treatment of detrusor-sphincter dyssynergia in spinal cord injury patients. *J. Urol.* **124,** 82–84.
53. Hackler, R. H., Broecker, B. H., Klein, F. A., and Brady, S. M. (1980) A clinical experience with dantrolene sodium for external urinary sphincter hypertonicity in spinal cord injured patients. *J. Urol.* **124,** 78–81.
54. Dykstra, D. D., Sidi, A. A., Scott, A. B., Pagel, J. M., and Goldish, G. D. (1988) Effects of botulinum A toxin on detrusor-sphincter dyssynergia in spinal cord injury patients. *J. Urol.* **139,** 919–922.

55. Berry, H. and Hutchinson, D. R. (1988) Tizanidine and ibuprofen in acute low-back pain: results of a double-blind multicentre study in general practice. *J. Intl. Med. Res.* **16,** 83–91.
56. Mojica, J. A., Mancao, B. D., Perez, L. P., Zamuco, M. A., and Lorenzana, G. (1994) A dose-finding therapeutic trial on tizanidine in Filipinos with acute muscle spasm. *Phil. J. Int. Med.* **12,** 141–145.
57. Lepisto, P. (1981) A comparative trial of tizanidine and placebo in patients with skeletal-muscle spasms after operation for herniated disc. *Curr. Therapeut. Res.* **30,** 141–146.
58. Fryda-Kaurimsky, Z. and Muller-Fassbender, H. (1981) Tizanidine (DS 103-282) in the treatment of acute paravertebral muscle spasm: a controlled trial comparing tizanidine and diazepam. *J. Intl. Med. Res.* **9,** 501–505.
59. Goei Thé, H. S. and Whitehouse, I. J. (1981) A comparative trial of tizanidine and diazepam in the treatment of acute cervical muscle spasm. *Clin. Trials J.* **19,** 20–28.
60. Hennies, O. L. (1981) A new skeletal muscle relaxant (DS 103-282) compared to diazepam in the treatment of muscle spasm of local origin. *J. Intl. Med. Res.* **9,** 62–68.
61. Roosen, H. (1981) A comparative study of a new skeletal muscle relaxant tizanidine (DS 103-282) and chlormezanone. *Clin. Trials J.* **18,** 321–332.
62. Fogelholm, R. and Murros, K. (1992) Tizanidine in chronic tension-type headache: a placebo controlled double-blind cross-over study. *Headache* **32,** 509–513.
63. Sakuta, M. and Takeda, K. (1991) Beneficial effect of tizanidine on the ischemic muscle contraction in chronic muscle contraction headache. *Cephalalgia* **11(Suppl. 11),** 339–340.
64. Shimomura, T., Awaki, E., and Kowa, H., et al. (1991) Treatment of tension-type headache with tizanidine hydrochloride: its efficacy and relationship to the plasma MHPG concentration. *Headache* **31,** 601–604.

9
Benzodiazepines

Herbert I. Karpatkin and Mindy Lipson Aisen

INTRODUCTION

Benzodiazepines are the oldest class of antispasticity drugs and continue to have widespread clinical use *(1)*. Although several more recently developed medications are now used more frequently than benzodiazepines, this class of drug still has a place in the management of spasticity, especially as adjunctive therapy and for the treatment of nocturnal spasms. The following will review the mechanisms of action and pharmacology, clinical trials, and administration of benzodiazepines, specifically as it relates to spasticity management.

HISTORY

Benzodiazepines were first synthesized in the 1930s but were not systematically evaluated until 20 years later. In the 1950s there was pharmaceutical-industry interest in developing muscle relaxants and anxiolytic agents. Based on the success of the drug myanesin in the animal model *(2,3)*, Sternbach and Reeder sought to create new compounds that produced more powerful sedative effects on humans. The first of the benzodiazepines, chlordiazepoxide, was formally marketed in 1960. Further investigation led to the development and introduction of diazepam, which proved to have a far greater spectrum of anxiolytic and muscle relaxant properties than chlordiazepoxide.

The first reported use of diazepam as an antispasticity agent was in 1961 by Randall and colleagues, who found a decrease in rigidity and flexor reflexes in decerebrate cats *(4)*. In 1964, Kendall described a significant reduction in resistance to passive movement of the lower extremities in humans with hemiplegia treated with diazepam *(5)*. Subsequently, Simpson *(6)* and Neil *(7)*, advocated the use of diazepam for the relief of spasticity owing to multiple sclerosis (MS) and spinal-cord lesions, respectively.

From: *Current Clinical Neurology: Clinical Evaluation and Management of Spasticity*
Edited by: D. A. Gelber and D. R. Jeffery © Humana Press, Inc., Totowa, NJ

A summary of clinical trials of benzodiazepines for the management of spasticity is detailed below.

MECHANISMS OF ACTION

The anxiolytic effects of the benzodiazepines have long been attributed to actions on supraspinal structures *(8)*. The locus and mechanism of action of their antispasticity properties have been more difficult to establish. Ngai and colleagues *(9)* administered diazepam in combination with several other central nervous system (CNS) depressants to midcollicular decerebrate cats, noting a blockade of elicited polysynaptic spinal reflexes. When the reflexes were then tested in the same animals following transaction of the cord at the cervical level, the drug showed no effect. The researchers concluded that diazepam's effect was predominantly supraspinal, probably within the reticular-activating system, and that the spinal cord was relatively resistant to diazepam.

Cook and Nathan *(10)* were the first to attempt to discern the site of action of diazepam on human subjects, administering 20 mg of intravenous (IV) Valium to 10 patients, 5 with clinically complete spinal lesions, 5 with some preservation of function below the level of injury. The drug appeared to have similar effects on patients with complete and incomplete lesions, and it was concluded that some of the antispastic effects of the drug must occur at the level of the spinal cord.

Verrier and colleagues *(11)* also examined the action of diazepam on complete and incomplete spinal lesions. They found greater inhibition of reflex activity in patients with incomplete lesions because of trauma or MS, supporting the hypothesis that diazepam enhances brainstem-reflex inhibition, when the appropriate descending pathways are intact. This trial assessed only neurophysiological measures of spasticity; therefore, it is unknown whether the clinical responses between the patient groups differed. In a later study, Verrier and colleagues *(12)* concluded that the effect of diazepam in patients with complete spinal lesions was caused by an action of the drug on the contractile mechanism of muscle. Outcome measures in this study were also limited to electrophysiologic findings.

A 1967 study by Schmidt and colleagues *(13)* showed that diazepam increased and prolonged presynaptic inhibition of the monosynaptic reflex in spinal cats without affecting postsynaptic inhibition. Schmidt postulated a spinal locus of action of benzodiazepines based on his findings, suggesting that the drug decreased dorsal-root potentials and depressed the ventral-root reflex. This was supported by later work of Haefley *(14)* who also showed that diazepam also affected presynaptic inhibition in the spinal cord. As gamma-amino butyric acid (GABA) has been shown to be the neurotransmitter responsible for presynaptic inhibition, it was assumed that benzodiazepines affected GABA-mediated presynaptic events. This point was further illustrated by Polc *(15)* who demonstrated that when spinal-cord levels of GABA were pharmacologically elevated, the effect of benzodiazepines on presynaptic inhibition were enhanced, while the blocking of GABA synthesis decreased the drug's inhibitory effect. Further evidence for the relationship between GABA and benzodiazepines was provided by the finding that benzodiazepines specifically increase GABAergic effects, but do not appear to affect events mediated by other neurotransmitters such as glycine *(16–18)*.

The study of the molecular mechanisms underlying the actions of benzodiazepines has contributed greatly to understanding the properties of these drugs. Biochemical studies have shown that benzodiazepines heighten the affinity of binding of GABA to $GABA_A$ receptors on presynaptic CNS membranes *(19,20)*. Enhanced GABA binding results in an increase in the frequency with which chloride channels open in response to a given amount of GABA *(21)*, resulting in an augmentation of the chloride current. Diazepam augments presynaptic inhibition in the spinal cord. In turn this results in a reduction in the release of excitatory transmitters from afferent sensory pathways, thus reducing the gain of the stretch reflex and decreasing spasticity *(22)*.

PHARMACOLOGY

Several different benzodiazepines have been used for the management of spasticity and associated spasms. These drugs have similar properties but differ in their pharmacokinetics.

Diazepam is the most commonly used benzodiazepine. It is well-absorbed following oral administration and peaks in the blood in 1 h *(23)*. It is 99% protein-bound *(8)*. Diazepam is metabolized by the liver into active products and has a half-life of 20–80 h *(23)*.

Clonazepam is most often used for the treatment of nocturnal spasms. It peaks in the blood in 1–2 h and is 86% bound to plasma proteins. The half-life is 18–28 h *(23)*.

Chlorazepate has a half-life of only 1–3 h; however, its active metabolite, desmethyldiazepam, has a half-life of over 100 h *(23)*. Its duration of antispasticity activity is longer than that of diazepam *(24)*.

CLINICAL TRIALS

Spinal-Cord Injury

An uncontrolled trial by Cook and Nathan in 1967 *(10)* examined the effects of intravenous diazepam on 10 patients with complete or incomplete spinal lesions. Measurement methods included surface electromyography

(EMG) following physical stimulus, and observation of movements and reactions. Results indicated clinical improvements with diazepam, with no difference in effectiveness between patients with complete and incomplete lesions.

In a double-blind study in 1972, Corbett et al. *(25)* administered diazepam, amytal, or placebo to 22 patients with traumatic spinal-cord injury. Diazepam proved to be superior in improving clinical measures of spasticity.

Multiple Sclerosis

Cartlidge *(26)* compared diazepam to baclofen in 34 MS patients. Each patient received both high and low doses of each drug. Efficacy was evaluated by clinical examination of spasticity and patient preference. Both drugs were equally effective in low doses for treating spasticity. Higher doses of both drugs were more successful in controlling spasticity. However, 11 patients could not tolerate the high dose of baclofen and 14 could not tolerate the high dose of diazepam. Seventeen of the patients preferred baclofen, 10 preferred diazepam.

From and Heltberg *(27)* compared diazepam and baclofen in 14 nonambulatory patients with MS in a double-blind crossover study. Clinical measures of spasticity, including muscle tone and clonus, improved equally for both drugs. Two ambulatory patients studied both experienced decreases in walking ability, one on each drug. No beneficial effect on bladder function was noted. Sedation was more prominent with diazepam. Patient and physician preference was much greater for baclofen.

Roussan et al. *(28)* compared clonazepam to baclofen in MS patients. Both drugs were found to be comparable in efficacy, with baclofen found to be more effective for patients with severe spasticity. Confusion, fatigue, and sedation were more common with clonazepam, often necessitating discontinuation of the drug.

Diazepam and dantrolene sodium have also been compared in patients with multiple sclerosis. Schmidt *(29)* treated 42 mostly ambulatory MS patients with high- and low-dose dantrolene and diazepam in a double-blind crossover study. Improvements in the subjects were equal at low doses for each drug, but increasing the dosage improved tone of the dantrolene group but not for the diazepam group. Greater weakness was experienced at both doses for dantrolene, while upper extremity incoordination, ataxia, and drowsiness were more frequent with diazepam.

Stroke

Kendall *(5)* administered diazepam to a small number of hemiplegic patients. A small reduction in resistance to passive movement was noted, but patients also developed a decrease in ambulation speed. In 1967, Cochiarella and colleagues *(30)* reported the results of a double-blind crossover study, on the effects of diazepam, phenobarbital, and placebo on 19 ambulatory hemiplegic patients, 16 with stroke. Measures included a time for extended knee drop from 180 to 90°, grip strength, and a timed maze walk. No significant change in the first measure was noted, but performance on the other two tests worsened on diazepam. Sedation was noted to be a significant side effect for those treated with diazepam.

Cerebral Palsy

Benzodiazepines have also been used to treat spasticity in children with cerebral palsy (CP). Engle *(31)* performed a double-bind crossover study of diazepam and placebo on 16 children with CP. Although 12 of the 16 appeared to improve on diazepam, the improvement appeared to be more behavioral than on their muscle tone. More recently, Dahlin et al. *(32)* reported significant reductions of spasticity in children with CP after being given a single low-dose intramuscular injection of clonazepam. Although improvements were noted in EMG activity decrease after stretch and measurement of passive restraint on a dynamic dynamometer during passive knee motion, no clinical measures of spasticity were included for analysis.

Traumatic Brain Injury

Benzodiazepines are not generally recommended for patients with traumatic brain injuries owing to their side effects of sedation and impairment of attention and memory *(1)*. However, they may be useful in persistently vegetative traumatic brain-injury patients who are not expected to make cognitive improvements and have not benefited from other antispasticity medications. In such patients it is recommended that the drug be tapered periodically in the possibility that some cognitive improvement has occurred in the interim *(33)*.

Mixed Populations

A double-blind crossover study published in 1966 by Wilson and McKechnie *(34)* examined the effect of diazepam on 21 paraplegic patients. A significant decrease in resistance to passive stretch was found when compared to placebo. No reduction in muscle strength was found. The results were not stratified by diagnosis.

Delwaide and colleagues *(35)* used clinical neurophysiological analysis in a group of 51 patients with spasticity owing to a variety of spinal and supraspinal diagnoses, in order to predict which patients would benefit more from four different antispasticity medications: diazepam, baclofen, tizandine, and idrocilamide. In some patients, diazepam enhanced vibratory inhibition of tendon reflexes, a normal phenomenon that is absent or reduced in patients with spasticity, whereas baclofen did not. In other patients, baclofen tended to normalize H-reflex recovery curves after stimulation of the tibial nerve at the ankle, whereas diazepam did not.

Glass and Hannah (36) treated a mixed population of patients with diagnoses including stroke, spinal-cord injury, MS, and CP, with dantrolene and diazepam. Global clinical assessment was best for combined treatment with both drugs, while improvement was equivalent for each drug used alone. Unfortunately, only 11 patients completed the trial, limiting the conclusions that can be drawn for this study.

In addition to spasticity, benzodiazepines have proven to be useful in treating other symptoms related to upper motor neuron (UMN) disease. Whyte and Robinson (1) report the usefulness of diazepam in the treatment of painful muscle spasms and reduction of clonus. Rudick et al. (37) reported clonazepam to be partially effective in the treatment of tremor and ataxia for some patients with MS.

ADVERSE EFFECTS

Benzodiazepines have a number of side effects that limit their chronic use. At doses generally required to treat spasticity, patients often develop light-headedness, slowed reaction time, lethargy, incoordination, ataxia, impaired attention and concentration, confusion, memory impairment, and dry mouth (8). Overdosage can result in excessive sedation and even coma (23). These effects may be worsened by concomitant use of alcohol or other CNS depressant medications.

A serious concern of chronic benzodiazepine use is the development of tachyphylaxis and habituation (38). Sudden discontinuation can lead to a florid withdrawal syndrome akin to that seen with alcohol. Symptoms include anxiety, agitation, sleep and dream abnormalities, progressing to acute psychosis and delirium. Seizures can also be precipitated by sudden benzodiazepine withdrawal (8). Patients at greatest risk for withdrawal symptoms are those who have taken benzodiazepines for more than 8 mo (23).

ADMINISTRATION

Diazepam is the benzodiazepine used most commonly in the management of spasticity. It is generally started at a low dose, 2–5 mg at night and slowly titrated upwards to a maximum of 60 mg/d, in divided doses. A single dose given at night may be all that is needed to manage nocturnal spasms. Diazepam can be used in the pediatric population at doses ranging from

0.12–0.8 mg/kg/d *(23)*. Clonazepam is typically started at 0.5–1 mg at bedtime and titrated up to a maximum of 6 mg split two to three times a day *(38)*.

CONCLUSIONS

Benzodiazepines are effective in the management of spasticity and spasms because CNS disorders, with efficacy similar to other antispasticity agents. Unfortunately, the use of benzodiazepines is limited by their side effects, including sedation, cognitive and motor impairments, and the development of tachyphylaxis and habituation. Abrupt discontinuation can lead to a severe withdrawal syndrome. With the recent development of equally efficacious but safer medications, benzodiazepines are probably now relegated to second-line treatment. Their use is best indicated as adjunctive therapy, perhaps in patients who can most benefit from the anxiolytic side effects, or for patients with unremitting nocturnal spasms.

REFERENCES

1. Whyte, J. and Robinson, K. M. (1990) Pharmacologic management, in *The Practical Management of Spasticity in Children and Adults* (Glen, M. B. and Whyte, J., eds.), Lea and Febiger, Philadelphia, pp. 210–226.
2. Ballenger, J. C. (1995) Benzodiazepines, in *The American Psychiatric Press Textbook of Psychopharmacology* (Schatzberg, A. F. and Nemeroff, C. B., eds.), American Psychiatric Press, Washington DC, p. 215.
3. Randall, L. O. (1982) Discovery of benzodiazepines, in *Pharmacology of Benzodiazepines* (Usdin, E., Skolnick, P., and Tallman, J. F., eds.), MacMillan Press, London, pp. 15–22.
4. Randall, L. O., Heise, G. A., and Schallek, W., et.al. (1961) Pharmacological and clinical studies on valium, a new psychotherapeutic agent of the benzodiazepine class. *Curr. Ther. Res.* **3**, 405–421.
5. Kendall, H. P. (1964) The use of diazepam in hemiplegia. *Ann. Phys. Med.* **7(6)**, 225–228.
6. Simpson, C. A. (1964) Use of diazepam for the relief of spasticity in multiple sclerosis. *Ann. Phys. Med.* **(Suppl.)**, 39–40.
7. Neill, R. W. K. (1964) Diazepam in the relief of muscle spasm resulting from spinal cord lesions. *Ann. Phys. Med.* **(Suppl.)**, 33–38.
8. Hardman, J. G. (1996) Drugs acting on the central nervous system, in *The Pharmacologic Basis of Therapeutics,* 9th ed. (Goodman, L. S. and Gilman, A. G., eds.), McGraw Hill, pp. 361–373.
9. Ngai, S. H., Tseng, D. T. C., and Wong, S. C. (1966) Effect of diazepam and other central nervous system depressants on spinal reflexes in cats: a study of site of action. *J. Pharm. Exp. Ther.* **153**, 344–351.
10. Cook, J. B. and Nathan, P. W. (1967) On the site of action of diazepam in spasticity in man. *J. Neurol. Sci.* **5**, 33–37.

11. Verrier, M., Ashby, P., and MacLeod, S. (1976) Effect of diazepam on muscle contraction in spasticity. *Am. J. Phys. Med.* **55,** 184–191.
12. Verrier, M., Ashby, P., and MacLeod, S. (1977) Diazepam effect on reflex activity in patients with complete spinal lesions and in those with other causes of spasticity. *Arch. Phys. Med. Rehabil.* **58,** 148–153.
13. Schmidt, R. F., Vogel, M. E., and Zimmermann, M. (1967) DieWirkung von diazepam auf die prasynaptische hemmung und andere ruckenmarksreflexe. *Naunyn Schmiedebergs Arch. Pharmacol* **258,** 69–82.
14. Haefely, W., Kulcsar, A., and Mohler, H., et al. (1975) Possible involvement of GABA in the central actions of benzodiazepines. *Adv. Biochem. Psychopharmacol.* **14,** 131–152.
15. Polc, P., Mohler, H., and Haefely, W. (1974) The effect of diazepam on spinal cord activities: possible sites and mechanisms of action. *Naunyn. Schmiedebergs. Arch. Pharmacol.* **284,** 319–339.
16. Curtis, D. R., Lodge, D., and Johnston, G. A. R., et al. (1976) Central actions of benzodiazepines. *Brain Res.* **118,** 344–347.
17. Macdonald, R. L. and Barker, J. L. (1978) Benzodiazepines specifically modulate GABA mediated postsynaptic inhibition in cultured mammalian neurones. *Nature* **267,** 720–721.
18. Costa, E. and Guidotti, A. (1979) Molecular mechanisms in the receptor action of benzodiazepines. *Ann. Rev. Pharmacol. Toxicol.* **19,** 531–545.
19. Skerritt, J. H. and Johnston, G. A. R. (1983) Enhancement of GABA binding by benzodiazepines and related anxiolytics. *Eur. J. Pharmacol.* **89,** 193–198.
20. Skerritt, J. H., Willow, M., and Johnston, G. A. R. (1982) Diazepam enhancement of low affinity GABA binding to rat brain membranes. *Neurosci. Lett.* **29,** 63–66.
21. Study, R. E. and Barker, J. L. (1982) Diazepam and pentobarbital: fluctuation analysis reveals different mechanisms for potentiation of gammaaminobutyric acid responses in cultured central neurons. *Proc. Natl. Acad. Sci. USA* **78,** 7180–7184.
22. Davidoff, R. A. (1985) Antispasticity drugs: mechanisms of action. *Ann. Neurol.* **17(2),** 107–116.
23. Gracies, J. M., Nance, P., Elovic, E., McGuire, J., and Simpson, D. M. (1997) Traditional pharmacologic treatments for spasticity Part II: general and regional treatments. *Muscle Nerve* **20(Suppl. 6),** S92–S120.
24. Lossius, R., Dietrichson, P., and Lunde, P. K. M. (1985) Effect of clorazepate in spasticity and rigidity: a quantitative study of reflexes and plasma concentrations. *Acta. Neurol. Scand.* **71,** 190–194.
25. Corbett, M., Frankel, H. L., and Michaelis, L. (1972) A double blind cross-over trial of valium in the treatment of spasticity. *Paraplegia* **10,** 19–22.
26. Cartlidge, N. E. F., Hudgson, P., and Weightman, D. (1974) A comparison of baclofen and diazepam in the treatment of spasticity. *J. Neurol. Sci.* **23,** 17–24.
27. From, A. and Heltberg, A. (1975) A double-blind trial of baclofen and diazepam in spasticity due to multiple sclerosis. *Acta. Neurol. Scand.* **51,** 158–166.
28. Roussan, M., Terrence, C., and Fromm, G. (1987) Baclofen versus diazepam for the treatment of spasticity and long-term follow-up of baclofen therapy. *Pharmatherapeutica* **4,** 278–284.

29. Schmidt, R. T., Lee, R. H., and Spehlman, R. (1976) Comparison of dantrolene sodium and diazepam treatment of spasticity. *J. Neurol. Neurosurg. Psychiatry* **39,** 350–356.
30. Cocchiarella, A., Downey, J. A., and Darling, R. C. (1967) Evaluation of the effect of diazepam on spasticity. *Arch. Phys. Med. Rehabil.* **49,** 393–396.
31. Engle, H. A. (1966) The effect of diazepam (Valium) in children with cerebral palsy: a double blind study. *Dev. Med. Child. Neurol.* **8,** 661–667.
32. Dahlin, M., Knutsson, E., and Nergardh, A. (1993) Treatment of spasticity in children with low dose benzodiazepine. *J. Neurol. Sci.* **117,** 54–60.
33. Glenn, M. B. (1986) Antispasticity medications in the patient with traumatic brain injury. *J. Head. Trauma Rehabil.* **1,** 71–72.
34. Wilson, L. A. and McKechnie, A. A. (1966) Oral diazepam in the treatment of spasticity in paraplegia. A double blind trial and subsequent impressions. *Scott Med. J.* **11,** 46–51.
35. Delwaide, P. J., Martinelli, P., and Crenna, P. Clinical neurophysiological measurement of spinal reflex activity, in *Spasticity: Disordered Motor Control* (Feldman, R. G., Young, R.R., and Koella, W. P., eds.), YearBook, Chicago, pp. 345–371.
36. Glass, A. and Hannah, A. (1974) A comparison of dantrolene sodium and diazepam in the treatment of spasticity. *Paraplegia* **12,** 170–174.
37. Rudick, R. A., Goodkin, D. E., and Ransohoff, R. M. (1992) Pharmacology of multiple sclerosis: current status. *Cleveland Clin. J. Med.* **59,** 267–277.
38. Gelber, D. A. and Jozefczyk, P. B. (1999) Therapeutics in the management of spasticity. *Neurorehabil. Neural Repair* **13,** 5–14.

10
Dantrolene

Walter S. Davis

INTRODUCTION

Dantrolene sodium is unique among medications used for the treatment of spasticity in that it acts directly at the level of the skeletal muscle. Historically, it has been best-known and most frequently used as a treatment for malignant hyperthermia, but it has found a permanent place in the treatment of spasticity for patients with brain injury, spinal-cord injury, and other neurologic disorders where increased muscle tone and spasticity are significant clinical features.

MECHANISM OF ACTION

Dantrolene sodium is a hydantoin derivative that produces direct muscle relaxation by affecting the response of the skeletal muscle fiber at a site beyond the myoneural junction *(1)*. Its primary pharmacological effect is to interfere with the release of calcium from the sarcoplasmic reticulum, therefore uncoupling sarcolemmal excitation and skeletal-muscle contraction *(2)*. It has no effect on neuromuscular transmission or the electrical properties of the muscle membrane itself *(3)*. Dantrolene affects both "fast" and "slow" twitch muscle fibers, but is more pronounced in fast fibers *(4)*.

Although dantrolene is available for intravenous administration, the oral form is more commonly used, and is prepared as a hydrated sodium salt to enhance absorption. Following an oral dose, absorption is relatively slow, with peak blood concentrations reached in 3–6 h, and is incomplete (approx 70%). Absorption primarily occurs in the small intestine. As a lipophillic molecule, dantrolene crosses cell membranes well and is widely distributed. Significant placental concentrations can be reached in pregnant patients. Liver metabolism is by mixed function oxidase and cytochrome P-450, and mild enhancement by other hepatically metabolized drugs is possible, though neither diazepam or phenobarbital appear to affect its metabolism significantly.

From: *Current Clinical Neurology: Clinical Evaluation and Management of Spasticity*
Edited by: D. A. Gelber and D. R. Jeffery © Humana Press, Inc., Totowa, NJ

INDICATIONS AND USAGE

As with all pharmacologic agents used to treat spasticity, treatment with dantrolene is indicated when it is likely to produce a significant reduction in disabling spasticity, when its use permits a significant reduction in the intensity or degree of nursing care required, or when it rids the patient of any of the complications of spasticity such as pain or sleep disturbance. In comparison with other agents, the side-effect profile and the patient's diagnosis and pattern of spasticity must be taken into account.

Placebo-controlled trials have shown that dantrolene reduces muscle tone, muscle-stretch reflexes, and grip strength, and increases passive range of motion (5,6). Dantrolene appears to be effective for severe episodes of clonus, which, for example, interferes with mobility skills such as transfers. Studies that have evaluated dantrolene in patients with spasticity of different etiologies have found that patients with stroke and spinal-cord injury tend to respond best to the drug (5).

Because of its peripheral site of action, dantrolene is not known to cause the degree of sedation and decreased intellectual functioning found with most other antispasmotic medications. Therefore, dantrolene may be an alternative for patients who have poor tolerance to the central nervous system (CNS) side effects of baclofen, diazepam, tizanidine, and other centrally acting drugs (7).

Unfortunately, because dantrolene acts at the level of the muscle, it causes weakness as a direct effect. The weakness is, of course, a direct result of dantrolene's action as an uncoupling agent of skeletal-muscle contraction, and it is precisely this activity that makes dantrolene useful for controlling widespread, intractable muscle tone and spasms. Treatment dosage is usually titrated for maximum reduction of spasticity with a minimum of weakness that interferes with function (7). It is especially important to avoid overtreating spasticity in patients who are using their tone for functional activities such as ambulation or transfers. It is also important that clinicians using dantrolene maintain a close, interactive relationship with the patient and other caregivers so that adjustments in drug dosage and decisions to discontinue use of the drug are based on a total picture of the patient's physical and functional status. Overall, because of the overriding problem with muscle weakness, dantrolene is used most often in nonambulatory patients with severe spastic quadriparesis who are already dependent on others for help with mobility and daily cares. As well, dantrolene may be an alternative for patients who are sensitive to the sedative and cognitive side effects of other medications.

The usual starting dose of dantrolene is 25 mg/d for the first week, 25 mg three times a day for the next week, then 50 mg three to four times a day and 100 mg three to four times a day for subsequent weeks. More than 400 mg/d is not generally recommended, but doses up to 800 mg/d have been used in some patients. Dosing for pediatric patients is as follows: 0.5 mg/kg/d for 7 d, then 0.5 mg/kg three times a day for 7 d, 1 mg/kg three times a day for 7 d, then 2 mg/kg three times a day thereafter. Further increases can be considered, but it is recommended that the maintenance dose be no higher than 100 mg four times a day *(8)*.

RISKS AND ADVERSE AFFECTS

Hepatotoxicity is by far the most significant adverse affect associated with the use of dantrolene. In a large cohort study of patients receiving dantrolene for more than 2 mo, the overall incidence of hepatotoxicity was 1.8%. Symptomatic hepatitis was seen in 0.6%, and fatal hepatitis in 0.3%. The greatest risk of hepatotoxicity was in female patients older than 30 yr of age who were taking more than 300 mg/d for more than 60 d. Laboratory monitoring of liver function should be done in all patients treated with dantrolene. The efficacy and safety of dantrolene in pregnant women has not been established.

Other reported, though less common, side effects of dantrolene include malaise, nausea, vomiting, diarrhea, and occasional drowsiness *(9)*. These effects appear to be dose-dependent and usually resolve with discontinuation of the drug.

SUMMARY

Dantrolene remains a useful addition to the pharmacologic management of spasticity in neurologic conditions. Its mechanism of action as an uncoupling agent in muscle contraction make it unique among antispasticity agents. Although sedation is usually less common with dantrolene compared to other antispasticity medications, global muscle weakness is a major limiting side effect and can impair functional recovery. In addition, hepatotoxicity, although relatively uncommon, can be life-threatening. For these reasons dantrolene is probably considered a second-line treatment and must be titrated and monitored carefully.

REFERENCES

1. Herman, R., Mayer, N., and Mecomber, S.A. (1972) Clinical Pharmacophysiology of dantrolene sodium. *Am. J. Phys. Med. Rehabil.* **51,** 296–311.
2. Ward, A., Chaffman, M. O., and Sorkin, E. M. (1986) Dantrolene. A review of its pharmacodynamic and pharmacokinetic properties and therapeutic use in malignant hyperthermia, the neuromalignant syndrome and an update of its use in muscle spasticity. *Drugs* **32,** 130–168.

3. Davidoff, R. A. (1985) Antispasticity drugs: mechanisms of action. *Ann. Neurol.* **17,** 107–116.
4. Mayer, N., Mecomber, S. A., and Herman, R. (1973) Treatment of spasticity with dantrolene sodium. *Am. J. Phys. Med. Rehabil.* **52(1),** 18.
5. Pinder, R. M., Brogden, R. N., and Speight, T. M., et al: (1977) Dantrolene sodium: a review of its Pharmacological properties and therapeutic efficacy in spasticity. *Drugs* **13,** 3–23.
6. Robinson, K. M. and Whyte, J. (1990) Pharmacogical management, in *The practical management of spasticity in children and adults* (Glenn and Whyte, eds.), Lea and Febiger, Philadelphia, pp. 1–26.
7. Rosenthal, Mitchell, et al. (eds.) (1983) *Rehab of the Adult and Child with Traumatic Brain Injury.* FA Davis, Co., Philadelphia, PA p. 597.
8. Cockrell, J. (1995) Pediatric brain injury rehabilitation, in *Medical Rehabilitation of Traumatic Brain Injury* (Horn and Zasler, eds.), Hanley & Belfus, Philadelphia, p. 183.
9. Schmidt, R. T., Lee, R. H., and Spehlman, R. (1976) Comparison of dantrolene sodium and diazepam in the treatment of spasticity. *J. Neurol. Neurosurg. Psychiatry* **39,** 350–356.

11
Alternative Pharmacologic Therapies

Joni Clark

INTRODUCTION

Current standard medical treatments for spasticity such as tizanidine, baclofen, diazepam, and dantrolene are not effective in all patients and may be limited by side effects. Alternative therapies that could be used as adjuvant or primary therapy are desirable, especially if side effects are minimal. Alternative classes of drugs that have been used or tested in cerebral or spinal spasticity include phenothiazines, alpha-receptor agonists and antagonists, anticonvulsants, gamma-amino butyric acid (GABA) agonists, N-methyl-D-aspartate (NMDA) antagonists, and several miscellaneous drugs. See Table 1 for a list of these drugs, dosages, and common side effects.

ALPHA$_2$-ADRENERGIC AGONISTS

Clonidine is an alpha$_2$-adrenergic agonist found to decrease spontaneous electromyographic (EMG) activity of flexor and extensor muscles in chronically spinalized rats (1). This finding led to studies of clonidine use in humans with spasticity secondary to spinal-cord injury. The mechanism of action is not entirely clear but clonidine may exert its action by suppressing sensory input from the substancia gelatinosa in the spinal cord (2) or by decreasing motor responses through occupation of the alpha$_2$-adrenergic receptor sites within the spinal cord (3). Its mechanism in spasticity associated with cerebral lesions may be secondary to reactive axonal sprouting, causing increased release of norepinephrine (4). Increased release of norepinephrine leads to overinhibition of Purkinje cells and ultimately hypertonia (5).

Clonidine relieves spasticity in some spinal cord-injured patients. Donovan et al. reported that clonidine used in conjunction with baclofen in 50 spinal cord-injured patients benefited 56% of the patients (6). The maximum

From: *Current Clinical Neurology: Clinical Evaluation and Management of Spasticity*
Edited by: D. A. Gelber and D. R. Jeffery © Humana Press, Inc., Totowa, NJ

Table 1
Doses of Alternative Agents

Drug	Initial dose	Maximum dose	Side effects
Chlorpromazine	25 mg	150 mg	Lethargy, tardive dyskinesia, parkinsonism
Clonidine	0.05 mg bid	0.4 mg daily	Postural hypotension, lethargy, dizziness
Clonidine patch	0.1 mg/wk	0.3 mg/wk	Orthostatic hypotension, skin allergy to the adhesive
Thymoxamine (IV)	0.1–0.15 mg/kg		Sedation
Valproic acid	250 mg tid		Nausea/vomiting
Gabapentin	400 mg tid	3600 mg/d	Drowsiness
Piracetam	50 mg/kg/d		Nausea/vomiting
Progabide	14.3–32.7 mg/kg Median dose: 1800 mg/d	45 mg/kg/d	Drowsiness, dizziness, nausea, elevation of liver enzymes
Orphenadrine citrate (IV)	60 mg		
Cyproheptedine heptadine	12 mg/d	24 mg/d	Sedation dry mouth
Cyclobenzaprine	30 mg/d	60 mg/d	
THC	5 mg or 10 mg		Long-term tolerance addiction

dose was 0.4 mg daily. Treatment was limited by side effects of postural hypotension, dizziness, and drowsiness. Three subjects suffered troubling side effects.

Objective measures of spasticity such as inhibition of the H-reflex by vibration, the Achilles deep tendon reflex, and duration of clonus were studied in six spinal cord-injured patients. These parameters were studied in patients before and after treatment with clonidine, clonidine plus desipramine, diazepam, and placebo (7). In normal human subjects, vibration of a limb suppresses or abolishes the tendon jerks and the H-reflex (8). The H reflex is not significantly reduced by vibration in humans with spasticity secondary to stroke, multiple sclerosis (MS), and spinal-cord injury (9,10). The vibratory inhibition index was significantly reduced from pre-treatment with clonidine alone (7). Patients in this small single-blind study noted subjective improvement. The authors hypothesized that this reduction in spasticity attributed to clonidine was owing to stimulation of the alpha$_2$-receptors in the spinal cord, thus restoring the noradrenergic inhibition lost following spinal-cord injury *(7)*.

In addition to oral clonidine, transdermal clonidine has been studied in spinal spasticity because of its improved side-effect profile. The most common side effect is a skin allergy to the adhesive. Its use as adjuvant therapy by Weingarden et al. revealed clinically significant relief of spasticity in 15 of 17 patients *(11)*. Twelve continued transdermal clonidine use after termination of the study. A case series by Yablon et al. reported similar results *(12)*.

ALPHA ADRENERGIC BLOCKING AGENTS

In two separate studies, thymoxamine, an alpha-adrenergic blocking agent, reduced spasticity after intravenous injection *(13,14)*. At a dose of 0.15 mg/kg, the drug depressed tendon reflexes and the amplitude of the H-reflex *(15)*. It also abolished the tonic vibration reflexes, clonus, and reduced tonic-stretch reflexes. In one study, thymoxamine (0.1 mg/kg), diazepam (0.05 mg/kg), and normal saline were injected on a double-blind, randomized basis on separate occasions in patients with severe spasticity *(14)*. All six patients had a striking reduction in the EMG response to muscle stretch after the injection of thymoxamine. Side effects included an increase in flexor spasms and slight sedation *(13,14)*.

ANTICONVULSANTS

Gabapentin

Anecdotal experience with the anticonvulsant gabapentin led to prospective, double-blind, placebo-controlled trials for treatment of spasticity in spinal-cord and head injury *(15)*. Gabapentin readily crosses the blood-brain barrier (BBB), does not bind plasma proteins, and is eliminated by the kidneys *(16)*. Gabapentin accumulates in the neocortex, hippocampus, and cerebellum *(16)*. However, it is unknown if this drug also has effects on the spinal cord.

In a study of 15 patients with MS, gabapentin was used as adjuvant therapy at a dose of 400 mg t.i.d. for 48 h. Administration of gabapentin resulted in significant reductions in the Visual Faces Scale rating, Ashworth score, and Kurtzke score when compared with baseline data *(15)*. The only side effect was drowsiness. This occurred in one patient.

This same group of investigators tested gabapentin in 25 patients with spinal-cord injury. Treatment with gabapentin resulted in an 11% reduction in the median Ashworth scale score and a 20% reduction in the median Likert Scale score when compared to placebo *(17)*.

One other study evaluated gabapentin in a double-blind placebo-controlled trial of seven patients *(18)*. This study utilized a quantitative brain motor-control assessment with surface EMG recordings. Only one subject obtained a clinically apparent and functionally apparent improvement in their spasticity. In an open-label extension of the study, patients who were titrated up to 3600 mg/d of gabapentin had clinically apparent improvement of spasticity.

The aforementioned studies show that gabapentin may be useful as adjuvant therapy for spasticity but the dose, length of treatment, and further clinical efficacy will need to be studied in larger clinical trials.

VALPROIC ACID

Valproic acid is an anticonvulsant that increases GABA in the brain. In a spastic mouse model, valproic acid was found to produce muscle relaxation *(19)*. Very few studies have been performed in humans but Finke reported good responses in 16 of 30 patients in a prospective trial *(20)*. Zachariah et al. described a case series of four patients, three with a history of spinal-cord injury and one with head injury who were treated with 250 mg of valproic acid t.i.d. *(21)*. Three of four patients showed marked improvement in spasticity and pain. Larger controlled studies will need to be undertaken to determine if this drug is truly an effective treatment.

DRUGS CHEMICALLY RELATED TO GABA

Piracetam

Piracetam is a drug chemically related to GABA, which crosses the BBB. It has been studied in a small group of patients with cerebral palsy (CP) at a dosage of 50 mg/kg/d *(22)* using a double-blind crossover technique. General spasticity, hand movement, hand function, and walking were assessed. On overall assessment, 8 out of the 16 patients revealed slight to moderate improvement in at least two categories while on piracetam, compared to no effect in the placebo group. Side effects were mild and included nausea and vomiting in one patient. No other studies have been pursued using piracetam.

Progabide

Progabide binds to both the $GABA_A$ and $GABA_B$ receptor. It has been studied in spasticity secondary to MS *(23,24)*. Spastic hypertonia was reduced in the patients on progabide (14/16) (median dose 1800 mg/d) along with a significant suppression of tendon reflexes and flexor spasms *(24)*. In another randomized, double-blind, placebo-controlled crossover study, progabide improved spasticity as measured by the Ashworth scale *(23)*. The minor side effects associated with progabide included drowsiness, dizziness, and nausea *(23)*. Elevation of the liver enzymes at doses of 45 mg/kg/d was seen in 23% of patients *(23)*, therefore limiting the usefulness of this drug.

NMDA-ANTAGONISTS

Orphenadrine citrate is an uncompetitive NMDA-type glutamate antagonist *(25)*. In a double-blind, crossover study of 11 patients with spastic hypertonia, the flexion-reflex threshold was compared before and after 60 mg IV of orphenadrine vs placebo *(26)*. In addition, spastic hypertonia of knee-flexor muscles was assessed by the Ashworth scale. In 10 patients orphenadrine increased the reflex threshold, thereby reducing the excitability of the flexon reflex at 30 min. There was statistical reduction of the clinical signs as revealed by the Ashworth scale at 60 min. No side effects were noted. It was suggested by the authors that this drug could potentially be used in the rehabilitation setting to prepare patients for physical therapy.

MISCELLANEOUS DRUGS

Cyproheptadine

Cyproheptadine is a seritonin antagonist that was evaluated in a small study of six patients with spasticity secondary to MS or traumatic injury to the spinal cord *(27)*. At a maximum dose of 24 mg/d, therapy varied from 4–24 mo. Cyproheptadine substantially reduced or abolished ankle clonus in all patients and spontaneous spasms in five patients. Cyproheptadine is thought to block the excitability on motor neurons from 5-HT *(27)*. Side effects may include sedation and dry mouth *(25)*.

Cyclobenzaprine

Cyclobenzaprine is a tricyclic amine related to amitriptyline. In a double-blind crossover trial, 15 patients with cerebral or spinal spasticity were treated with cyclobenzaprine 60 mg/d vs placebo. Treatment was crossed over after 2 wk. Clinical assessments and EMG activity were studied *(28)*. Cyclobenzaprine was no more effective than placebo in the treatment of spasticity. In one patient who was treated with 150 mg/d, there was a reduction in the frequency of spasms and a 63% reduction in reflex EMG compared to placebo. No trials at the higher dose have been performed. The only significant side effect was a rash in one patient.

Phenothiazines

Phenothiazines are thought to exert their effect by reducing the discharge of fusimotor fibers *(29)*. They have been found to abolish the hypertonia of cats decerebrated by intercollicular section *(30)*. Their site of action has been hypothesized to be the brainstem reticular formation, on the bulbospinal noradrenergic pathway *(31,32)*. Phenothiazines with the greatest alpha-adrenergic blocking action are the most effective *(30)*. In a small study, chlorpromazine was found to reduce muscular tone *(33)*. Patients who received the drug also noted modest subjective improvement. Greater benefits were seen, though, when chlorpromazine was used in combination with phenytoin *(33)*. Phenytoin was used because it depresses afferent discharges from muscle spindles *(34)*. The authors hypothesized that this synergistic effect of phenytoin and chlorpromazine was owing to decreased responsiveness of the muscle spindle *(33)*. A major drawback of chlorpromazine use is the side effect of lethargy *(33)*. In addition, it has the potential long term side effect of tardive dyskinesia and parkinsonism. Other phenothiazine derivatives such as dimethothiazine have demonstrated some clinical benefit but side effects such as phototoxicity limit clinical usefulness *(35)*.

Cannabinoids

Marijuana or its synthetic derivatives may reduce spasticity in patients with spasticity of spinal-cord origin. Most of the literature consists of anecdotal reports or reports including a very small number of patients. A survey taken by spinal-cord injured males at the Miami VA Hospital reported 10 patients who had used marijuana. Five patients reported a decrease in spasticity, whereas there was no effect in three *(36)*. In a double-blind pilot study, nine patients were given either 10 mg, 5 mg, or no synthetic Δ^9-tetrahydrocannabinol (THC) *(37)*. Deep tendon reflexes, muscular resistance to stretch in the legs, spasticity score, and EMG-interference pattern were evaluated. The differences between the groups in regards to change in spasticity score was significant ($p < 0.01$) *(37)*. Side effects were minimal at these dosages. The long-term tolerance and addictive effects of these agents may limit their use and beneficial effects need to be proven in large clinical trials.

CONCLUSION

The treatment of spasticity is often limited by the side effects of the medications. All patients will not be able to benefit from or tolerate the standard medical treatments but there are alternative classes of drugs as discussed in this chapter that may prove useful as adjuvant or primary therapy.

REFERENCES

1. Tremblay, L. E. and Bedard, P. J. (1986) Effect of Clonidine on motorneuron excitability in spinalized rats. *Neuropharmacology* **25,** 41–46.
2. Unnerstall, J. R., Kopajtic, T. A., and Kuhar, M. J. (1984) Distribution of alpha$_2$-agonist binding sites in rat and human central nervous system: analysis

of some functional, anatomic correlates of pharmacologic effects of clonidine and related adrenergic agents. *Brain Res.* **319**, 69–101.
3. Naftchi, N. E. (1982) Functional restoration of the traumatically injured spinal cord in cats by clonidine. *Science* **217**, 1042–1044.
4. Boyeson, M. G., Jones, J. L., and Harmon, R. L. (1994) Sparing of motor function after cortical injury: a new perspective on underlying mechanisms. *Arch. Neurol.* **51**, 405–414.
5. Dall, J. T., Harmon, R. L., and Quinn, C. M. (1996) Use of clonidine for treatment of spasticity arising from various forms of brain injury: a case series. *Brain Inj.* **10**, 453–458.
6. Donovan, W. H., Carter, R. E., Rossi, D., and Wilkerson, M. A. (1998) Clonidine effect on spasticity: a clinical trial. *Arch. Phys. Med. Rehabil.* **69**, 193–194.
7. Nance, P. W., Shears, A. H., and Nance, D. M. (1989) Reflex changes induced by clonidine in spinal cord injured patients. *Paraplegia* **27**, 296–301.
8. DeGail, P., Lance, J. W., and Neilson, P. D. (1966) Differential effects on tonic and phasic reflex mechanisms produced vibration of muscles in man. *J. Neurol. Neurosurg. Psych.* **29**, 1–11.
9. Burke, D. and Ashby, P. (1972) Are spinal 'presynaptic' inhibitory mechanisms suppressed in spasticity? *J. Neurol. Sci.* **15**, 321–326.
10. Taylor, S., Ashby, P., and Verrier, M. (1984) Neurophysiological changes following traumatic spinal lesions in man. *J. Neurol. Neurosurg. Psychiatry* **47**, 1102–1108.
11. Weingarden, S. I. and Belen, J. G. (1992) Clonidine transdermal system for treatment of spasticity in spinal cord injury. *Arch. Phys. Med. Rehabil.* **73**, 876–877.
12. Yablon, S. A. and Sipski, M. L. (1993) Effect of transdermal clonidine on spinal spasticity: a case series. *Am. J. Phys. Med. Rehabil.* **72**, 154–157.
13. Mai, J. (1978) Depression of spasticity by alpha-adrenergic blockade. *Acta. Neurol. Scand.* **57**, 65–76.
14. White, C. and Richens, A. (1974) Thymoxamine and spasticity. *Lancet* **i(859)**, 686–687.
15. Mueller, M. E., Gruenthal, M., Olson, W. L., and Olson, W. H. (1997) Gabapentin for relief of upper motor neuron symptoms in multiple sclerosis. *Arch. Phys. Med. Rehabil.* **78**, 521–524.
16. McLean, M. J. (1994) Clinical pharmacokinetics of gabapentin. *Neurology* **44**, S17–S22.
17. Gruenthal, M., Mueller, M., Olson, W. L., Priebe, M. M., Sherwood, A. M., and Olson, W. H. (1997) Gabapentin for the treatment of spasticity in patients with spinal cord injury. *Spinal Cord* **35**, 686–689.
18. Priebe, M. M., Sherwood, A. M., Graves, D. E., Mueller, M., and Olson, W. H. (1997) Effectiveness of gabapentin in controlling spasticity: a quantitative study. *Spinal Cord* **35**, 171–175.
19. Biscoe, T. J. and Fry, J. P. (1982) Some pharmacological studies on the spastic mouse. *Br. J. Pharmacol.* **75**, 23–35.
20. Finke, J. (1978) Therapy of spasticity using sodium valproate. *J. Medizinischewelt* **29**, 1579–1581.

21. Zachariah, S. B., Borges, E. F., Varghese, R., Cruz, A. R., and Ross, G. S. (1994) Positive response to oral divalproex sodium (Depakote) in patients with spasticity and pain. *Am. J. Med. Sci.* **308,** 38–40.
22. Maritz, N. G., Müller, F. O., and Pompe Van Meerdervoort H.F. (1978) Piracetam in the management of spasticity in cerebral palsy. *S. Afr. Med. J.* **53,** 889–891.
23. Rudick, R.A., Breton, D., and Krall, R. L. (1987) The GABA-agonist progabide or spasticity in multiple sclerosis. *Arch. Neurol.* **44,** 1033–1036.
24. Mondrup, K. and Pedersen, E. (1984) The clinical effect of the GABA-agonist, progabide, on spasticity. *Acta. Neurol. Scand.* **69,** 200–206.
25. Gracies, J. M., Elovic, E., McGuire, J., and Simpson, D. (1997) Traditional pharmacological treatments for spasticity Part II: general and regional treatments. *Muscle Nerve* **20(Suppl. 6),** S92–S119.
26. Casale, R., Glynn, C. J., and Buonocore, M. (1995) Reduction of spastic hypertonia in patients with spinal cord injury: a double-blind comparison of intravenous orphenadrine citrate and placebo. *Arch. Phys. Med. Rehabil.* **76,** 660–665.
27. Barbeau, H., Richards, C. L., and Bedard, P. J. (1982) Action of cyproheptadine in spastic paraparetic patients. *J. Neurol. Neurosurg. Psychiatry* **45,** 923–926.
28. Ashby, P., Burke, D., Rao, S., and Jones, R. F. (1972) Assessment of cyclobenzaprine in the treatment of spasticity. *J. Neurol. Neurosurg. Psychiatry* **35,** 599–605.
29. Davidoff, R. A. (1985) Antispasticity drugs: mechanisms of action. *Ann. Neurol.* **17,** 107–116.
30. Keary, E. M. and Maxwell, D. R. (1967) A comparison of the effects of chlorpromazine and some related phenothiazines in reducing the rigidity of the decerebrate cat and in some other central actions. *Br. J. Pharmaacol. Chemother.* **30,** 400–416.
31. Maxwell, D. R. and Sumpter, E.A. (1972) Noradrenergic receptors and the control of fusimotor activity. *J. Physiol.* **222,** 173–175.
32. Maxwell, D. R. and Sumpter, E. A. (1974) A comparison of the actions of some drugs on decerebrate rigidity, muscle spindle activity, and alpha-adrenoreceptors. *Br. J. Pharmacol.* **50,** 355–363.
33. Cohan, S. L., Raines, A., Panagakos, J., and Armitage, P. Phenytoin and chlorpromazine in the treatment of spasticity. *Arch. Neurol.* **37,** 360–364.
34. Anderson, R. J. and Raines, A. (1976) Suppresion of decerebrate rigidity by phenytoin and chlorpromazine. *Neurology* **26,** 858–862.
35. Matthews, W. B., Rushworth, G., and Wakefield, G. S. (1972) Dimethothiazine in spasticity: a further attempt at pharmacological control. *Acta. Neurol. Scand.* **48,** 635–644.
36. Dunn, M. and Davis, R. (1974) The perceived effects of marijuana on spinal cord injured males. *Paraplegia* **12,** 175.
37. Petro, D. J. and Ellenberger, C. (1981) Treatment of human spasticity with Δ^9-tetrahydrocannabinol. *J. Clin. Pharmacol.* **21,** 413S–416S.

12
Nerve Blocks

David S. Rosenblum

INTRODUCTION

Spasticity is one of the greatest challenges impacting functional independence for many individuals, and it can greatly affects one's quality of life. In conditions affecting the central nervous system (CNS) such as spinal-cord injury, multiple sclerosis (MS), brain injury, stroke, and cerebral palsy (CP), the spasticity can be diffuse or focal. In diffuse spasticity, a generalized increase in muscle tone affects a variety of different muscle groups. In focal spasticity, a localized region of increased muscle tone is appreciated. In either case, the general initial treatment principles involve avoidance and reduction of any noxious/nociceptive stimuli, treatment of underlying infections, proper positioning, splinting, and frequent stretching. Medications may be indicated for significant generalized spasticity. However, for patients with focal spasticity, nerve blocks are an excellent alternative treatment, one that avoids the systemic adverse effects often seen with oral medications.

NERVE BLOCKS

Nerve blocks generally involve chemical neurolysis, which impairs nerve conduction by temporarily destroying part of the nerve. It is appropriate to help individuals with focal spasticity reach specific goals. To identify the issues, the evaluator must do a careful and thorough examination, functional history, and functional assessment. The extent and severity of spasticity, as well as which specific muscle groups are affected, must be identified. The functional impact of the muscles impaired by spasticity must be queried and assessed. It is important to specifically assess the impact and effect of spasticity, clonus, hyperreflexia, weakness, pain, and decreased range of motion of affected joints on issues such as self-care, mobility, and gait. As well, it is important to determine the severity of spasticity and if the spastic muscle has any voluntary control. The presence of focal spasticity does not always

From: *Current Clinical Neurology: Clinical Evaluation and Management of Spasticity*
Edited by: D. A. Gelber and D. R. Jeffery © Humana Press, Inc., Totowa, NJ

necessitate treatment. Rather, efforts should be made to control spasticity if it is adversely affecting one's function and quality of life.

BENEFITS OF NERVE BLOCKS

Nerve blocks are indicated to decrease focal spasticity in order to improve seating, positioning, bed mobility, transfers, gait, and self-care. For example, spasticity of the elbow flexors and forceful spastic gripping of the hand both may be effectively treated with nerve blocks to improve the ability to perform self-care, and lessen the need for assistance from caregivers. Nerve blocks can also aid in treatment and prevention of skin maceration, which can result from clenched fists and flexed elbows. The focal relief of spasms may lessen pain, improve sleep, and contribute to improvements in self esteem. Better mobility, positioning, and posture helps protect the skin from pressure ulcers and may additionally aid in healing by making pressure relief possible. Volitional function may improve as well: decreasing tone of one muscle may allow better use and control of all the muscles crossing a particular joint. Sexual function may be improved by selective reduction of spasticity in the adductors. Serial casting, a technique that slowly and gently increases the range of motion across a joint, can be greatly facilitated by selective nerve block prior to casting. Gait can also be improved by blocking the ankle and toe plantar flexors if clonus and plantar-flexor spasticity interferes with foot positioning. Additionally, blocking the hip adductors can decrease scissoring of the legs during gait. Finally, nerve blocks may allow for more efficient use of an orthosis. Whether the orthosis is designed for positioning (i.e., wrist hand orthosis [WHO]) or for function (i.e., ankle foot orthosis [AFO]), the ability to more effectively take advantage of orthotic intervention has clear benefits.

TIMING OF NERVE BLOCKS

Although nerve blocks can be initiated at any time after injury, there are specific advantages to considering this intervention during the first 12–18 mo. Shortly after neurologic injury, during a time of potential neurologic improvement, it is prudent to avoid definitive surgical procedures to treat spasticity, such as tendon transfers, tendon lengthening, and muscle releases. This will avoid early procedures that may not be needed after there is neurologic improvement. In contrast, nerve blocks are particularly useful early because their effects are temporary. Selective use of nerve blocks during initial rehabilitation may allow work towards goals that would not otherwise be possible. For example, early and temporary focal treatment of wrist-flexor spasticity may allow aggressive grasp and hand activities otherwise

Nerve Blocks

not possible or appropriate for the individual with a flexed nonfunctional spastic wrist. Additionally, following selective nerve blocks, range of motion and stretching may be more easily performed, helping prevent the development of contractures. Because nerve blocks will not be effective once the joint the spastic muscle crosses is frozen or contracted, early assessment and intervention is critical in maintaining and improving joint mobility.

PHENOL

Phenol has been used as a neurolytic agent for over 60 years and specifically for the management of spasticity for more than 30 years *(1,2)*. Early uses of phenol included using low concentrations as a local anesthetic agent. By 1959, intrathecal and epidural injections were used for the treatment of cancer pain *(3)*. Additionally, phenol was used for sympathectomies *(2)*. Although initially used intrathecally or epidurally to treat spasticity, more recently phenol has been used in the form of peripheral nerve blocks for management.

Phenol, or carbolic acid, is a local anesthetic at concentrations of 1–2% *(3)*. At concentrations of more than 5%, it denatures protein, causes necrosis, and is neurolytic within 1 h of injection *(4–6)*. The usual limit on dose per day is 20 cc of a 5% solution (1 g), although the toxic dose in adults (systemic LD-50) is 8.5 g *(7)*. The lethal dose in children is 0.1–0.2 g/kg *(8)*. For clinical use, considerably less phenol is required; e.g., 1–2 cc of a 6% solution may be effective for a peripheral nerve block.

Phenol acts by chemically destroying axons and myelin at concentrations higher than 5% *(4)*. Although the large axons take longer to be destroyed, all nerve fiber sizes are affected and undergo Wallerian degeneration *(9)*. The destroyed axons do regenerate over time; this accounts for the temporary effect of phenol. As well, there may be reinervation of denervated muscles by motor neurons other than those that originally innervated them *(10)*. Intramuscular nerve blocks or motor-point blocks with phenol additionally causes muscle necrosis; muscle and nerve regeneration is complete by 3 mo *(6,11)*.

The clinical duration of effect of phenol nerve blocks is quite variable, ranging from 1 mo to 1 yr, but generally lasts several months *(2,5,7,10,12)*. A number of variables may be important in considering the wide range of reported durations of efficacy, such as technique used, concentration of phenol used, volume used, the severity of the spasticity before treatment and, importantly, the timing of administration after injury.

ETHANOL

Ethanol is also a neurolytic agent but has not been used for spasticity treatment to the extent that phenol has *(8)*. Similar to phenol, ethanol has an effect on both motor and sensory nerves *(4)*. At low concentrations, 5–10% ethanol acts as a local anesthetic by interfering with sodium and potassium conduction *(4)*. At higher concentrations, ethanol denatures protein and destroys both axons and myelin; concentrations of 35–60% are effective for spasticity treatment *(6,13,14)*. Ethanol can also be combined with 0.5% lidocaine and administered intramuscularly to treat spasticity *(6)*. Although its efficacy has not been directly compared to phenol or botulinum toxin, ethanol appears to be an effective and inexpensive alternative as a temporary chemical neurolytic agent.

LOCAL ANESTHETICS

Local anesthetics can be used as short-acting nerve-blocking agents. They act by decreasing sodium-channel permeability resulting in a block of transmission of the nerve signal. The most commonly used local anesthetics for the treatment of spasticity include lidocaine, etidocaine, and bupivicaine. Each has its own relative risks, side effects, and dosing parameters. Temporary nerve block with a local anesthetic allows the individual to experience, for a few hours, the effect of focal control of spasticity. The longer-acting agents are sometimes used for blocks to allow time for a detailed functional assessment before the block wears off. These blocks can also be used diagnostically to help the clinician differentiate between contracture and severe spasticity. If the nerve block is successful, then repeat nerve block with a longer-acting neurolytic agent, such as phenol, may be appropriate. It is important to let the patient know that the clinical results of the neurolytic agent will not be identical to the effect of the anesthetic agent.

POTENTIAL ADVERSE EFFECTS OF NERVE BLOCKS

In order to perform nerve blocks safely, technical expertise is required, and a thorough knowledge of anatomy and applied kinesiology is necessary. Nerve blocks should not be performed on spastic muscles that are needed for function unless there are overriding considerations, such as pain. This is a most important issue because if one requires use of a spastic muscle for functional activities and that muscle is weakened by a nerve block, then function is likely to be compromised. Additionally, a decrease in spasticity may unmask underlying weakness resulting in joint instability, muscle sprains, and strains.

A side effect of nerve blocks is local infection, although this is less common with phenol and alcohol because of their antibacterial action *(15)*. Dependent edema may result as muscle tone is decreased, especially in the lower extremities, and this may last for 1–2 wk *(4,7)*. Venous thrombosis from phenol injections has been reported, but is unusual *(16)*. One must be careful to avoid intravascular injections of phenol. Systemic toxicity of phenol includes CNS depression, CNS stimulation, convulsions, and cardiogenic shock *(3,7)*.

Chemical neurolysis of mixed sensorimotor nerves may produce painful dysesthesias in the distribution of the sensory part of the nerve. This does not occur with motor-nerve blocks (motor-branch or motor-point blocks). The incidence of neuropathic pain following blocks of mixed nerves ranges from 2–32% *(4,6,7)*. Patients experience burning pain, parasthesias, or allodynia in the area corresponding to the blocked sensory nerve. Although the pain can be severe, it is more commonly mild and self-limited, and generally resolves in a few weeks *(4)*. Rarely, it can last for many months. There is no correlation between neuropathic pain and the quantity or concentration of phenol used *(4)*. If the pain is mild, then observation alone is generally appropriate. However, if treatment of the pain is required, initial options include gentle compression of the affected area with stockings or gloves, and transcutaneous electrical nerve stimulation (TENS). Capsaicin applied topically in concentrations of 0.025–0.075% may also be effective. Pharmacologic options include gabapentin, low-dose tricyclic antidepressants, carbamazepine, and nonsteroidal anti-inflammatory drugs. If the pain is severe, then a short course of corticosteroids may be useful *(4,7)*. For severe neuropathic pain that persists despite aggressive local and pharmacological treatment, surgical neurolysis or repeat neurolysis with phenol may be effective *(4,17,18)*.

TYPES OF NERVE BLOCKS AND TECHNIQUES
Percutaneous Closed Nerve Trunk Blocks

With this technique, mixed sensorimotor nerves are blocked. After a thorough static, dynamic, and functional assessment, the specific spastic muscle and its corresponding nerve supply is identified. Informed consent should be obtained after the potential risks and benefits of the procedure are discussed. If necessary, surface stimulation may be used to help localize the nerve. The specific approach used depends on the nerve and the corresponding anatomy. Universal precautions should be observed. Proper positioning is critical to ensure adequate access, comfort for the patient, and to ensure control of the spastic limb. Aseptic technique is used. The skin should be punctured in a quick and smooth way to minimize discomfort. Pulling the skin taut before puncture may also minimize the pain of needle entry. A small-gauge needle, such as 22-gauge, may be used. The needles used are coated with Teflon to allow electrical stimulation to localize the nerve; the needle tip is uncoated. When the needle is in the vicinity of the nerve, electrical stimulation results in contraction of the muscle. The amperage is reduced as the needle is advanced closer to the nerve. As the needle approaches the nerve, the muscle contracts vigorously with less stimulation. Very small advances and rotation of the needle allows for accurate localization. When minimal stimulation (approx 1 milliampere) produces the best possible muscle contraction of the spastic muscle, the agent is injected. One should aspirate before injection to ensure the needle is not in an intravascular space. The patient may feel a burning sensation during the injection. The amount of phenol injected depends on the size of the nerve and the goal of the block, but is usually from one to a few cubic centimeters. Results are generally apparent within a few minutes after the block. However, the full potential of an alcohol or phenol block may not be seen until 2 to 3 days after the block. During this time, aggressive stretching to the treated area should be avoided. The patient should be advised to take extra care with activities because the biomechanics of mobility may be significantly altered.

Motor-Point Blocks

Motor-point blocks involve injecting the motor nerve terminals in the spastic muscle. With this technique, the sensory nerves are avoided, and therefore the side effect of neuropathic pain is avoided. Motor point blocks have been used since the 1960s and are the most common nerve-block technique performed today *(19)*. Although phenol is used most often, alcohol can be used as an inexpensive and effective alternative *(4,20)*. The motor-point technique with phenol or alcohol utilizes electrical-surface stimulation over the targeted muscle to find the areas where minimal stimulation causes maximal muscle response. This area is called the motor point. These electrically sensitive points are believed to be where the motor-nerve approaches the surface of the muscle, or the endplate zone *(3,13)*. An understanding of the general location of clusters of endplates within a given muscle may help facilitate localization of the motor points and injection of these points. The concentration of phenol used is 2–7%, with volumes of 0.1 to several cubic centimeters *(4,21)*. Ethanol is commonly diluted between 35–60% for motor-point blocks *(6)*. Multiple injections are often required to multiple motor points. As such, patient tolerance may be a limiting factor. Swelling and pain may occur after motor-point blocks. Initially, the use of ice and avoidance of both repetitive motion and aggressive stretching is helpful. Motor-point blocks may be used in conjunction with sensorimotor-nerve blocks.

Open Nerve Blocks

This technique involves surgical exposure of a nerve with injection specifically of the motor branches *(22)*. The incidence of dysesthesias is lower because the sensory nerves are not injected *(23)*. The risks of the procedure include those related to the surgery and anesthesia. This technique is not utilized as much as the percutaneous blocks because it requires operative exposure of nerves. The duration of effect from this type of block is generally less than 6 mo *(24)*.

PATIENT SELECTION AND EVALUATION

Because nerve blocks are indicated for the treatment of focal spasticity, it is important to additionally consider the musculoskeletal, functional, and kinesiological issues impacted by the spasticity. Specific goals beyond simple relief of spasm are helpful in considering the planning of postinjection interventions. The relative advantages of nerve blocks over medications, such as the absence of cognitive side effects and the temporary effect, should be weighed against the potential side effects. The evaluation of the potential nerve block candidate should include consideration of the diagnosis/natural history of the disorder, timing after injury, severity and location of spasticity, relative strength of the affected muscle and other muscles also impacting the spastic joint, the active and passive range of motion of the affected joint, and the potential level of function attainable if the block is successful. It is important to assess the individual's pain and pain tolerance, as well as to understand the impact of any psychological issues such as anxiety, before doing a nerve block. Tolerance to the procedure and any adverse reactions from prior nerve blocks should be assessed. Importantly, one should review the success, efficacy, duration, and functional consequences of previous blocks.

Comprehensive rehabilitation is well-suited to provide specific, goal-directed care and evaluation before and after nerve blocks to ensure that the many multifaceted issues are addressed: maximal functional independence for self-care; mobility; current and potential equipment and orthotic needs; psychological, social, and vocational support; and continuity of care. Preinjection rehabilitation provides education to the individual, provides the physician with extensive insight into the patient's current functional status and what the specific barriers to further independence are, and ensures good continuity of care pre- and postblock. For example, after a block the individual may need a different program for stretching, strengthening, and functional-mobility training. Personal-care needs and equipment needs may change.

Lower-Extremity Nerve Blocks

Obturator Nerve

Patients with cerebral palsy, spinal-cord injuries, and traumatic brain injuries often have increased hip-adductor spasticity, which can cause scissoring of gait and difficulty with perineal hygiene. In these individuals, specifically blocking the obturator nerve may be of benefit *(25,29)*. Motor-point blocks to the adductor muscles (adductor longus, brevis, magnus, pectineus, gracilis) is difficult with phenol because of the number of injections that are necessary, the associated pain, and unpredictable outcome. They may be useful, however, in supplementing the nerve block. The anterior branch of the obturator nerve supplies the adductor longus, brevis, and gracilis. The posterior branch innervates the adductor magnus. One may target either branch, and the techniques available to block the obturator nerve are well-described and effective *(4,26–28)*.

Tibial Nerve

Patients with spasticity of the ankle plantar flexors, such as that seen in hemiplegia secondary to cerebrovascular accident (CVA), may benefit from a tibial nerve block. Plantar-flexion spasticity interferes with gait, transfers, self-care activities such as dressing, and may be painful. Whereas motor-point blocks with phenol require multiple injections to relatively large muscles, a nerve block can be done easily for diagnostic purposes with a local anesthetic or therapeutically with chemically denervating agents. The block is simple, effective, and may eliminate clonus, decrease or eliminate resistance to passive stretch of the ankle dorsiflexors, improve ambulation and orthotic fitting, and prevent equinus deformity *(30–32)*. Care must be taken to avoid the popliteal artery, which is medial to the nerve. The peroneal nerve is lateral to the tibial nerve in the popliteal fossa, and is usually avoided unless everter spasm is also present.

The tibial nerve also innervates tibialis posterior, which acts as a primary inverter of the foot. Spasticity of the foot inverters interferes with gait. In addition to blocking the branches of the tibial nerve to the tibialis posterior, it is possible to provide direct motor blocks to the muscle. Similarly, although tibial nerve block may be useful for toe-flexor spasticity, the flexor digitorum longus may be specifically treated by direct motor-point block.

Sciatic Nerve

It may be appropriate to consider a nerve block of the sciatic nerve in patients with knee-flexor spasms secondary to spasticity of the hamstrings muscles. The knee flexors are primarily the semimembranosis, semitendinosis, and the long head and short head of biceps femoris. However, the gracilis, gastrocnemius, popliteus, and plantaris also cross the knee and assist in knee flexion. It is therefore difficult to effectively control severe knee-flexion spasticity with motor-point blocks alone. It is important to realize that the long head of the biceps femoris, semitendinosus, and semimembranosis all originate from part of the ischial tuberosity. They therefore cross the hip joint, and assist in extension of the hip. Blocking the nerve to these muscles may decrease hip-extensor tone, which could make pre-existing hip-flexor spasticity unopposed and therefore more apparent and dysfunctional. The sciatic nerve is usually blocked in the area of the gluteal fold midway between the ischial tuberosity and the greater trochanter *(4)*.

Femoral Nerve

The femoral nerve can be blocked to decrease knee-extensor spasticity. The risk of decreasing function and gait by decreasing extensor tone and unmasking underlying weakness should be considered. Knee buckling and loss of ambulation is a potential consequence. The femoral nerve supplies the rectus femoris, vastus lateralis, medialis, and intermedius. The nerve is located just below the inguinal ligament *(4)*. Motor-point blocks to selected knee extensors may be effective, but one must consider the size of the muscle, number of motor points requiring injection, and the tolerance of the patient.

Hip Flexor Spasticity

Patients with hip-flexor spasticity may be eligible for paravertebral lumbar-spine nerve blocks *(26,33)*. Other muscles that can be blocked using the paravertebral lumbar-spine blocks include the hip adductors, hamstrings, and quadratus lumborum *(4)*.

Hip-flexor spasticity is often painful, interferes with sitting, standing, ambulation, and activities of daily living. Although the major hip flexor is the iliopsoas, many other muscles cross the hip and assist hip flexion such as the rectus femoris, sartorius, and even the adductors *(34)*. Motor-point block of the psoas major and minor under ultrasound monitoring can be effective for hip-flexor spasticity, may improve gait, lessen pain, ease skin care, and improve sitting and positioning *(35)*.

Upper-Extremity Nerve Blocks

Musculocutaneous Nerve

These blocks may be helpful in patients with elbow-flexor spasticity because the primary elbow flexors, biceps and brachialis, are supplied by the musculocutaneous nerve *(36,37)*. However, complete paralysis of the elbow flexors does not occur after block to the musculocutaneous nerve because of the radially innervated brachioradialis, which is also an elbow flexor. Motor-point injections may be used in conjunction with musculocutaneous nerve blocks for added benefit *(37)*. The technique is safe, effective, and particularly well-suited for individuals with significant elbow-flexor tone who may potentially show further neurologic improvement *(37,38)*.

Median Nerve

Median nerve blocks may be used to treat focal spasticity of the wrist and finger flexors *(5)*. Median nerve innervated muscles include flexor digitorum profundus (digits 2 and 3), first and second lumbricals, flexor digitorum sublimis, flexor carpi radialis (FCR), flexor pollicis longus, palmaris, and part of the flexor pollicis brevis. Flexion of the wrist is mainly by FCR and flexor carpi ulnaris (FCU), although many other muscles cross this joint. Although chemical denervation of the median nerve may affect all these muscle groups and cause relaxation of the wrist and fingers, one should also consider the risk of dysesthetic pain possible with a median nerve block. Motor-point blocks to the appropriate wrist of finger flexors can be effectively done with good results. Motor-point blocks to the FCR and FCU, for example, are generally well-tolerated and can be very effective for decreasing wrist-flexor spasticity. Phenol motor-point blocks to spastic forearm-flexor muscles in patients with head injury has been shown to be effective in relaxing muscle tone and in improving active wrist extension *(39)*.

Subscapularis

This muscle is a primary internal rotator of the shoulder. Spasticity in the subscapularis is commonly seen in hemiplegia and is partially responsible for the typical shoulder position of adduction and internal rotation of the shoulder. The tightness in internal rotation causes pain and also limits external rotation, abduction, and flexion of the shoulder; motor-point block to the subscapularis for the painful hemiplegic shoulder has been described *(40)*. Phenol blocks of the nerves to the subscapularis in patients with hemiplegia has also been shown to be safe, effective in improving range of motion, and helpful for decreasing pain *(41)*.

CARE AFTER NERVE BLOCK

After a nerve block, the patient may apply ice for up to 20 min a few times a day as needed. Specific strengthening to the treated muscle, as well as stretching, should be avoided for the first 1–2 days. Although there may be an early response to phenol injection, the maximum response usually takes a few days. Therefore, the patient may experience changes over time. Rehabilitation after the block is performed may address the changing functional issues and is well-suited to help the individual meet new functional goals made possible by the nerve block. Specific bracing needs, wheelchair and seating needs are just a few examples of the issues that are often appropriate to address after a block.

SUMMARY

Nerve blocks are an effective therapeutic intervention for the treatment of focal spasticity. In contrast to botulinum toxin, the agents most commonly used for nerve blocks, including phenol, ethanol, and the local anesthetics, are relatively inexpensive and have a rapid onset of action. Conversely, there is more skill required to perform nerve blocks. Unfortunately, comparative studies between these agents have not yet been performed.

The clinician considering recommending a block should carefully evaluate the individual for spasticity and ensure that any contributing factors/noxious stimuli are addressed. A thorough neurologic, musculoskeletal, and kinesiologic evaluation will assist in the selection of the appropriate nerves or muscles to be treated and will aid in anticipating the potential positive and negative functional consequences. The goals of treatment should be specific and clearly oriented towards functional independence and quality-of-life issues. Rehabilitation assessment and treatment before and after a block can be very useful. For the appropriate individual, well-planned nerve blocks or motor-point blocks can be a powerful tool in assisting individuals with focal spasticity to achieve their goals.

REFERENCES

1. Khalili, A. A., Harmel, M. H., Foster, S., and Benton, J. G. (1964) Management of spasticity by selective peripheral nerve block with dilute phenol solutions in clinical rehabilitation. *Arch. Phys. Med. Rehabil.* **45,** 513–519.
2. Botte, M. J., Abrams, R. A., and Bodine-Fowler, S. C. (1995) Treatment of acquired muscle spasticity using phenol peripheral nerve blocks. *Orthopedics* **18(2),** 151–160.
3. Wood, K. M. (1978) The use of phenol as a neurolytic agent: a review. *Pain* **5,** 205–229.
4. Glenn, M. B. (1990) Nerve blocks, in *The Practical Management of Spasticity in Children and Adults.* Lea & Febiger, Philadelphia, pp. 227–258.
5. Katz, R. T. (1988) Management of spasticity. *Am. J. PM&R* **67(3),** 108–116.
6. Gracies, J. M. and Simpson, D. (1999) Neuromuscular blockers. *Phys. Med. Rehabil. Clin. North Am.* **10(2),** 357–383.
7. Glenn, M. B. and Elovic, E. (1997) Practice protocol. Chemical denervation for the treatment of hypertonia and related motor disorders: phenol and botulinum toxin. *J. Head Trauma Rehabil.* **12(6),** 40–62.
8. Formley, M. E. (1999) Management of spasticity in children: Part I: chemical denervation. *J. Head Trauma Rehabil.* **14(1),** 97–99.

9. Burkel, W. E. and McPhee, M. (1970) Effect of phenol injection into peripheral nerve of rat: electron microscope studies. *Arch. Phys. Med. Rehabil.* **51,** 391–397.
10. Bodine-Fowler, S., Allsing, S., and Botte, M. (1996) Time course of muscle atrophy and recovery following phenol-induced nerve block. *Muscle Nerve* **19,** 497–504.
11. Halpern, D. (1977) Histological studies in animals after intramuscular neurolysis with phenol. *Arch. Phys. Med. Rehabil.* **58,** 438–443.
12. Khalili, A. A. and Bets, H. B. (1967) Peripheral nerve block with phenol in the management of spasticity. *JAMA* **200(13),** 103–105.
13. Tardieu, G., Tardieu, C., Hariga, J., and Gagnard, L. (1968) Treatment of spasticity by injection of dilute alcohol at the motor point or by epidural route. *Dev. Med. Child. Neurol.* **10,** 555–568.
14. Carpenter, E. B. and Seitz, D. G. (1980) Intramuscular alcohol as an aid in management of spastic cerebral palsy. *Dev. Med. Child. Neurol.* **22,** 497–501.
15. Felsenthal, G. (1974) Pharmacology of phenol in peripheral nerve blocks: a review. *Arch. Phys. Med. Rehabil.* **55,** 13–16.
16. Macek, C. (1983) Venous thrombosis results from some phenol injections. *JAMA* **249,** 1807.
17. Petrillo, C. R., Chu, D. S., and Davis, S. W. (1980) Phenol block of the tibial nerve in the hemiplegic patient. *Orthopedics* **3,** 871–874.
18. Braun, R. M., Hoffer, M. M., and Mooney, V., et al. (1973) Phenol nerve block in the treatment of acquired spastic hemiplegia in the upper limb. *J. Bone Joint Surg.* **55A,** 580–585.
19. Cain, H. D., Glass, A., Spiegler, J., Liebgold, H., and Mead, S. (1966) Peripheral nerve and motor point blocks for spasticity. *Paraplegia* **4,** 166–167.
20. Kimura, J. (1989) *Electrodiagnosis in Diseases of Nerve and Muscle: Principles and Practice,* 2nd ed. FA Davis Co., Philadelphia, p. 631.
21. Copp, E. P. and Keenan, J. Phenol nerve and motor point block in spasticity. *Rheum. Phys. Med.* **11,** 287–292.
22. Moore, T. J. and Anderson, R. B. (1991) The use of open phenol blocks to the motor branches of the tibial nerve in adult acquired spasticity. *Foot Ankle* **11(4),** 219–221.
23. Garland, D. E., Lucie, R. S., and Waters, R. L. (1982) Current uses of open phenol block for adult acquired spasticity. *Clin. Orthop. Relat. Res.* **165,** 217–222.
24. Braun, R. M., Hoffer, M. M., Mooney, V., McKeever, J., and Roper, B. (1973) Phenol nerve block in the treatment of acquired spastic hemiplegia in the upper limb. *JBJS* **55(31),** 580–585.
25. Koffman, M. (1981) Proximal femoral resection in total hip replacement in severely disabled cerebral-spastic patients. *Orthop. Clin. North. Am.* **12,** 91–100.
26. Awad, E. A. (1972) Phenol block for control of hip flexor and adductor spasticity. *Arch. Phys. Med. Rehabil.* **53(12),** 554–557.
27. Felsenthal, G. (1974) Nerve blocks in the lower extremities: anatomic considerations. *Arch. Phys. Med. Rehabil.* **55,** 504–517.
28. Wassef, M. R. (1993) Interadductor approach to obturator nerve blockage for spastic conditions of adductor thigh muscles. *Reg. Anesth.* **18(1),** 13–17.

29. Trainer, N., Bowser, B. L., and Dahm, L. (1986) Obturator nerve block for painful hip in adult cerebral palsy. *Arch. Phys. Med. Rehabil.* **67,** 819–830.
30. Petrillo, C. R., Chu, D. S., and Davis, S. W. (1980) Phenol block of the tibial nerve in the hemiplegic patient. *Orthopedics* **3(9),** 871–874.
31. Kempthorne, D. M. and Brown, T. C. K. (1984) Nerve blocks around the knee in children. *Anaesth. Intens. Care.* **12,** 14–17.
32. Kirazli, Y., Yagiz, A., Kismali, B., and Aksit, R. (1998) Comparison of phenol block and botulinus toxin type A in the treatment of spastic foot after stroke. *AJRM* **77(6),** 510–515.
33. Meelhuysen, F. E., Halpern, D., and Quast, J. (1968) Treatment of flexor spasticity of hip by paravertebral lumbar spine nerve blocks. *Arch. Phys. Med. Rehabil.* **49,** 717–722.
34. Warfel, J. (1985) *The Extremities,* 5th ed. Lea & Febiger, Philadelphia, pp. 72–74.
35. Koyama, H., Murakami, K., Suzuki, T., and Suzuki, K. (1992) Phenol block for hip flexor muscle spasticity under ultrasonic monitoring. *Arch. Phys. Med. Rehabil.* **73,** 1040–1043.
36. Wainapel, S. F., Haigney, D., and Labib, K. (1984) Spastic hemiplegia in a quadriplegic patient: treatment with phenol nerve block. *Arch. Phys. Med. Rehabil.* **65,** 786–787.
37. Keenan, M. A. E., Tomas, E. S., Stone, L., and Gersten, L. M. (1990) Percutaneous phenol block of the musculocutaneous nerve to control elbow flexor spasticity. *JHS* **15A(2),** 340–346.
38. Braun, R. M., Hoffer, M. M., Mooney, V., McKeever, J., and Roper, B. (1973) Phenol nerve block in treatment of acquired spastic hemiplegia in upper limb. *J. Bone Joint Surg.* **55,** 580–585.
39. Garland, D. E., Lilling, M., and Keenan, M. A. (1984) Percutaneous phenol blocks to motor points of spastic forearm muscles in head injured adults. *Arch. Phys. Med. Rehabil.* **65,** 243–245.
40. Chironna, R. and Hecht, J. S. (1990) Subscapularis motor point block for the painful hemiplegic shoulder. *Arch. Phys. Med. Rehabil.* **71,** 428–429.
41. Hecht, J. S. (1992) Subscapular nerve block in the painful hemiplegic shoulder. *Arch. Phys. Med. Rehabil.* **73,** 1036–1039.

13
Botulinum Toxins

Lauren C. Seeberger and Christopher F. O'Brien

INTRODUCTION

In recent years, there has been a dramatic increase in the use of botulinum toxin for the management of spasticity. Botulinum toxin is a unique compound, effective for a variety of conditions in which the predominant clinical feature is abnormal muscle contraction. Since 1989, a number of reports have demonstrated the usefulness of botulinum toxin injections to improve spasticity and reduce painful muscle spasms. Although use of botulinum toxin for spasticity is approved in many European countries, it is still considered "off-label" for use in spasticity in the United States.

MECHANISM OF ACTION

Botulinum toxin is a potent neurotoxin produced by the bacteria, Clostridium botulinum. There are seven immunologically distinct serotypes, including A, B, C, D, E, F, and G. Type A has been the best-studied to date and likely has the longest duration of biological activity *(1)*. There are two formulations of Botulinum toxin type A available commercially, Botox® (Allergan Inc., Irvine, CA) and Dysport (Ipsen Products Pharmaceuticals Ltd, Maidenhead, Berkshire, UK). Clinically, the activity of 1 unit (U) of Botox is roughly equivalent to 3–4 U of Dysport® *(2)* although some controversy continues about how to best measure toxicity in contrast to clinical effect. A formulation of botulinum toxin type B, Myobloc®, has recently been FDA approved and is now available for clinical use (Elan Pharmaceuticals, San Francisco, CA). For the purpose of this Chapter, Botulinum toxin type A will be abbreviated as BTX-A and will refer to the Allergan product, Botox.

The botulinum toxin is synthesized as a single polypeptide chain with a molecular weight around 150,000 Daltons *(3)*. There is little potency in this

From: *Current Clinical Neurology: Clinical Evaluation and Management of Spasticity*
Edited by: D. A. Gelber and D. R. Jeffery © Humana Press, Inc., Totowa, NJ

state but then it is cleaved to its active form, a two-chained compound, composed of a heavy chain and light chain held by a disulfide bond. The heavy chain specifies binding to the acetylcholine receptor and the light chain is responsible for intracellular toxicity *(4)*.

Botulinum toxin avidly binds to presynaptic cholinergic nerves and blocks the release of acetylcholine. It does this through a three-step process including binding, internalization by endocytosis, and ultimately, inactivation of acetylcholine release by disruption of vesicle-docking proteins *(5)*. Although all botulinum-toxin types have a similar mechanism of action ultimately, i.e., blocking release of acetylcholine, the external binding proteins are unique to each serotype and the site of intracellular activity may also differ between toxins. The effect of BTX-A depends on the high affinity of the type A toxin to receptors on the human neuromuscular junction *(6)*. There is no alteration in synthesis or storage of acetylcholine in these nerve endings *(7)*. The lack of transmission of acetylcholine results in a functional denervation and subsequent muscle atrophy occurs within 10–14 d. There will be continued atrophy over the ensuing 4–6 wk *(8)*. Axonal sprouting occurs after BTX-A injection resulting in a reestablishment of neuromuscular junctions and reversal of BTX-A effects *(9)*. Short-term recovery of muscle-fiber diameter is seen 4–6 mo after the blockade and muscle studies after repeated injections continue to show good recovery of diameter size *(10)*. Long-term studies of muscle and nerve effects are underway.

Some patients lose their beneficial response to BTX-A after repeated injection. Although the most common reason for "lack of benefit" is most likely poor muscle choice or an inappropriate dose of BTX-A, some patients develop secondary nonresponsiveness. This can be ascertained by examining the injected muscle 2–3 wk after giving the BTX-A. If there is no atrophy, weakness, or electromyographic (EMG) evidence of denervation, one can conclude that the BTX-A did not have the desired effect. It is assumed that such nonresponsiveness is owing to blocking antibodies against the type A toxin *(11)*. Studies to date clearly demonstrate the presence of such antibodies, but clinical correlation between resistance and antibody titer is not clear. Some patients have measurable antibodies and continued responsiveness. Other nonresponders lack such serologic findings *(12,13)*. This riddle may reflect insensitive assay techniques, e.g. biologic mouse assay *(14)*, limited enzyme-linked immunosorbent assay (ELISA) assays *(15)*, or the reality that several mechanisms are responsible for resistance.

If the patient is felt to be resistant to the toxin, a simple test can be performed by injecting 15 U of Botox into the corrugator muscle unilaterally and examining the patient 2 wk later for the presence of muscle weakness. Hanna and Jankovic have shown good correlation between assay results, patient clinical status, and unilateral brow injections that supports the use of this test to assess BTX responsiveness *(16)*.

Despite our ignorance, guidelines have emerged from clinical practice. Greene and colleagues found the resistant patients were more likely to have received BTX-A in doses greater than 250 U per injection or at intervals of less than 12 wk *(11)*. Thus, it is recommended that injections be given no more frequently than at 12-wk intervals and that doses be limited to no more than 300–400 U per 3-mo period.

Botulinum toxin type B, Myobloc®, has been shown to be safe and efficacious in type A resistant cervical dystonia patients and offers a therapeutic alternative *(17)*. Botulinum toxin type B (BTX-B) has a duration of benefit, similar to type A, of 12–16 wk *(18)*. It must be kept in mind that the biological potency, as expressed in mouse units, is different from BTX-A. BTX-B recently received FDA approval and is available in 2,500-, 5,000-, and 10,000-U vials.

PREPARATION OF BTX-A FOR INJECTION

BTX-A is a lyophilized, freeze-dried preparation that is stored at $-5°$ centigrade. It must be diluted using normal saline without preservative prior to injection. The most common dilution is 100 u/mL. It is not recommended to refreeze prepared solution or to use the toxin after being at room temperature for more than 4 h. In contrast, BTX-B is a liquid preparation that is refrigerated (2–8°C) and is stable for approx 6 mo.

INJECTION TECHNIQUES

Although some muscles may be easily injected via palpation technique, experience suggests that more accurate placement of botulinum toxin may be achieved with localization techniques. In a busy clinical practice, methods to improve efficiency and efficacy of any treatment technique are valuable. Botulinum toxin injection is a good example of a treatment that requires significant time commitment and skill development on the part of the injector. Fortunately, the avid binding of botulinum toxin to pre-synaptic neuron terminals and the diffusion characteristics of the medication allow relative ease of administration. However, for many clinical applications, efficacy may be improved and adverse effects reduced, by more precise targeting of the muscles to be injected. This is particularly important for regions where target muscles are adjacent to muscles for which no BTX effect is desired (e.g., the flexor carpi and flexor digitorum in the forearm). Palpation technique is still an option for simple muscles with easily identified surface landmarks in a region with low-risk for diffusion-related adverse effects. At the present time, our understanding of the role of electrophysiologic guidance is in the early stages of development.

Electromyography

EMG may be used to assess muscle activity in patients with dystonia and spasticity (19,20). It may also be used as a localization technique to aid the injector with placement of botulinum toxin, phenol, or local anesthetic). A discussion of EMG for diagnosis of dystonia or spasticity is beyond the scope of this article, therefore, attention will be directed towards localization methods.

EMG for localization of target muscles can be quite straightforward. The objective is to record motor unit potentials (MUPs) that are in close proximity to the needle tip as assessed by MUP morphology or acoustic properties. Subsequent elicitation of MUPs by various passive and active maneuvers confirms needle-tip placement within the desired muscle fascicle/tendon/joint group. Similar active and passive maneuvers are then used to confirm that needle placement does not risk injection of BTX into nontarget muscles.

Proximity of the needle tip to the muscle fascicle can be demonstrated by the presence of full-sized bi- or tri-phasic MUPs with fast rise times. Such MUPs have the acoustic property of a "crisp" sound. If low amplitude, poorly defined units are seen (or low-amplitude "muffled" units are heard), the needle can be repositioned in order to achieve optimal placement. Occasionally, the "sea shell" sound is encountered, which may reflect miniature end-plate potentials of the neuromuscular junction.

Crisp MUPs do not, however, signify correct placement of the needle in a target muscle, only proximity of tip to a contracting fascicle. Confirmation of placement in a target muscle must be accomplished by either active contraction or passive movement. This can be difficult in patients with patterns of mass action (i.e., spasticity following a stroke) or in young children. The steps outlined below represent a typical sequence for injection of an awake, cooperative patient.

1. Target muscle selection based on clinical assessment.
2. Palpation of local anatomy for belly and tendon of target muscle.
3. Palpation of local anatomy for belly and tendon of nontarget muscles.
4. Passive range of motion (ROM) of target muscle/tendon/joint unit.
5. Passive ROM of nontarget muscle/tendon/joint units.
6. Voluntary activation of target muscle/tendon/joint unit.
7. Voluntary activation of nontarget muscle/tendon/joint units.

At this point, the Teflon-coated, hollow EMG needle is inserted into the target muscle and the EMG device turned on. Table 1 lists the most com-

Table 1
Equipment Requirements for Botulinum Toxin Injections

Teflon-coated, hollow EMG needle
Reference lead with surface electrode
EMG machine (standard or portable)
Electrical stimulation (in EMG machine or portable unit)
Alcohol skin cleanser
Syringe
Preservative-free 0.9% saline
Botulinum toxin

monly employed equipment items. If MUP activity is present, one attempts to relax the patient with gentle stretching, encouragement, and so on. Once relatively quiet, electrode-tip location is assessed with passive and active maneuvers. The primary objective is, of course, to obtain crisp MUPs corresponding only with the target muscle/tendon/joint unit.

8. Move target joint through passive ROM and monitor EMG for MUP activation (these may reflect spasm triggered by the movement or insertion potentials).
9. Move nontarget joint through passive ROM and monitor EMG for MUP activation (they should be absent or minimal in nontarget areas).
10. Have patient activate target muscle and monitor EMG for MUP activation.
11. Have patient activate nontarget muscles and monitor EMG for MUP activation (they should be absent or minimal in nontarget areas).

The steps outlined here can be quite effective in isolating small, deep muscles such as individual fascicles of the finger flexors. For example, one can demonstrate flexor carpi ulnaris activity independent of flexor digitorum profundus with passive and active flexion/extension of wrist and fingers. The steps are equally useful for large, deep muscles such as the tibialis posterior. Table 2 lists common muscle groups for which EMG localization is helpful prior to botulinum toxin injection. Short-acting sedation may be given by an anesthesiologist in an appropriate out-patient setting in patients unable to co-operate or intolerant of these procedures. Obviously, the injector must use the passive ROM technique or electrical stimulation as the patient would be unable to voluntarily activate muscles while sedated.

The main problem associated with EMG is separation of target vs compensatory muscle MUPs. Choosing which muscle to inject is a clinical decision. One can use EMG during patient movement to delineate primarily

Table 2
Muscle Groups Typically Localized by EMG Guidance

Forearm flexors (e.g., flexor digitorum profundus, flexor carpi radialis, pronator teres, flexor digitorum superficialis)
Wrist and digit extensors (e.g., extensor digitorum communis, extensor carpi radialis)
Thumb adductors, opponens pollicis, flexor pollicis longus
Interossei and lumbricals
Hip flexors
Posterior tibialis
Extensor hallucis longus

---

overactive muscles from compensatory activity. However, in patients with spasticity or dystonia, co-contraction of agonists and antagonists may confound the assessment.

Electrical Stimulation

In contrast to EMG, electrical stimulation (ES) may be used to activate an entire muscle via large-nerve stimulation, or to activate small fascicles within the muscle belly. The first technique is referred to as motor-nerve stimulation, and is used primarily in phenol neurolysis (nerve blocks). The second technique, referred to as motor-point stimulation, reflects stimulation of small motor-nerve branches within the belly of the muscle. Motor-point stimulation is useful for BTX in that needle placement is, in theory, within a region of a high density of neuromuscular junctions. Such placement would presumably allow BTX to be applied as close to the presynaptic nerve terminals as possible. Whether this affords maximal effect at reduced doses remains intriguing but unproven in humans; studies to address this are underway *(10)*.

The basic technique of motor-point stimulation is similar to that for EMG. After the initial palpation and passive ROM steps, the Teflon-coated, hollow EMG needle is inserted into the target muscle. Stimulation is initiated at an intensity sufficient to produce a visible contraction or fascicle twitch. Initial intensity is often in the 1–3 milli-amperage (mA) range. The primary objective at this point is to reposition the tip with successive reductions in stimulus intensity such that maximum twitch is produced from the minimum stimulus. The final target stimulus intensity is typically in the 0.025–0.5 mA range. A variety of stimulators may be employed. Most high-quality EMG/NCV machines have a stimulator used for nerve-conduction studies. A reference lead with surface electrode is plugged in and the surface electrode located above the muscle/tendon junction. The lead from the injection needle is plugged into the stimulator. Alternatively, a portable, battery-powered stimulator may be purchased or manufactured. The advantages include cost, portability, and ease of use.

Other techniques, including fluoroscopy, computed tomography (CT), and ultrasound, used in conjunction with EMG or ES may help identify and access muscles for botulinum toxin injections.

PHENOL VS BOTULINUM TOXIN

Chemodenervation can be accomplished by phenol or botulinum toxin injections. Phenol causes its effect by neurolysis of the motor nerve. Single motor-nerve blocks can be quite successful for excess elbow flexion or thigh adduction. In contrast, neurolysis of a mixed nerve, i.e., containing both motor and sensory branches, may produce transient or permanent dysesthesias owing to injury of the myelin sheath surrounding the sensory nerve. Phenol injections can be undertaken without this risk if primarily motor nerves are selected, such as the obturator nerve or the musculocutaneous nerve.

There are potential drawbacks to the use of phenol. There can be marked decrease in muscle tone after phenol injections. In those patients who need some degree of spasticity to function, the decrease in tone may be excessive, actually worsening functional skills. In addition, injections using phenol require a high degree of technical proficiency.

The advantages of botulinum toxin over phenol include a lack of sensory side effects, relative ease of administration and a dose-dependent, graded decrease in muscle tone.

MUSCLE SELECTION AND DOSE RANGES

Despite various etiologies, there are several common clinical patterns of spasticity that are amenable to botulinum toxin injections. These common elements allow a systematic approach to the selection of muscles involved. Some dosage guidelines have been established for sets of muscles depending on the clinical findings and treatment objectives (*see* Table 3) *(21)*.

TREATMENT OBJECTIVES

Criteria influencing outcome of treatment with botulinum toxin are listed in Table 4. The treatment objectives are based on the functional goals of the patient, therapist, and physician. Explicit, concrete, patient-specific goals are set prior to injecion. Input from physical and occupational therapists is invaluable in realistic goal setting. Pre- and post-treatment assessments help refine treatment. Some common assessments include rating of tone (e.g., the

Table 3
Suggested Adult Botulinum Toxin A Dosing

Clinical pattern	Potential muscles involved	Average starting dose/units	BOTOX® dose units/visit	Number of injection sites
Upper limbs				
Adducted/internally rotated shoulder	Pectoralis complex	100	75–150	4
	Latissimus dorsi	100	50–150	4
	Teres major	50	25–75	1
	Subscapularis	50	25–75	1
Flexed elbow	Brachloradialis	50	25–75	2
	Biceps	100	50–200	4
	Brachialis	50	25–75	2
Pronated forearm	Pronator quadratus	25	10–50	1
	Pronator teres	40	25–75	1
Flexed wrist	Flexor carpi radialis	50	25–100	2
	Flexor carpi ulnaris	40	10–50	2
Thumb-in-palm	Flexor pollicis longus	15	5–25	1
	Adductor pollicis	10	5–25	1
	Opponens	10	5–25	1
Clenched fist	Flexor digitorum superficialis	50	25–75	4
	Flexor digitorum profondus	15	25–100	2
Intrinsic plus hand	Lumbricales interossei	15	10–50/hand	3
Lower limbs				
Flexed hip	Illacus	100	50–150	2
	Psoas	100	50–200	2
	Rectus femoris	100	75–200	3
Flexed knee	Medial hamstrings	100	50–150	3
	Gastrocnemius (as knee flexor)	150	50–150	4
	Lateral hamstrings	100	100–200	3
Adducted thighs	Adductor brevis/longus/magnus	200/leg	75–300	6/leg
Stiff (extended) knee	Quadriceps mechanism	100	50–200	4
Equinovarus foot	Gastrocnemius medial/lateral	100	50–200	4
	Soleus	75	50–100	2
	Tibialis posterior	50	50–200	2
	Tibialis anterior	75	50–150	3
	Flexor digitorum longus/brevis	75	50–100	4
	Flexor hallucis longus	50	25–75	2
Striatal toe	Extensor hallucis longus	50	20–100	2

Table 3 (*continued*)

Clinical pattern	Potential muscles involved	Average starting dose/units	BOTOX® dose units/visit	Number of injection sites
Neck				
	Sternocleidomastoid (SCM)*	40	15–75	2
	Scalenus complex	30	15–50	3
	Splenius capitis	60	50–150	3
	Semispinalis capitis	60	50–150	3
	Longissimus capitis	60	50–150	3
	Trapezius	60	50–150	3
	Levator scapulae	80	25–100	3

*The dose should be reduced by 50% if both SCM muscles are injected.
Dosing guidelines:
Total maximum dose per visit = 400 Units.
Maximum dose per injection site = 50 Units.
Maximum volume per site = 0.5mL, except in select situations.
Reinjection >3 mo.

Table 4
Criteria Influencing Outcome of Treatment with Botulinum Toxin

Features associated with favorable outcome	Features associated with poor outcome
Well-defined short- and long-term treatment objectives	Poorly defined treatment objectives
Spastic muscles well-defined	Severe generalized spasticity with extensive upper motor neuron deficits
Preservation of agonist/antagonist muscle activity	Loss of functional agonist/antagonist groups
Absence of contractures	Fixed contractures
Superficial, easily accessible target muscles	Anatomically "risky" injection sites
Acute or subacute spasticity	Chronic spasticity

Ashworth scale), range of motion (e.g., joint goniometry), or function (e.g., the 9-hole peg test). Correlation between alterations of tone or range of motion and functional benefits depend upon severity and chronicity of spasticity and the upper motor neuron syndrome. The most likely measure of success is percentage of set-goal attainment. For example, a specific goal such as speed of dressing or ability to groom independently is set and then success of intervention gauged by accomplishment of the task. In the context of a clinical trial, in addition to recognized, validated scales to measure spasticity, an individual goal tailored for each patient and percentage achieved would be important to assess functional outcome.

Botulinum toxin injections should be combined with a rehabilitation program focusing on stretching and strengthening. This program should begin within 2 wk of the injections to capitalize on a period of maximal improvement and continued as long as the patient makes steady gains. Strengthening of opposing muscle groups while overactive muscles are weakened will optimize motor ability. Also, range of motion will be more easily achieved and should be done to fullest benefit. The patient must be taught to avoid old habits for coping with spasticity while learning to work with improved range of motion and newly reduced tone.

CLINICAL TRIALS

Botulinum toxin has been evaluated for the treatment of focal spasticity secondary to a variety of neurologic disorders, including multiple sclerosis (MS), stroke, cerebral palsy (CP), and spinal-cord injury. A number of series have been published, including case reports, open-label and double-blind trials *(22–39)*. All have shown some improvement of spasticity (by various measures) after botulinum toxin injections. An overview of clinical trials to date permits some generalizations and uncovers several problems with the use of BTX-A. First, the injections are safe and well tolerated but typically provide only 2–6 mo of benefit. As a result, concomitant treatments or repeat injections may be needed to maintain benefit. Second, there are limitations on the total dose of BTX-A that can be injected per session. This may limit the number of muscles that can be injected for patients with severe generalized spasticity. Third, botulinum toxin injections are effective for reducing tone but may not significantly improve function in some patients. Fourth, there continues to be debate on whether the injection technique alters effectiveness of the intervention (i.e., EMG guidance vs palpation).

CONTRAINDICATIONS

The use of botulinum toxin is contraindicated in patients with known neuromuscular junction disease such as myasthenic-like syndrome or myasthenia gravis. In addition, it should not be administered to patients with motor-neuron disease or patients taking aminoglycosides as it may exacerbate weakness. Botulinum toxin is not recommended for use during pregnancy owing to lack of sufficient data *(5)*.

Table 5
Future Research Issues: Botulinum Toxin and Spasticity

Injection techniques
Timing of injections
Role of PT/OT
Quantitative Assessments of results, e.g., gait laboratory
Combined interventions
    BTX and oral medications
    BTX and phenol
    BTX and casting
    BTX and surgery
Alternate toxin types
Combined toxin types
Secondary nonresponsiveness
Cost/benefit analysis

PT, physical therapy; OT, occupational therapy.

FUTURE RESEARCH IN SPASTICITY

Many questions remain to be answered regarding optimal use of botulinum toxin in the management of spasticity. Table 5 lists several questions worthy of additional study. The selection of patients, timing of injections, ideal injection technique, and optimal integration of therapies all must be studied in detail. The role of electrophysiology with BTX injections must be better-defined. Whether EMG guidance or ES results in greater efficiency (i.e., equal or greater effect with a lower dose of toxin) is unclear; this would have important implications for patients requiring injections at multiple sites (e.g., spastic quadraparesis following traumatic brain injury). It also may be important in terms of dose of BTX/antigen exposure and secondary nonresponsiveness *(8,11)*. Further study is also needed as to which response parameters are most altered when EMG or ES are compared to palpation technique. For example, localization with ES may alter extra-fusal fibers disproportionately. Finally, the many issues of good clinical-trial design must be addressed. Double-blind studies comparing EMG, ES, and palpation techniques should include equivalent subjects, not an easy task given the clinical variability in spasticity patients. Finally, biochemical modifications of the different serotypes of toxin may allow development of more site-specific medication less likely to cause resistance, increase or decrease diffusion properties, and perhaps permit formulation of more tailored treatments for individual patients.

REFERENCES

1. Simpson, L. L. (1980) Kinetic studies on the interaction between botulinum toxin type A and the cholinergic neuromuscular junction. *J. Pharmacol. Exp. Ther.* **212,** 16–21.
2. Poewe, W., Schelosky, L., Kleedorfer, B., Heinen, F., Wagner, M., and Deuschl, G. (1992) Treatment of spasmodic torticollis with local injections of botulinum toxin. One year follow up in 37 patients. *J. Neurol.* **239,** 21–25.
3. DasGupta, B. R. (1994) Structures of botulinum neurotoxin, its functional domains, and perspectives on the crystalline type A toxin, in *Therapy with Botulinum Toxin* (Jankovic, J. and Hallett, M., eds.), Marcel Dekker, New York, pp. 15–39.
4. DasGupta, B. R. and Tepp, W. (1993) Protease activity of botulinum neurotoxin type E and its light chain: cleavage of actin. *Biochem. Biophys. Res. Commun.* **190,** 470–474.
5. Brin, M. F. (1997) Botulinum toxin: chemistry, pharmacology, toxicity, and immunology. *Muscle Nerve* **20(Suppl. 6),** S146–S168.
6. Coffield, J. A., Considine, R. V., and Simpson, L. L. (1994) The site and mechanism of action of botulinum neurotoxin, in *Therapy with Botulinum Toxin* (Jankovic, J. and Hallet, M., eds.), Marcel Dekker, New York, pp. 3–13.
7. Simpson, L. L. (1989) Peripheral actions of the botulinum toxins, in *Botulinum Neurotoxin and Tetanus Toxin* (Simpson, L. L., ed.), Academic Press, New York, pp. 153–178.
8. Borodic, G., Johnson, E., Goodnough, M., and Schantz, E. (1996) Botulinum toxin therapy, immunologic resistance, and problems with available materials. *Neurology* **46,** 26–29.
9. Alderson, K., Holds, J. B., and Anderson, R. L. (1991) Botulinum induced alteration of nerve muscle interactions in the human orbicularis oculi following treatment for blepharospasm. *Neurology* **41,** 1800–1805.
10. Borodic, G. E., Ferrante, R., Pearce, L. B., and Smith, K. (1994) Histologic assessment of dose-related diffusion and muscle fiber response after therapeutic botulinum A toxin injections. *Mov. Disord.* **9,** 31–39.
11. Greene, P., Fahn, S., and Diamond, B. (1994) Development of resistance to botulinum toxin type A in patients with torticollis. *Mov. Disord.* **9,** 213–217.
12. Greene, P. E. and Fahn, S. (1996) Response to botulinum toxin F in seronegative botulinum toxin A resistant patients. *Mov. Disord.* **11,** 181–184.
13. Janovic, J. and Schwartz, K. (1995) Response and immunoresistance to botulinum toxin injections. *Neurology* **45,** 1743–1746.
14. Hatheway, C. H., Snyder, J. D., Seals, J. E., Edell, T. A., and Lewis, G. E. (1984) Antitoxin levels in botulism patients treated with trivalent equine botulism antitoxin to toxin types A, B, and E. *J. Infect. Dis.* **150,** 407–412.
15. Doellgast, G. J., Beard, G. A., Bottoms, J. D., Mheng, T., Roh, B. H., Roman, M. G., et al. (1994) Enzyme-linked immunosorbent assay and enzyme-linked-coagulation assay for detection of Clostridium botulinum neurotoxin A, neurotoxin B, and neurotoxin E and solution phase complexes with dual label antibodies. *J. Clin. Microbiol.* **32,** 105–111.

16. Hanna, P. A. and Jankovic, J. (1998) Mouse bioassay versus western blot assay for botulinum toxin antibodies-correlation with clinical response. *Neurology* **50,** 1624–1629.
17. Brin, M. F., Lew, M. F., and Adler, C. H. (1999) Safety and efficacy of Neurobloc (botulinum toxin type B) in type A-resistant cervical dystonia. *Neurology* **53,** 1431–1438.
18. Brashear, A., Lew, M. F., Dykstra, D. D., Comella, C. L., Factor, S. A., and Rodnitzky, R. L. (1999) Safety and efficacy of Neurobloc (botulinum toxin type B) in type A responsive cervical dystonia. *Neurology* **53,** 1439–1446.
19. Comella, C. L., Buchman, A. S., Tanner, C. M., Brown-Toms, N. C., and Goetz, C. G. (1992) Botulinum toxin injection for spasmodic torticollis: increased magnitude of benefit with electromyographic assistance. *Neurology* **42,** 878–882.
20. Geenen, C., Consky, E., and Ashby, P. (1996) Localizing muscles for botulinum toxin treatment of focal hand dystonia. *Can. J. Neurol. Sci.* **23,** 194–197.
21. Brin, M. F. and the Spasticity Study Group. (1997) Dosing, administration, and a treatment algorithm for use of botulinum toxin A for adult-onset spasticity. *Muscle Nerve* **20(Suppl. 6),** S208–S220.
22. Benecke, R. (1994) Botulinum toxin for spasms and spasticity in the lower extremities, in *Therapy with Botulinum Toxin* (Jankovic, J. and Hallett, M., eds.), Marcel Dekker, New York, pp. 557–565.
23. Borg-Stein, J., Pine, Z. M., Miller, J. R., and Brin, M. F. (1993) Botulinum toxin for the treatment of spasticity in multiple sclerosis: new observation. *Am. J. Phys. Med. Rehabil.* **72,** 364–368.
24. Snow, B. J., Tsui, J. K. C., Bhatt, M. H., Varelas, M., Hashimoto, S. A., and Calne, D. B. (1990) Treatment of spasticity with botulinum toxin: a double blind study. *Ann. Neurol.* **28,** 512–515.
25. Dykstra, D. D. and Sidi, A. A. (1990) Treatment of detrusor-sphincter dyssynergia with botulinum A toxin: a double-blind study. *Arch. Phys. Med. Rehabil.* **71,** 24–26.
26. Bohlega, S., Chaud, P., and Jacob, P. C. (1995) Botulinum toxin A in the treatment of lower limb spasticity in hereditary spastic paraplegia. *Mov. Disord.* **10,** 399 (Abstract).
27. Takanega, S., Kawahigashi, Y., Sonoda, Y., Horikiri, T., Hirata, K., Arimura, K., and Osame, M. (1995) Treatment of spastic paraparesis with botulinum toxin with reference to beneficial effects, disease severity and long-term treatment. *Rinsho Shinkeigaku* **35,** 251–255.
28. Koman, L. A., Mooney, J. F., Smith, B., Goodman, A., and Mulvaney, T. (1993) Management of cerbral palsy with botulinum -A toxin: preliminary investigation. *J. Pediatr. Orthop.* **13,** 489–495
29. Cosgrove, A. P. and Graham, H. K. (1992) Botulinum toxin A in the management of spasticity with cerebral palsy. *Br. J. Surg.* **74,** 135–136.
30. Chutorian, A. and Root, L. (1994) Management of spasticity in children with botulinum A toxin. *Intl. Pediatr.* **9,** 35–43.
31. Chutorian, A., Root, L., and BTA Study Group. (1995) A multicentered, randomized, double-blind placebo-controlled trial of botulinum toxin type A in the

treatment of lower limb spasticity in pediatric cerebral palsy. *Mov. Disord.* **10,** 364(Abstract).
32. Corry, I. S. (1997) Botulinum toxin A in the hemiplegic upper limb: a double-blind trial. *Dev. Med. Child. Neurol.* **39,** 185–193.
33. Das, T. K. and Park, D. M. (1989) Effect of treatment with botulinum toxin on spasticity. *Postgrad. Med. J.* pp. 208–210.
34. Memin, B., Pollack, P., Hommel, M., and Perret, J. (1992) Effects of botulinum toxin on spasticity. *Rev. Neurol.* **148,** 212–214.
35. Grazko, M. A., Polo, K. B., and Jabbari, B. (1995) Botulinum toxin A for spasticity, muscle spasms, and rigidity. *Neurology* **45,** 712–717.
36. Dengler, R., Neyer, U., Wohlfarth, K., Bettig, U., and Janzik, H. H. (1992) Local botulinum toxin in the treatment of spastic drop foot. *J, Neurol.* **239,** 375–378.
37. Jabbari, B., Polo, K. B., Ford, G., and Grazko, M. A. (1995) Effectiveness of botulinum toxin A in patients with spasticity. *Mov. Disord.* **10,** 379(Abstract).
38. Simpson, D. M., Alexander, M. D., O'Brien, C. F., Tagliati, M., Aswad, A., Leon, J. M., et al. (1996) Botulinum toxin type A in the treatment of upper extremity spasticity: A randomized, double-blind, placebo-controlled trial. *Neurology* **46,** 1306–1310.
39. Yablon, S. A., Agana, B. T., Ivanhoe, C. B., and Boake, C. (1996) Botulinum toxin in severe upper extremity spasticity among patients with traumatic brain injury: an open-labeled trial. *Neurology* **47,** 939–944.

14
Intrathecal Medications

Randall T. Schapiro

INTRODUCTION

As has been discussed in previous chapters, the management of spasticity generally involves a stepwise approach, beginning with the removal of noxious stimuli and the initiation of a therapeutic exercise program including stretching and range-of-motion exercises. If spasticity persists, the addition of oral antispasticity medications is often necessary.

If the aforementioned measures fail to control the spasticity, more procedurally oriented treatments become appropriate. These include orthopedic and neurosurgical procedures (reviewed elsewhere in this text), nerve blocks, and botulinum toxin injections, and intrathecal administration of medications.

The major advantage of intrathecal administration of antispasticity agents is that this permits the use of minute amounts of medications to be directed closely to the sensorimotor pathways in the spinal cord that modulate muscle tone, allowing for control of even the most resistant spastic abnormalities. Pharmacokinetic studies have shown that the cisternal cerebrospinal fluid (CSF) drug level is much lower than the lumbar CSF level during continuous infusion into the lumbar space of various agents. Radionuclide techniques have been utilized to determine the distribution of agents in the intrathecal space when delivered over 72 h with implanted drug pumps. Over a 20-cm distance of the thoracic cord, radionuclide counts decreased gradually showing at T2 43% of that seen at T12 *(1)*. Because most patients with spasticity caused by spinal-cord disorders have preferentially increased tone in the lower extremities, there is an inherent advantage to this distribution of substances in this manner. Furthermore, because of the gradient of distribution of medication delivered by intrathecal pump favors lower cerebral concentrations, behavioral and cognitive side effects of medication is limited.

From: *Current Clinical Neurology: Clinical Evaluation and Management of Spasticity*
Edited by: D. A. Gelber and D. R. Jeffery © Humana Press, Inc., Totowa, NJ

HISTORY OF INTRATHECAL MEDICATIONS

The use of intrathecal medication for spasticity antedated the invention of the intrathecal pump for administration of medication by several decades. Intrathecal phenol has been used for the treatment of intractable spasticity since the late 1950s. At that time, clinical studies were lacking and its use tended to be reserved for patients with nonfunctional lower extremties, i.e., those who had severe pain in conjunction with spastic paraplegia. In 1975, two cases of patients with multiple sclerosis (MS) who had paraplegia in flexion with painful muscles spasms were described. The use of intrathecal phenol in glycerin converted the spastic paralysis into a flaccid one. This resulted in a marked reduction of pain and allowed the patients to be better-positioned *(2)*. The benefits of this chemical myelotomy and rhizolysis were again described in a case report in1985 *(3)*.

In the 1960s the use of methylprednisolone acetate by intrathecal spinal injection became popular for the treatment of MS exacerbations. There have been a number of reviews of the procedure, both pro and con *(4-6)*. Although there are no actual clinical studies categorizing the effect of methylprednisolone on spasticity when given intrathecally (80 mg), many of us who had experience with this treatment were struck with the decrease in muscle tone experienced by those who received the medication. The greatest drawback to the use of intrathecal corticosteroids is that because they were typically delivered in a polyethylene glycol (PEG) preparation, comprised of both alcohol and detergent, there was the potential development of arachnoiditis *(5)*. It was feared that over time the potential arachnoiditis might actually worsen the spasticity. Because of this, intrathecal administration of corticosteroids is now discouraged.

In the 1980s the use of morphine intrathecally became more popular for the treatment of intractable pain of various causes. It was also found that spasticity could be controlled with implantable continuous-flow morphine given intrathecally in doses of 1–2 mg by bolus followed by continuous delivery of approx 2 mg/d *(7,8)*. There was concern that the patients would become tolerant to the morphine but that did not prove to be the usual case.

CLINICAL TRIALS OF INTRATHECAL BACLOFEN

In 1984, Penn studied the effects of intrathecal bolus injections of baclofen in two patients with spinal-cord injury *(9)*. A significant reduction in lower-extremity spasticity was noted, with the effect lasting 5–8 h. Penn performed a subsequent randomized, double-blinded cross-over study of 20 patients with intractable spasticity secondary to MS or spinal-cord injury *(10)*. In this series, an implantable pump was filled with either saline or baclofen, and then delivered intrathecally to the lumbar subarachnoid space via a catheter for 3 d. Then the other treatment was adminstered for 3 d. No improvement in spasticity was seen with saline, whereas 90% of patients improved with baclofen. Improvement in activities of daily living, including dressing, feeding, and bowel and bladder management was also reported for the patients treated with intrathecal baclofen (ITB) *(11)*.

Penn has also reported the results of long-term study of 66 patients treated with ITB *(12)*. Patients were followed for an average of 30 mo; painful lower-extremity spasms and spasticity were reduced in 97% of patients and the medication was generally well-tolerated *(12,13)*.

ITB has also been shown to be effective in the treatment of spasticity secondary to cerebral causes, including traumatic brain injury and cerebral palsy (CP) *(14–17)*. In addition, an improvement in lower-extremity tone and spasms, reductions in upper-extremity spasticity, spasms, and muscle-stretch reflexes have also been reported, especially when the catheter is threaded more rostrally, to an approximate T10 level *(18)*. A recent study reported even greater relief of upper-extremity spasticity, without loss of effect on the lower extremities, when the tip of the intrathecal catheter was placed at the T6-T7 level in children with spastic quadriparesis *(19)*. ITB has also been shown to be of benefit in patients with traumatic brain injury or stroke with spastic hemiplegia. In a recent study of 6 hemiparetic patients, ITB resulted in a significant reduction of muscle tone on the affected side without adversely affecting the "normal" side *(20)*. ITB is also of benefit in the treatment of stiff-man (person) syndrome *(21)*.

PATIENT SELECTION

ITB is formally approved for the treatment of intractable spasticity and spasms owing to disorders of brain and spinal cord. Treatment is beneficial in adults and children with guidelines allowing treatment in patients as young as age 4 *(22)*. ITB therapy is indicated for spasticity that is clinically severe (≥3 on the Ashworth scale) *(23)* (*see* Table 1) and affects functional activities, such as mobility, daily cares, urinary catheterization, or hygiene.

Candidates for ITB should have had adequate trials of oral antispasticity medications. Failures are characterized by ineffective relief of spasticity and spasms, or inability to tolerate medications because of side effects *(16)*. Although ITB therapy can be initiated at any time in a patient's course, it is generally recommended that one wait at least 1 yr before considering pump implantation in individuals with traumatic brain injury. Patients and families must be reliable and responsible to manage the pump long-term. As with any treatment, specific clinical and functional goals of ITB treatment should be discussed in detail with the patient and family prior to implementation.

Table 1
The Ashworth Scale

Score	Degree of muscle tone
1	No increase in tone
2	Slight increase in tone, giving a "catch" when the affected part is flexed or extended
3	More marked increase in tone, but affected part is easily flexed
4	Considerable increase in tone; passive movement difficult
5	Affected part rigid in flexion or extension

The presence of a systemic infection is a contraindication to pump placement; increasing the risk of surgical complications. A history of an allergic reaction to oral baclofen is also a direct contraindication to ITB therapy. The presence of a ventriculoperitoneal shunt, gastrostomy tube, or other implantable devices, such as cardiac pacemakers and spine stimulators, are not contraindications to ITB therapy.

PUMP-IMPLANTATION PROTOCOL

Prior to implantation of a pump, patients must respond favorably to a screening trial of ITB. The standard procedure is to test-dose the individual by administering 50 μg of baclofen intrathecally via a spinal tap or catheter. This bolus is administered slowly over 5 min. Onset of drug action is within 30–60 min and lasts 4–8 h. It should be discussed with the patient that the baclofen bolus can cause transient muscle weakness but that this will not necessarily occur with the "smoother" administration of the computerized pump. Prior to administration, an Ashworth scale score is determined for hip abductors, hip flexors, knee flexors, and ankle dorsiflexors bilaterally *(11)*. An average Ashworth score is calculated by adding these scores and dividing by the number of muscle evaluated. A Spasm scale score is also recorded (*see* Table 2). These scores are reassessed at 1,2,4, and 8 h. A positive response is defined as a 1 point decrease in either the average Ashworth score or spasm score *(24)*. If the 50 μg dose is inneffective, the test bolus is repeated at 75 or 100 μg on successive days. If the patient responds favorably the pump is implanted. If there is no response to a 100 μg test dose the pump should not be implanted and alternative treatments should be considered. However, it is rare to see a failure with testdosing.

The surgical implantation involves placement of the medication pump subcutaneously in the abdominal wall connected to a catheter that is tunneled subcutaneously around to the back where it is passed into the in-

Table 2
The Spasm Scale

Score	Frequency of spasms
0	No spasms
1	No spontaneous spasms; vigorous sensory and motor stimulation result in spasms
2	Occasional spontaneous spasms and easily induced spasms
3	One to 10 spontaneous spasms per hour
4	More than 10 spontaneous spasms per hour

trathecal space at the L3-4 level. In most cases the catheter tip is threaded to approx the T10 level. Although there are pumps manufactured by various manufactures that can deliver baclofen intrathecally there is only one (Medtronic) that is programmable and approved by the Food and Drug Administration (FDA) for this use. Cordis and Infusaid have nonprogrammable systems (25).

At the time of implantation, the pump is usually set at twice the test bolus that produced a positive effect. For example, if the patient responded to a test dose of 50 µg the pump administration is started at 100 µg per 24 h. Adjustment over several days to weeks is required, with dosage increases of 10–20% at a time (usually no more than 50 µg per day), until a satisfactory response is obtained. The effective dose of ITB varies between patients and ranges from 50–2000 µg per day. The pump is usually programmed to deliver medication continuously; however, depending on the pattern of the individual's spasticity, boluses may be administered at specific times of the day as necessary. The pump is refilled percutaneously every 4–12 wk depending on the dosage administered and type of reservoir used.

COMPLICATIONS

Complications related to the surgical procedure itself or device malfunctions have been well-reported (see Table 3). In a long-term follow-up study of 75 patients with implanted pumps, two developed erosion of the pump pocket, necessitating either surgical repair or pump replacement (13). One patient developed a superficial wound infection that responded to antibiotics; another suffered a deep pump-pocket infection resulting in removal of the pump. Mechanical pump failures occurred in three individuals, necessitating replacement of the pump. Catheter malfunctions occurred in 18 patients. These included kinking, dislodgment, cuts, breaks, or disconnection of the catheter tubing (13).

Table 3
Complications of Intrathecal Baclofen Pump

Surgical complications
Infection
Problems with the device
  Battery failure
  Pump failure
  Catheter disruption or kinking
Overmedication
  Drowsiness
  Dizziness
  Seizures
  Respiratory depression
  Coma
Baclofen withdrawal (pump failure)
  Increased spasticity and spasms
  Irritability
  Tachycardia
  Fever

In this same long-term study *(13)*, 12% of patients developed drug-related side-effects. These included respiratory depression and seizures, which occurred in the setting of inadvertent drug overdosage. Physostigmine has been advocated to reverse the muscle weakness and respiratory failure but is not effective in all cases *(13,26)*. Hypotension, depression, and drowsiness are also seen in patients receiving ITB *(13)*. A reduced bladder capacity and relaxation of the external urinary sphincter (potentially leading to leakage of urine) have also been reported *(27)*, as has the loss of the ability to achieve and maintain penile erections *(28)*.

Tolerance to ITB may develop during the initial 12 mo following pump implantation; often requiring upward adjustments of pump dosage over time; this is thought to be owing to gamma-amino butyric acid (GABA)-receptor downregulation *(28)*. However, the tolerance that develops is generally less than that seen with intrathecal administration of opiods *(29)*.

OTHER INTRATHECAL MEDICATIONS

As discussed earlier, morphine may also be administered intrathecally via an implantable pump. Morphine has been shown to inhibit polysynaptic spinal-cord reflexes through its action on opiate receptors located in the dorsal horns *(30)*. Intrathecal morphine has been used most commonly in the treatment of intractable pain, but has also been shown to improve spasticity associated with spinal-cord injuries. However, its use is limited because of the development of tolerance and habituation, and is generally considered as an option only for refractory cases of spasticity *(7)*.

Intrathecal tizanidine has been evaluated in the rat model and shown to be effective in pain reduction *(31)*. Clonidine is an alpha$_2$-adrenergic agonist similar to tizanidine, has been used intrathecally for postoperative analgesia *(32)*. There are ongoing studies of in both rats and dogs evaluating the analgesic and hemodynamic effects of tizanidine and clonidine administered intrathecally *(33)*. The addition of clonidine to baclofen in a baclofen pump was reported to decrease spasticity and neuropathic pain following a spinal-cord injury *(34)*. Other neurochemical agents including GABA, glycine, taurine, and beta-alanine are being studied in animals looking for potential new intrathecal agents *(35)*.

SUMMARY

For patients with intractable spasticity secondary to cerebral or spinal-cord injury, intrathecal administration of medications, such as baclofen, have been shown to be safe and efficacious. Because these medications are delivered directly to the intrathecal space, they are administered in much lower doses than when given orally, and have less central nervous system (CNS) sedative and cognitive side effects. Although intrathecal baclofen tends to have greater effect on lower-extremity spasticity and spasms, it is also effective in reducing upper-extremity tone, and newer techniques with placement of the catheter more rostrally in the thoracic spine may be proven to be even more effective in this regard. Other medications, including tizanidine and clonidine, which are used as oral antispaticity medications, are currently being evaluated in intrathecal form and may be an option for intractable spasticity in the future. Although the cost of intrathecal treatment is high, cost-benefit studies do demonstrate cost savings by preventing potential complications of spasticity *(36)*. Overall, the management of intractable spasticity has been revolutionized by the addition of intrathecal therapy. It would appear that we are just scratching the surface of this mode of therapy; the future of treatment should be bright.

REFERENCES

1. Kroin, J. S., Ali, A., and York, M., et al. (1993) The distribution of medication along the spinal canal after chronic intrathecal administration. *Neurosurgery* **32**, 226–230.
2. Browne, R. A. and Catton, D. V. (1975) The use of intrathecal phenol for muscle spasms in multiple sclerosis. A description of two cases. *Can. Anaesth. Soc. J.* **22**, 208–218.

3. Scott, B. A., Weinstein, Z., and Chiteman, R., et al. (1985) Intrathecal phenol and glycerin in metrizamide for treatment of intractable spasms in paraplegia. Case report. *J. Neurosurg.* **63,** 125–127.
4. Nelson, D. A. (1988) Dangers from methylprednisolone acetate therapy by intraspinal injection. *Arch. Neurol.* **45,** 804–806.
5. Wilkinson, H. A. (1992) Intrathecal depo-medrol: a literature review. *Clin. J. Pain.* **8,** 49–56.
6. Nelson, D. A. (1993) Intraspinal therapy using methyl prednisolone acetate. Twenty three years of clinical controversy. *Spine* **18,** 278–286.
7. Erickson, D. L., Blacklock, J. B., Michaelson, M., Sperling, K. B., and Lo, J. N. (1985) Control of spasticity by implantable continuous flow morphine pump. *Neurosurgery* **16,** 215– 217.
8. Erickson, D. L., Lo, J., and Michaelson, M. (1989) Control of intractable spasticity with intrathecal morphine sulfate. *Neurosurgery* **24,** 236–238.
9. Penn, R. D. and Kroin, J. S. (1984) Intrathecal baclofen alleviates spinal cord spasticity. *Lancet* **1,** 1078.
10. Penn, R. D., Savoy, S. M., Corcos, D. M., Latash, M., Gottlieb, G., Parke, B., Penn, B., and Kroin, J. S. (1989) Intrathecal baclofen for severe spinal spasticity. *N. Engl. J. Med.* **320,** 1517–1521.
11. Parke, B., Penn, R. D., Savoy, S., and Corcos, D. (1989) Functional outcome after delivery of intrathecal baclofen. *Arch. Phys. Med. Rehabil.* **70,** 30–32.
12. Penn, R. D. (1990) Intrathecal baclofen for spasticity of spinal origin: seven years of experience. *J. Neurosurg.* **77,** 236–240.
13. Coffey, J. R., Cahill, D., Steers, W., Parke, T. S., Ordia, J., Meythaler J., et al. (1993) Intrathecal baclofen for intractable spasticity of spinal origin: results of a long-term multicenter study. *J. Neurosurg.* **78,** 226–232.
14. Albright, A. L., Barron, W. B., Fasick, M. P., Polinko, P., and Janosky, J. (1993) Continuous intrathecal baclofen infusion for spasticity of cerebral origin. *JAMA* **270,** 2475–2477.
15. Meythaler, J. M. (1996) Pharmacology update: Intrathecal baclofen for spastic hypertonia in brain injury. *J. Head. Trauma Rehabil.* **12,** 87–90.
16. Meythaler, J. M., McCary, A., and Hadley, M. N. (1997) Prospective assessment of continuous intrathecal infusion of baclofen for spasticity caused by acquired brain injury: a preliminary report. *J. Neurosurg.* **87,** 415–419.
17. Becker, R., Alberti, O., and Bauer, B. L. (1997) Continuous intrathecal baclofen infusion in severe spasticity after traumatic or hypoxic brain injury. *J. Neurol.* **244,** 160–166.
18. Meythaler, J. M., DeVivi, M. J., and Hadley, M. (1996) Prospective study on the use of bolus intrathecal baclofen for spastic hypertonia due to acquired brain injury. *Arch. Phys. Med. Rehabil.* **77,** 461–466.
19. Grabb, P. A., Guin-Renfroe, and Meythaler, J. M. (1999) Midthoracic catheter tip placement for intrathecal baclofen administration in children with quadriparetic spasticity. *Neurosurgery* **45,** 833–837.
20. Meythaler, J. M., Guin-Renfroe, S., and Hadley, M. (1998) Continuously infused intrathecal baclofen (ITB) for dystonic hemiplegia. *Am. J. Phys. Med. Rehabil.* **77,** 173–174.

21. Silbert, P. I., Matsumoto, J. Y., and McManis, P. G., et al. (1995) Intrathecal baclofen therapy in stiff-man syndrome: a double-blind, placebo-controlled trial. *Neurology* **45(10),** 1893–1897.
22. Albright, A. L. (1996) Baclofen in the treatment of cerebral palsy. *J. Child. Neurol.* **11,** 77–83.
23. Ashworth, B. (1964) Preliminary trial of carisoprodol in multiple sclerosis. *Practitioner* **192,** 540–542.
24. Albright, A. L. (1995) Spastic cerebral palsy. Approaches to drug treatment. *CNS Drugs* **4,** 17–27.
25. Gardner, B., Jamous, A., Teddy, P., et al. (1995) Intrathecal baclofen: a multicentre clinical comparison of the Medtronics Programmable, Cordis Secor and Constant Infusion Infusaid drug delivery systems. *Paraplegia* **33,** 551–554.
26. Müller-Schwefe, G. and Penn, R. D. (1989) Physostigmine in the treatment of intrathecal baclofen overdose. Report of three cases. *J. Neurosurg.* **71,** 273–275.
27. Nanninga, J. B., Frost, F., and Penn, R. (1989) Effect of intrathecal baclofen on bladder and sphincter function. *J. Urol.* **142,** 101–105.
28. Meythaler, J. M., Steers, W. D., Tuel, S. M., Cross, L. L., and Haworth, C. S. (1992) Continuous intrathecal baclofen in spinal cord spasticity. *Am. J. Phys. Med. Rehabil.* **71,** 321–327.
29. Loubser, P. G., Narayan, R. K., Sandin, K. J., Donovan, W. H., and Russell, K. D. (1991) Continuous infusion of intrathecal baclofen: Long-term effects on spasticity in spinal cord injury. *Paraplegia* **29,** 48–64.
30. Rossi, P. W. (1994) Treatment of spasticity, in *The Handbook of Neurorehabilitation* (Good, D. C. and Couch, J. R., eds.), Marcel Dekker, New York, pp. 197–218.
31. McCarthy, R. J., Kroin, J. S., Lubenow, T. R., et al. (1990) Effect of intrathecal tizanidine on antinocieption and blood pressure in the rat. *Pain* **40,** 333–338.
32. Eisenach, J. C., Tong, C., and Limauro, D.(1992) Intrathecal clonidine and the response to hemorrhage. *Anesthesiology* **77,** 522–528.
33. Kroin, J. S., McCarthy, R. J., Penn, R. D., et al. (1996) Intrathecal clonidine and tizanidine in conscious dogs: comparison of analgesic and hemodynamic effects. *Anesth. Analg.* **82,** 627–635.
34. Middleton, J. W., Siddall, P. J., Walker, S., et al. (1996) Intrathecal clonidine and baclofen in the management of spasticity and neuropathic pain following spinal cord injury: a case study. *Arch. Phys. Med. Rehabil.* **77,** 824–826.
35. Larson, A. A. (1989) Intrathecal GABA glycine, taurine, or beta-alanine elicits dyskinetic movements in mice. *Pharmacol. Biochem. Behav.* **32,** 505–509.
36. Nance, P., Schryvers, O., and Schmidt, B., et al. Intrathecal baclofen therapy for adults with spinal spasticity: therapeutic efficacy and effect on hospital admissions. *Can. J. Neurol. Sci.* **22,** 22–29.

15
Orthopedic Interventions for the Management of Limb Deformities in Upper Motoneuron Syndromes

Mary Ann E. Keenan and Patrick J. McDaid

INTRODUCTION

Neuro-orthopedics is the field of orthopedic surgery that treats limb deformities resulting from neurologic disease or injury. In this chapter we present the neuro-orthopedic perspective on managing patients with upper motor neuron (UMN) dysfunction. UMN dysfunction commonly follows injuries to the brain from stroke, traumatic brain injury, anoxia, infections of the brain, and perinatal trauma (i.e., cerebral palsy [CP]or static encephalopathy) *(1–5)*. The approach to management of limb dysfunction follows the same principles regardless of etiology. A number of common patterns of movement dysfunction are seen in patients with UMN dysfunction *(see* Table 1). These patterns typically develop against a background of weakness, impaired voluntary and postural motor control, spasticity, and contracture that comes with the territory of UMN dysfunction.

Many complications result from spasticity *(see* Table 2) *(5–71)*. Some of these are not obvious. The most common complications are extremity contractures. Limb contractures lead to skin maceration, difficulty with hygiene, and decubitus ulcers. In brain-injured patients with fractures, uncontrolled spasticity can lead to fracture malunions. Extremes of limb position often result in peripheral-nerve lesions such as cubital tunnel or carpal-tunnel syndrome *(22,23,37,52,64,72–74)*. With severe spasticity, joint subluxation or dislocation can develop. Hip dislocation occurs with severe long-standing adductor spasticity. Posterior subluxation of the knee can occur in the presence of hamstring spasticity. Iatrogenic fractures can happen in the presence of spasticity and contracture. The humerus is vulnerable to spiral fracture when attempting to put the arm in a shirt sleeve, if a shoulder adduction and

From: *Current Clinical Neurology: Clinical Evaluation and Management of Spasticity*
Edited by: D. A. Gelber and D. R. Jeffery © Humana Press, Inc., Totowa, NJ

Table 1
Common Upper Motoneuron Extremity Deformities

Upper extremity	Lower extremity
Adducted shoulder	Adducted hip
Flexed elbow	Flexed hip
Pronated forearm	Flexed knee
Flexed wrist	Stiff knee gait
Clenched fist	Equinovarus foot
Thumb-in-palm	Claw toes or cavus foot
	Valgus foot

Table 2
Complications of Spasticity

Contractures
Decubitus ulcers
Hygiene difficulties
Fracture malunion
Joint subluxation or dislocation
Heterotopic ossification
Peripheral neuropathy

internal rotation contracture is present. Heterotopic ossification (HO) is also thought to be in part stimulated by the mechanical tension caused by the spasticity.

In the past, UMN dysfunction patterns have been facilely attributed to increased "muscle tone" in specific groups of reflexly excitable musculature but "muscle tone" is not a simple construct. It depends on complex mechanisms of which hyperexcitable reflexes are just one part. The biomechanics of joint motion, the active contractile and passive properties of muscle, tendon, skin, and subcutaneous connective tissue, all contribute to the resistance the examiner appreciates as "muscle tone." They also contribute to the resistance that the patient with UMN dysfunction works against when trying to generate a voluntary movement. For rehabilitation clinicians, manifestations of spasticity, muscle stiffness, and contracture become intertwined with the issue of how much motor control has been spared and how much will recover. These factors are important determinants of how a patient with UMN dysfunction will function. They are also pertinent for establishing clinical goals.

Although neurological damage after acquired brain injury is obviously central in nature, neuro-orthopedic interventions are based on the idea that central damage generates altered and unbalanced forces in peripheral actuators and the latter may be manipulated neuro-orthopedically. Centrally mediated UMN dysfunction features such as paresis, spasticity and impaired motor control ultimately alter the ability of peripheral actuators to generate movement. Using a variety of techniques that aim at components of peripheral actuators such as tendons, nerves, bones, and joints, neuro-orthopedic interventions aim to rebalance deforming forces, thereby enabling some degree of functional restoration that, for all intents and purposes, is not dependent on central neurological recovery.

Philosophy of Neuro-Orthopedic Surgery

Wellness promotion has become an objective of our general medical care. This of course cannot mean the complete prevention of disease, injury, and disability. In the physically disabled population, wellness promotion means maximizing function and mobility in order to avoid the complications of their chronic incapacity. Potential complications of physical immobility include decubiti, infection, pain, social isolation, and physical and emotional dependence. For society this results in a costly loss of productivity for the patient and often family members as well.

The effects of injury or disease of the brain extend beyond the confines of the skull. The musculoskeletal system is profoundly effected by brain dysfunction. The converse is also true. The brain is strongly affected by dysfunction of the musculoskeletal system. Just as the shoulder and elbow function to position the hand for grasping and manipulating objects, the musculoskeletal system gives mobility to the brain and positions it to observe and interact with the world environment.

Professionals working in the field of neurologic rehabilitation are generally very aware and knowledgeable about cognitive and behavioral deficits. It has been our experience that less attention or importance has been given to the musculoskeletal impairment that occurs concomitantly. The subsequent penalties of these musculoskeletal limitations for the individual can be devastating. Improving an individual's physical mobility is often therapeutic leading to increases in their cognitive, behavioral, and emotional capacities.

When to Operate: What to Expect

When evaluating persons with central nervous system (CNS) dysfunction, questions often arise as to the indications for corrective limb surgery, the cost of providing such treatment, what type of outcome to expect, and the practicality of this approach. General principles have been delineated that can serve as guidelines for decision-making.

1. Operate early, before deformities are severe and fixed.

Surgery is a powerful rehabilitation tool. It is often the only treatment that will correct a limb deformity or improve function. Surgery should not be considered a treatment of last resort when "conservative" measures have failed. Physical and occupational therapy cannot effect a permanent change in motor control. Drug therapy for increased muscle tone has generalized effects and cannot be targeted to specific offending muscles. Even intrathecal baclofen (ITB) is not directed at specific muscles. Phenol blocks and botulinum toxin injections provide temporary modulation of tone. When a permanent treatment is needed to decrease muscle tone or redirect muscle force, surgery should be considered. The results of surgical intervention are improved when deformities are corrected early. Early surgery preserves maximum muscle strength, joint capsule and ligament flexibility, and articular cartilage integrity.

2. Better underlying motor control means better function for the extremity.

Clearly orthopedic surgery cannot impart neurologic control to a muscle. Lengthening a dyssynergic or spastic muscle can improve its function by diminishing the overactive stretch response and uncovering the control, which was present all along. The key to success is a careful evaluation prior to surgery. Here we attempt to determine the amount of volitional control pres-ent in each individual muscle that might be effecting the limb posture and movement.

Surgery, however, should not be reserved only for patients with severe impairment and deformity. Persons with milder degrees of impairment can benefit greatly from relatively simple procedures such as myotendinous lengthening of the extrinsic finger flexors and regain sufficient fine motor control to perform more intricate hand functions. The amount of improvement correlates best with the degree of underlying motor control and not the severity of the deformity.

3. Distinguish between the function of the extremity and the function of the individual.

We speak of "functional" and "nonfunctional" surgical procedures. These terms refer to expected outcomes for a limb but do not indicate the overall outcome for the individual person. An example is a hemiplegic patient with severe spasticity in the shoulder, elbow, wrist, and finger muscles who holds the arm in a flexed and internally rotated position. There is no underlying volitional control of movement but the arm has no fixed contractures and can be gradually stretched into extension. When the patient attempts to put on a shirt, he is unable to get his arm into the sleeve because he cannot hold both the shirt and his hemiplegic arm. Surgical releases of the dynamic flexion deformities of the upper extremity will position the arm in a more relaxed posture and allow the patient to be independent in dressing even though the arm itself remains nonfunctional. Similar "nonfunctional" procedures are often done to allow positioning of the hand and forearm on a walker to improve ambulation.

4. Consider the cost of not correcting limb deformities.

The cost of motor-control evaluation using dynamic electromyography (EMG) is relatively modest for the benefits it provides. The cost of performing an incorrect surgical procedure that fails to correct or worsens a limb deformity is much greater. The cost of performing a surgical procedure is limited when compared to a lifetime of attendant care, medications, orthotics, complications such as skin ulceration and infection, and lost productivity for the patients and their caretakers.

EVALUATION OF SPASTIC-LIMB DEFORMITIES

Extremity function requires complex and highly sophisticated mechanisms working together in unison. Improving extremity function requires careful systematic evaluation before surgery. The goals of surgery must be practical and clearly understood by the patient and the family. Assessment includes an evaluation of cognition and communication skills *(1–5,35,70,75–83)*.

Intact sensation is essential to functional use of the hand. The basic modalities of pain, light touch, and temperature must be present. It is helpful to observe the patient's spontaneous use of the hand. A patient with impaired sensation will often use a hand on request, by relying on visual feedback. The patient, however, may not necessarily use the extremity in activities of daily living. Visual perceptual deficits add increased problems involving motion of the limb and even awareness of the limb itself. In the lower extremity the ability to maintain balance and ambulate is dependent on adequate sensation in the foot and ankle. Proprioception and kinesthetic awareness of the limb in space are important *(84)*.

Diffuse axonal injury, multi-focal vascular pathology and diffuse hypoxic encephalopathy lead to a large variety of post-traumatic motor phenomena, many of which are functionally significant. Lesions affecting the corticospinal system, the cerebellum and its pathways, and the extrapyramidal system are common. Many patients, especially during the early recovery stage from head injury, reveal mixed signs such as spasticity combined with tremor and ataxia. Hemiballismus has been reported after head injury, though frank parkinsonism is said to be rare. Peripheral neuropathy is, of course, quite common after head injury, and focal dystonia, though unusual, is also seen. Because so many different aspects of the motor-control system may be affected by a head injury, we present a system of organizing the unwieldy array of clinical signs and symptoms that result from a damaged nervous system. The perspective taken is a functional one, namely taking into account the impact of restricted or excessive movement disorders on the patient's ability to function in real-life.

Treatment of spasticity is most effective when functional problems are formulated and described in focal rather than diffuse terms. For example, a patient may have spastic musculature across all joints of the upper extremity, which some might consider sufficient justification for the use of a systemic agent to reduce tone in the arm as a whole. A closer inspection of the patient might reveal that function of one joint in particular is most important. Treatment of focal problems lends itself well to surgical intervention that can target particular muscles. Surgical lengthening, transfer, or release of targeted muscles can provide very effective solutions to problems of function that are clearly identified from the outset. In large part, the localizing approach is useful because it forces the clinician to indicate the desired outcome in advance because the outcome is based on an analysis that identifies the specific spastic muscles responsible for the problem. If the clinical problem is an adducted shoulder that hinders access to the axilla for purposes of bathing and deodorant application, blocking the pectoralis major or surgically releasing it will not solve the problem if teres major and latissimus dorsi are the culprits responsible for the problem. If the clinical problem is an equinovarus foot that inhibits walking, surgically lengthening or transferring the tibialis posterior will not solve the problem if tibialis anterior and gastroc-soleus muscles are the muscles responsible for the problem. Identifying the specific offending muscles is critically important to localized strategies of intervention.

In a neurologically impaired patient it is frequently difficult to distinguish between the many potential causes of limited joint motion. The possibilities include increase muscle tone, a myostatic contracture, the presence of periarticular HO, an undetected fracture or dislocation, joint subluxation, pain, or the lack of patient cooperation secondary to diminished cognition. Bony deformities may not exhibit an obvious clinical deformity but can be detected by radiography.

CLINICAL EVALUATION OF MOTOR CONTROL

In broad terms, evaluation of spasticity focuses on identification of three factors: 1) the clinical pattern of motor dysfunction, 2) the patient's ability to control muscles involved in the clinical pattern, and 3) the role of muscle stiffness and contracture in relation to the functional problem. For purposes of convenience, we have identified 13 clinical patterns of motor dysfunction that are most commonly seen, organized by joint or limb segment, that are typically found in patients with UMN lesions (*see* Table 1). Other variations of motor dysfunction occur less commonly.

Various muscles may contribute to motor dysfunction across joints and limb segments in these clinical patterns. Evaluation focuses on the following characteristics of the involved muscles: A) voluntary or selective control, B) spastic reactivity, C) rheologic stiffness, and D) contracture. There are five specific questions asked. 1) Does the patient have voluntary control over a given muscle? 2) Is the muscle spastic to passive stretch? 3) Is the muscle, as an antagonist, activated during active movement generated by an agonist? 4) Does the muscle have increased stiffness when stretched? 5) Does the muscle have fixed shortening (contracture)? When many muscles cross a joint, the characteristics of each muscle may vary. Because each muscle may contribute to motion and movement of the joint, information about each muscle's contribution is useful to the assessment as a whole. Treatment depends on such information *(3,5)*. Spasticity often masks underlying motor control. In the upper extremity the most common pattern of spasticity is one of flexion. In the lower extremity it is one of extension. Passive range of motion of each joint should be established first. This is tested by slow extension of the joint to avoid the velocity-sensitive response of the muscle spindle. When spasticity is significant and passive joint motion is incomplete, it is necessary and advisable to perform an anesthetic nerve block to assess whether a myostatic contracture is present *(32,85)*.

Differentiating between the relative contributions of pain, increased muscle tone, and contracture to a limb deformity can be difficult. Anesthetic nerve blocks are extremely useful in assessing joint range of motion. The blocks can be easily performed without the use of special devices. By temporarily eliminating pain and muscle tone, patient cooperation is gained and the amount of myostatic contracture can be determined. Using local anesthetic blocks, the strength and motor control of the antagonistic muscle group can also be evaluated. In order to evaluate passive joint motion in the entire upper extremity, a brachial plexus block using a local anesthetic is performed. To evaluate passive joint motion in the entire lower extremity combined femoral and sciatic nerve blocks using a local anesthetic are performed. Alternately, the patient can be examined while under general anesthesia. This is usually done only when the patient is going to surgery for another reason.

Unmasking of primitive patterning reflexes further contributes to the motor impairment. Spasticity (hyperactive response to quick stretch), rigidity (resistance to slow movement), or movement dystonias may be present *(1,3,5,77,78,86–88)*. The degree of spasticity within selected muscles can be

Table 3
Clinical Scale of Motor Control

Grade	Motor control	Description
1	Flaccid	Hypotonic, no active motion
2	Rigid	Hypertonic, no active motion
3	Reflexive mass pattern (synergy)	Mass flexion or extension in response to stimulation
4	Volitional mass pattern	Patient-initiated mass flexion or extension movement
5	Selective with pattern overlay	Slow volitional movement of specific joints. Physiologic stress results in mass action
6	Selective	Volitional control of individual joints

graded clinically in response to a quick stretch as mild, moderate, or severe. There is surprising consistency between observers using this simple grading system. Another method of quantifying muscle tone, which is readily accessible and easily performed at the bedside, is to measure the amount of intramuscular pressure generated by a passive quick stretch or during functional use of the limb. Intramuscular pressure can be measured using a wick or slit catheter technique. The pressure generated within the muscle is proportional to the force of contraction *(89,90)*.

Motor control can be graded in the extremity using a clinical scale (*see* Table 3) *(1,2,78,86)*. The extremity may be hypotonic or flaccid and without any volitional movement (Grade 1). A spastic extremity may be held rigidly without any volitional or reflexive movement (Grade 2). Patterned or synergistic motor control is defined as a mass flexion or extension response involving the entire extremity. This mass-patterned movement may be reflexive in response to a stimulus but without volitional control (Grade 3). The patient (Grade 4) can also volitionally initiate the mass-patterned movement. Although patterned movement can often be volitionally initiated, it is a neurologically primitive form of motor control and of no functional use in the upper extremity. Selective motor control with pattern overlay is defined as the ability to move a single joint or digit with minimal movement in the adjacent joints when performing an activity slowly (Grade 5). Grade 5 motor control is the most common but also the most widely variable pattern seen in those patients with potential for functional improvement from orthopedic surgery. Rapid movements or physiologic stress make the mass pattern more pronounced. Selective motor control is defined as the ability to volitionally move a single joint or digit independently of the adjacent joints (Grade 6). The patient should be observed clinically in a variety of functional tasks.

LABORATORY ASSESSMENT OF MOTOR CONTROL

Clinical examination supported by laboratory studies is the gold standard of evaluation. The clinical questions of interest regarding a given muscle (that might be targeted for localized intervention) include the following: 1) Does the patient have selective voluntary control over the given muscle? 2) Is the muscle activated dyssynergically (i.e., in antagonism to movement) when the patient attempts to move the relevant joint? 3) Is the muscle resistive to passive stretch? 4) Does the given muscle have fixed shortening (i.e., contracture: limited range of motion that is attributed, in large measure, to fixed shortening of the given muscle crossing its joint)? 5) Given the degree of clinical effort, patient morbidity and procedural costs involved in treating complicated movement dysfunction in patients with UMN syndrome, clinical examination alone is not sufficient to answer these questions with a high degree of confidence.

Technology-driven laboratory assessments that include formal gait and motion analysis, dynamic EMG studies, and nerve blocks are helpful *(24,34,35,38,39,49,53,70,74,91–118)*. Laboratory gait analysis is performed preoperatively on all patients using a standard laboratory protocol. This consists of bi-directional, slow-motion video recordings. Ground-reaction forces are recorded from a force plate mounted into the walkway. Ground-reaction forces are displayed using a laser vector superimposed on the video. The force plate consists of a rigid platform suspended on strain-gauge transducers fitted with strain gauges. Each supporting corner has three sensors set at right angles to one another and the vertical load, horizontal shear force, and the mediolateral direction are measured. Temporospatial parameters obtained include walking velocity, cadence, stride time and measurements of symmetry of gait.

Dynamic multi-channel EMG is acquired with simultaneous measurements of joint motion (kinematics) in the upper and lower extremities and with ground-reaction forces (kinetics) obtained from force-plate measurements in the lower extremities. Kinetic, kinematic, and dynamic EMG data assist the clinician in interpreting whether voluntary function (effort-related initiation, modulation, and termination of activity) is present in a given muscle and whether that muscle's behavior is also dyssynergic (sometimes referred to as "out of phase" behavior). In addition, responses to different rates of passive stretch of muscle before and after local anesthetic nerve block can help the clinician distinguish between the dynamic, velocity-sensitive reflex resistance of spasticity vs passive muscle-tissue stiffness and contracture. Somatosensory-evoked potentials (SEPs) and motor-evoked potentials (MEPs) provide information on the integrity of the sensory and motor pathways and may be helpful in predicting recovery of motor function after stroke *(119)*. Combined with clinical information, laboratory measurements of muscle function often provide the degree of detail and confidence necessary for making conservative and surgical treatment decisions.

Combining the findings in several previous studies of spastic patients the following classification of EMG activity was devised to standardize terminology and may be used for either the upper or lower extremity *(98,120,121)*. Class I constitutes a normal phasic pattern with appropriate on and off electromyographic activity. Class II consists of EMG activity that, although phasic, begins prematurely and continues for a short period beyond the normal duration of activity for that muscle. This is more commonly seen in the lower extremity. Class III consists of phasic activity with prolongation beyond the normal timing of the muscle. Class III activity can be further subdivided into three patterns depending on the degree of prolongation. Class IIIA consists of phasic activity with a short period of low intensity EMG activity extending into the next phase of the flexion-extension cycle secondary to mild spasticity. Class IIIB consists of phasic activity with prolongation extending for at least half of the next phase of motion. This is indicative of a moderate amount of spasticity. Class IIIC represents a severely spastic muscle and consists of phasic activity with severe prolongation in which EMG activity is continued throughout the next phase of motion at a high intensity but the underlying phasic nature of the muscle activity is still distinguishable. Class IV consists of continuous EMG activity without phasic variations. Class V consists of EMG activity seen only in response to a quick stretch by the antagonist muscles. There is no volitional activation of the muscle. This pattern is common in the finger extensors *(98,121)*. Class VI consists of absent EMG activity.

Clinical Examples

Spastic Elbow-Flexion Deformity

The usual clinical picture is one of cogwheel motion on attempted extension of the elbow. Elbow extension range is often limited with a very prolonged period of extension. Elbow flexion is relatively normal. Laboratory examination utilizing dynamic EMG helps to confirm the presence of volitional capacity as well as dyssynergy during movement for each of the elbow flexors. Dynamic recordings are obtained from biceps, brachialis, brachioradialis, lateral, medial, and long head of the triceps. Dynamic EMG combined with electrogoniometric measurement of elbow motion of stroke and traumatic brain-injured patients has revealed a consistent pattern of muscle activity responsible for this clinical picture *(120–122)*. The pattern most commonly seen is that all three heads of the triceps muscle are operating in a normal phasic pattern. The brachioradialis muscle most frequently shows continuous spastic activity *(120–122)*. One or both heads of the biceps muscle is also spastic. Less frequently, some spasticity is observed in the brachialis muscle. This pattern of muscle activity is also common in patients with CP. Armed with this information, a rational surgical plan can be devised to improve elbow control.

Equinovarus Foot Deformity

Dynamic EMG performed during walking illustrates the motor pattern responsible for the spastic equinovarus deformity *(76,93,94,96,107,108,112, 117,123–139)*. Foot switches are used to record the swing and stance phases of gait for each foot. The gastrocnemius and soleus muscles are firing continuously (Class IV) throughout stance and swing phase causing the equinus posture of the foot. The peroneus brevis is also firing continuously. The peroneus longus muscle is active prematurely and for a prolonged period (Class II). The tibialis anterior shows continuous activity and results in the varus position of the foot seen primarily during swing. In stroke and brain injury, the tibialis posterior muscle is less commonly an offending force. When the tibialis posterior is over-active, excessive heel varus is seen. The flexor digitorum longus, flexor hallucis longus, and intrinsic muscles of the foot are also commonly spastic, resulting in curled toes.

Spastic Valgus Foot

Spastic valgus deformities of the foot are less common in stroke and brain-injured patients but can easily be missed. The valgus deformity may occur alone as a result of overactivity of the peroneus longus or brevis muscle *(117)*. It may also occur during stance phase in combination with an equinovarus deformity that occurs during the swing phase of gait.

Stiff-Knee Gait

Inadequate knee flexion during the swing phase of gait causes the patient to hike the hip and circumduct the leg in order to clear the foot. This is a very energy-consuming gait deviation. Because equinus of the ankle will result in an extension thrust at the knee, it is first necessary to rule out either a static contracture or dynamic equinus posturing as a cause.

Normally the knee begins to flex in the pre-swing phase of gait marked by the point at which the opposite foot contacts the ground and double stance begins. Knee flexion is a passive event caused by the forward momentum of the body rather than by contraction of the knee-flexor muscles.

Dynamic EMG studies during gait have shown that patients with a spastic stiff-legged gait exhibit inappropriate activity of the quadriceps during early swing that blocks knee flexion *(3–5,11,57,91,108,111,122,125,138, 140–154)*. In 13% of head-injured patients, there is isolated firing of the rectus femoris during early swing. There is no clinical test to determine the pattern of muscle activity within the quadriceps. Dynamic EMG gait analysis is required for surgical decision-making.

Differentiating between the relative contributions of pain, increased muscle tone, and contracture to a limb deformity can be difficult. Anesthetic nerve blocks are extremely useful in assessing joint range of motion. The blocks can be easily performed without the use of special devices. By temporarily eliminating pain and muscle tone, patient cooperation is gained and the amount of myostatic contracture can be determined. Using local anesthetic blocks the strength and motor control of the antagonistic muscle group can also be evaluated.

The following sections illustrate how to apply strategies of focal evaluation and localized treatment, using a joint by joint approach in spastic patients with familiar patterns of UMN dysfunction.

ORTHOPEDIC MANAGEMENT OF COMMON DEFORMITIES

General Considerations

The patterns of limb spasticity seen in CP, stroke, anoxia, and traumatic brain injury are very similar. Therefore the same principles or evaluation and the same orthopedic procedures can be used. We will describe the orthopedic-treatment interventions together. However, these procedures are not applied equally to all patient groups. The degree of spasticity, the timing of neurologic recovery, and the pattern of spontaneous neurologic recovery are different between patients.

Orthopedic Surgical Techniques

Several techniques to modify muscle function are available to the orthopedic surgeon. These include denervation, release, lengthening, and transfer. Denervation is used to eliminate a dynamic deforming force when that muscle has been shown to have no potential for function. Denervation is not helpful if there is a fixed myostatic contracture. Release of a muscle or tendon can be done when the muscle is a deforming force with no function. Tendon or muscle release will correct both a static contracture and a spastic dynamic deformity. Lengthening of a muscle-tendon unit is done when the muscle exhibits volitional control with dyssynergy. Fractional (myotendinous) lengthening is preferred whenever possible in spastic muscles. This allows the underlying tone and strength of the muscle to determine the amount of lengthening rather than having the surgeon estimate this elusive quantity. Lengthening over the muscle belly eliminates the need for suturing and this diminished the amount of scarring that occurs. A new tendon reforms and fills in the gap within several months. The fractional lengthening technique allows the patient to begin gentle active motion immediately after surgery because the muscle-tendon unit remains intact. By contrast, a Z lengthening technique requires immobilization for a minimum of 4 wk to allow healing of the relatively avascular tendon and prevent inadvertent rupture. A tendon transfer is done when it is desirable to redirect a muscle force.

Shoulder

The paretic shoulder deserves special attention because it is a common source of pain. A variety of different factors contribute to the painful, immobile shoulder: reflex sympathetic dystrophy, brachial plexitis, inferior subluxation, spasticity with adduction, internal rotation contracture, adhesive capsulitis, spastic abduction, heterotopic ossification, and traumatic lesions such as rotator cuff tears or fractures and dislocations.

Adhesive Capsulitis

Adhesive capsulitis is commonly seen in patients following stroke and in those with reflex sympathetic dystrophy *(22,50,61,65,102,106,155–162)*. They have a characteristically painful shoulder with limited glenohumeral motion. The treatment in this group of patients is similar to that for the general population. Nonsteroidal anti-inflammatory drugs, physical therapy, and intra-articular injections are all useful. Selected cases may benefit from manipulation under anesthesia. Arthroscopic capsular release may be performed for adhesive capsulitis.

Inferior Subluxation

Inferior subluxation of the shoulder is a common occurrence in patients with flaccid paralysis of the shoulder girdle. This is most commonly seen in stroke patients or in brain-injured patients with concomitant brachial plexus trauma. The subluxation is usually self-limiting but occasionally, the shoulder will chronically be subluxated, causing pain *(1–3,5,75,78,86,156, 158,163–166)*. The patients typically have no functional use of the extremity. Patients complain of increased pain when upright. The pain may be owing to chronic stretch on the shoulder capsule or from traction on the brachial plexus. Physical examination shows a positive sulcus sign with little to no active motion of the involved shoulder. There is a prominence of the acromion and atrophy of the deltoid. There may be contracture of the shoulder in adduction and internal rotation. Subacromial or intraarticular injections of local anesthetics do not relieve the symptoms. Radiographs show inferior subluxation of the humerus on the glenoid. Brachial plexopathy must be ruled out by using diagnostic EMG.

Conservative treatment may include electrical stimulation to the deltoid and supraspinatus muscles but commonly and pragmatically the arm is placed in a sling. This relieves the symptoms by elevating the humeral head in the glenoid. Although usually successful in the short run, this is frequently unacceptable to the patient as a permanent solution.

Shoulder arthrodesis has been performed but is not well-accepted by the patient because it produces a rigid joint that interferes with passive positioning, hygiene, and nursing care. The procedure we prefer is to convert the long head biceps tendon to a proximally based suspensory ligament. The biceps-suspension procedure preserves passive shoulder motion while correcting the subluxation *(60)*. Because only the tendon is being used, there is no opportunity for paretic muscle to develop laxity and for the deformity to recur. The repair is protected in a sling for 3 mo to allow bone to tendon healing.

Spastic Abduction

Over activity of the supraspinatus muscle can cause spastic abduction posturing. The deformity is usually dynamic, becoming more prominent with ambulation, transfers, or other attempted activities. The affected arm is held in an abducted posture, making balance while ambulating difficult. Patients complain that their balance is thrown off because of bumping into furniture, doorways, and people in crowds. Diagnosis requires examination of the patient at rest and during a variety of activities. It is also helpful to elicit from caretakers or family members any history of activities that trigger this posture. Dynamic EMG is used to confirm that spasticity of the supraspinatus muscle is causing the deformity.

The Supraspinatus Slide

It is possible to effectively lengthen the supraspinatus by means of a slide procedure *(75)*. This procedure has been used successfully to correct spastic abduction deformity. The patient is placed in the lateral decubitus position with the affected extremity uppermost. An axillary roll is placed in the unaffected axilla to protect the brachial plexus and all bony prominences are well-padded. A 10–15 cm incision is made parallel to the scapular spine. The trapezius insertion is detached from the spine of the scapula, leaving a cuff of fascia for later reattachment. The deltoid is retracted laterally. Using a small periosteal elevator, the origin of the supraspinatus is elevated subperiosteally from the medial border of the scapula. The dissection is continued laterally, with care being taken to avoid injury to the neurovascular pedicle at the suprascapular notch. The muscle is then allowed to slide laterally. The trapezius is then reattached to the scapular spine. The remainder of the closure is performed in routine fashion. The patient is allowed full, unrestricted postoperative motion.

The Adducted/Internally Rotated Shoulder

The arm is adducted tightly against the lateral chest wall and shoulder internal rotation causes the forearm to lie against the middle of the chest. The tendon of pectoralis major is often prominent when the examiner attempts to abduct and externally rotate the shoulder but other muscles contribute to the deformity as well. The glenohumeral joint normally functions as a universal joint, enabling the hand to reach an almost spherical volume of locations in three-dimensional space. When patients attempt to reach forward, spastic adductors and internal rotators can severely restrict acquisition of targets in the environment and on the body. The patient's ability to stabilize, push, or apply force to an object is also compromised. From the perspective of passive function goals such as skin care and axillary hygiene, spastic adductors and internal rotators hinder efforts of caregivers to gain access to the axilla to provide needed care. Restricted motion may impair dressing, washing, and bathing and promote skin irritation and maceration. Passive manipulation of the shoulder during personal care may cause pain when motion and contact trigger spastic resistance in reactive muscles.

Muscles that contribute to spastic adduction/internal rotation dysfunction of the shoulder include latissimus dorsi, teres major, the clavicular and sternal heads of pectoralis major and subscapularis. Involvement of latissimus dorsi and teres major should be considered when hyperextension posturing of the shoulder is observed. Antagonistic activity in these muscles may be masking a patient's potential for active flexion. Diagnostic lidocaine block to the thoracodorsal nerve and/or lower subscapular nerve may unmask that voluntary potential.

Release of all four muscles may be required to relieve the deformity in a nonfunctional extremity *(1,2,17,75,77,78,167)*. In patients who have evidence of underlying control of muscle function despite the presence of dyssynergy, the pectoralis major, latissimus dorsi, and teres major muscles can be fractionally lengthened at their muscle-tendon junctions. Alternately, the teres major muscle can be partially released from its origin on the scapula and allowed to slide distally in the same manor as the supraspinatus slide. Postoperatively, an aggressive mobilization program is instituted following skin healing. Gentle range of motion exercises are employed to correct any remaining contracture. Careful positioning of the limb in abduction and external rotation is necessary for several months to prevent recurrence.

Elbow

Spastic Flexion

Upright posture favors hypertonia in the "antigravity" elbow flexors of the upper limb. In the patient without motor control, severe flexion posturing can lead to skin maceration in the antecubital fossa, malodor, and skin breakdown. In reality, a continuum of volitional control is seen. Many patients complain that their elbows persistently "ride up" when they stand up and walk. They also complain that their flexed elbow hooks door frames and other people. Putting on a shirt or jacket is a struggle. Kinesiologically, the elbow lengthens and shortens the upper extremity. Consequently, active dysfunction is characterized by impaired reaching for objects in the environment, placing them elsewhere or bringing them to the body.

Control of limb placement depends on both shoulder and elbow control. Smooth control of elbow flexion and extension is frequently impaired. The usual clinical picture is one of cogwheel motion on attempted extension of the elbow. Elbow-extension range is often limited with a very prolonged period of extension. Elbow flexion is relatively normal. Laboratory examination utilizing dynamic EMG helps to confirm the presence of volitional capacity as well as dyssynergy during movement for each of the elbow flexors. Dynamic recordings are obtained from biceps, brachialis, brachioradialis, lateral, medial, and long head of the triceps. Dynamic EMG combined with electrogoniometric measurement of elbow motion of stroke and traumatic brain-injured patients has revealed a consistent pattern of muscle activity responsible for this clinical picture *(3,5,35,76,98,101,120,122,167,168)*. The pattern most commonly seen is that all three heads of the triceps muscle are operating in a normal phasic pattern. The brachioradialis muscle most frequently shows continuous spastic activity. One or both heads of the biceps muscle is also spastic. Less spasticity is observed in the brachialis muscle. This pattern of muscle activity is also common in patients with CP. Armed with this information, a rational surgical plan can be devised to improve elbow control.

FUNCTIONAL ELBOW LENGTHENING

Fractional (myotendinous) lengthening is preferred whenever possible in spastic muscles. This allows the underlying tone and strength of the muscle to determine the amount of lengthening rather than having the surgeon estimate this elusive quantity. Lengthening over the muscle belly eliminates the need for suturing and this diminished the amount of scarring that occurs. A new tendon reforms and fills in the gap within several months. The fractional lengthening technique allows the patient to begin gentle active motion immediately after surgery because the muscle tendon unit remains intact. By contrast, a Z lengthening technique requires immobilization for a minimum of 4 wk to allow healing of the relatively avascular tendon and prevent inadvertent rupture.

Three methods are available to decrease tone in a spastic brachioradialis. Surgical lengthening of the brachioradialis can be used if volitional control is demonstrated on EMG *(75)*. If little or no control is demonstrated, release of the severely spastic brachioradialis muscle at the level of the elbow may be performed *(2,3,5,75,78,122)*. Lengthening of the spastic biceps and brachialis muscles as indicated by dynamic EMG is also performed to improve elbow motion and hand placement. Meals has advocated neurectomy of the radial nerve branches to the brachioradialis *(169)*. This technique would not correct an established contracture of the brachioradialis and does not preserve use of the muscle if volitional control is present.

In arms where there is potential for function our preferred technique is to fractionally lengthen the long and short heads of the biceps in the upper arm. When the elbow deformity is greater than 90°, it is usually necessary to Z lengthen the biceps at its tendon distally. The brachialis muscle is fractionally lengthened above the antecubital space and the brachioradialis is lengthened in the upper forearm.

When the biceps has been lengthened proximally, no immobilization is needed. The drain is removed within the first 24 h following surgery and active exercises are started. No resistive exercises are allowed for 3 wk to prevent over-lengthening of the muscles with resulting weakness. When a Z lengthening of the biceps tendon was done distally, the patient is placed in a posterior splint with the elbow in 90° of flexion for 4 wk to protect the biceps tendon repair. Functional elbow-flexor lengthening has significantly enhanced the fluid control of elbow motion and improved hand placement in properly selected patients.

NONFUNCTIONAL ELBOW RELEASE

Persistent spasticity of the elbow flexors causes a myostatic contracture and flexion deformity of the elbow. This results in skin maceration and breakdown of the antecubital space *(5,15,16,32,35,47,49,52,57,66,67,70, 100,101,110,120,122,170–173)*. This position of severe elbow flexion also predisposes the ulnar nerve to an acquired compression neuropathy by increasing the vulnerability to direct pressure and decreasing the cross-sectional area of the cubital tunnel *(37,62,64)*. When no functional use is expected, surgical release of the biceps tendon and brachioradialis muscle combined with lengthening or release of the brachialis is performed depending on the severity of the contracture. The joint capsule is generally not released. Gradual extension of the elbow with serial casting or physical therapy corrects the pre-operative deformity and decreases the ulnar-nerve compression. Anterior transposition of the ulnar nerve may be necessary to further improve ulnar-nerve function. Serial casting or drop out casts can be used to obtain further correction over the ensuing weeks *(12,15,32,35,49)*.

Spastic Extension

Spastic extension of the elbow is much less common than spastic flexion. These patients have frequently had a brain-stem infarct or injury. They complain of difficulty reaching their face for activities of daily living.

TRICEPS LENGTHENING

Experience with triceps lengthening for spasticity is limited because it is an uncommon problem. When needed, however, good results have been reported with surgical lengthening *(172)*. A V-Y triceps plasty allows improved flexion range of motion, with a cost of decreased extension power and extensor lag. This procedure should be used with caution in patients who rely on their arms to assist with ambulation or transfers because strength is lost with any lengthening procedure.

Ulnar Neuropathy

Ulnar neuropathy occurs commonly in spastic patients for a number of reasons. Prolonged elbow flexion with traction on the nerve can lead to decreased volume of the cubital tunnel resulting in nerve compression. Support of the torso by leaning on a chronically flexed elbow may result in direct compression of the nerve. Heterotopic ossification in any location about the elbow, but particularly in a posterior location, can cause ulnar neuropathy secondary to the intense inflammatory reaction. The patients are often limited in their ability to complain about ulnar-nerve symptoms because of limited cognitive and communicative abilities. The diagnosis is usually suspected because of intrinsic atrophy, and confirmed using nerve-conduction studies. A 2.5% incidence has been shown in patients with traumatic brain injury *(22,37,64,72)*.

Treatment is ulnar nerve transposition, often at the same time as elbow-flexor lengthenings, flexor releases, or resection of heterotopic ossification. Subcutaneous transposition is preferred to avoid stimulation of heterotopic ossification formation.

Forearm

Supination and pronation deformities are commonly associated with elbow spasticity, wrist spasticity, or both. Pronation deformities are much more common. These deformities are most often treated together with the associated deformities. They seldom require treatment individually.

Spastic Pronation

Pronation deformity of the forearm in an UMN lesion is more common than supination deformity. Pronation bias makes it difficult for a person to reach for a target underhand whereas supination deformity impairs reaching for targets that require overhand reach. Many activities of daily living depend on active supination. The use of feeding and grooming utensils and clothes fasteners becomes problematic when spastic or contracted pronators restrict supination. Physical examination reveals a fully pronated resting position of the forearm. When passive supination range of motion exceeds active supination range, the possibility of pronator muscle dyssynergy during active supination should be suspected. Muscles that potentially contribute include pronator teres and pronator quadratus. Dynamic EMG studies of pronator teres, pronator quadratus and biceps greatly augment clinical examination. Clinical examination does not easily predict which of the pronators might be retaining volitional capacity and which might be spastic. Both pronator muscles may show varying degrees of volition and spasticity. Interestingly, flexor spasticity of the powerful biceps often coexists with a pronated forearm deformity.

Surgical lengthening of pronator teres and pronator quadratus may be performed depending on their individual voluntary capacities and the clinical goal is to improve active supination function by reducing pronator dyssynergy. The possibility of lengthening pronator teres has long been recognized, but fractional lengthening of the pronator quadratus is of recent vintage *(75)*.

Release of the flexor-pronator origin was previously a common operation. We do not advocate this procedure because it does not target the individual muscles responsible for deformities. When an excessive amount of the pronator teres origin was released or when there was no function in the pronator quadratus muscle, an iatrogenic supination deformity occurred. The supination deformity was much less functional than a pronated forearm. When the pronators are contracted and not active volitionally, muscle releases may be considered, though passive functional advantages, other than cosmesis, may be hard to come by.

Spastic Supination

Spastic supination is a far less common deformity but is also associated with elbow-flexion deformities. Most often this deformity is seen as a complication of the surgical flexor-pronator origin release *(75)*. The biceps, supinator, or both may cause supination deformity. Physical examination supplemented by dynamic EMG may be used to determine the relative contribution of each.

Correction of the supination deformity is performed in conjunction with correction of the elbow flexion deformity. As described previously, in the functional extremity a biceps lengthening is performed. In a nonfunctional extremity a distal biceps release is performed. Often at the conclusion of this, the arm is able to achieve a functional range of pronation. If not, attention must be turned to the supinator. Elevating the insertion from its radial insertion lengthens the supinator. Once elevated, the supinator is allowed to slide. It will subsequently reattach in a lengthened position.

Wrist

A flexed wrist is common after traumatic brain injury but hyperextension deformity may also be seen. Patients complain of difficulty inserting their hand into shirts, jackets, and other narrow openings. They frequently have pain on passive motion. They may also have symptoms of carpal-tunnel syndrome secondary to compression of the median nerve against the transverse carpal ligament by taut flexor tendons *(64,73)*. In severe cases, wrist subluxation may be present. Radial or ulnar deviation and a clenched fist are often present as well.

Spastic Flexion

Muscles that potentially contribute to wrist flexion include the flexor carpi radialis (FCR), flexor carpi ulnaris (FCU), palmaris longus (PL), flexor digitorum sublimis (FDS), and flexor digitorum profundus (FDP). Singly or in combination, these muscles may have variable features of spasticity, contracture, and voluntary control. Because they have a larger cross-sectional area, wrist-flexor muscles are generally stronger than their extensor counterparts. Despite a net balance of forces favoring flexion, the extent to which a patient may have voluntary control over wrist extensors should be investigated. Dynamic EMG studies and temporary diagnostic motor-point blocks are helpful. When wrist-hyperextension deformity is present, wrist extensors are typically volitional and spastic, wrist flexors are often poorly volitional and mildly spastic, and the fingers are tightly clenched into the palm.

Clinical examination begins by observing resting posture of the wrist. FCR, FCU, or both may bowstring across the wrist and radial or ulnar deviation suggests their respective involvement. A clenched fist points to extrinsic finger flexors as having a role. If fingernails dig into the palm, FDP is likely to be involved. If the PIP joint is markedly flexed but the DIP joint is not, involvement of FDS is likely.

Laboratory examination of the flexed wrist deformity includes recordings from FCR, FCU, ECR, ECU, FDS, and FDP *(3,5,35,52,70,75,76,78–80, 82,83,87,95,98,109,110,121,153,154,168,175–178)*. Kinesiologic study includes 'isolated' muscle group testing along with whole-limb movements such as reaching, grasping, and releasing objects. In addition, passive stretch of the wrist flexors and finger flexors provides an indication of spastic reactivity as seen electromyographically. Dynamic EMG findings are not easily predictable from clinical examination. Some patients show extensive activation of wrist extensors during extension and reaching efforts. Nevertheless, the wrist remains flexed because tension in the wrist flexors and finger flexors overbalances extensor forces. EMG activity in FCR is often pres-ent during attempts at wrist extension and activity in FDS or FDP may be present. In patients with ulnar deviation, EMG activity is typically seen in FCU on reaching effort but "isolated" testing also suggests that patients can often activate FCU voluntarily. Because EMG activity is not correlated with force production, diagnostic nerve blocks are often helpful in unmasking movement. Temporary chemical "weakening" of a dyssynergic wrist flexor may unmask strength in the wrist extensors sufficient to improve active wrist motion. A similar hypothesis can be used for the extrinsic finger flexors after dynamic EMG reveals whether FDS and/or FDP are generating antagonistic activity acting to restrain wrist extension. Motor-point block of the target muscle group or median and/or ulnar-nerve blocks at the elbow may be performed to examine for active wrist extension during reach. Combined median and ulnar-nerve blocks at or above the elbow will also reveal the presence of muscle contracture.

When a patient has underlying voluntary control, surgical treatment for flexed and hyperextended wrists are myotendinous lengthenings (Fig. 1). Selective muscle releases, wrist fusion, and proximal row carpectomy can be considered in the presence of severe deformities (Fig. 2). Subtotal carpectomy combined with radio-carpal or radio-metacarpal fusion has been suggested for the treatment of severe flexion contracture either not amenable to, or refractory to, soft-tissue releases alone *(52,109)*.

In patients with a severely contracted hand, a single-stage procedure consisting of superficialis to profundus (STP) transfer, wrist-flexor release, flexor pollicus longus (FPL) lengthening, wrist arthrodesis, carpal-tunnel release, and ulnar motor-branch neurectomy or intrinsic release can provide

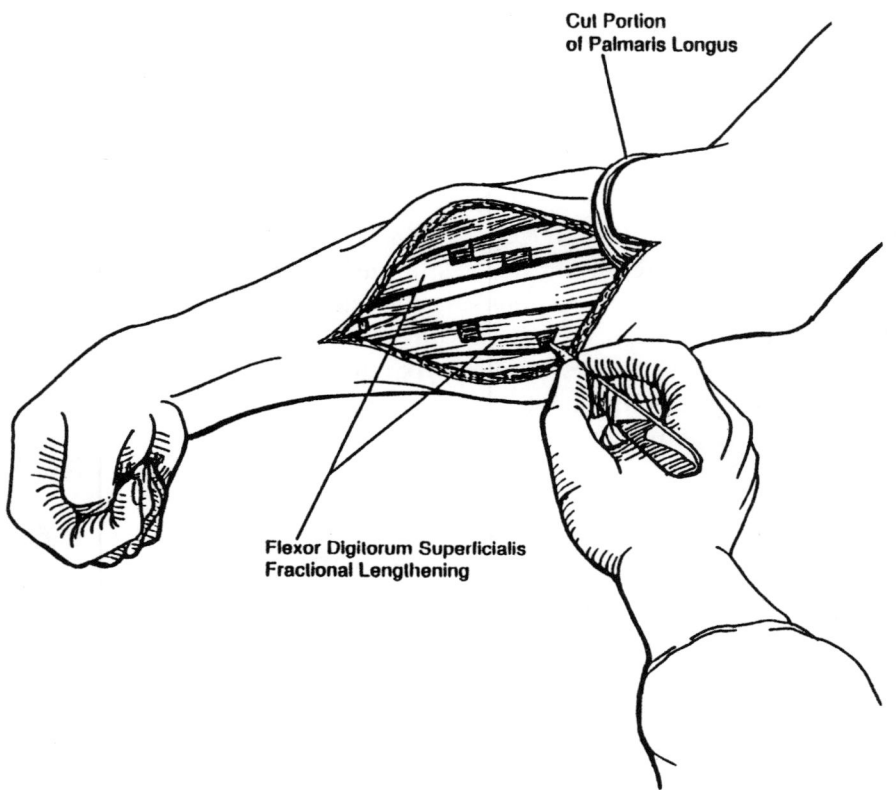

Fig. 1. Myotendinous lengthening of the extrinsic finger flexors in the forearm. Reprinted with permission from ref. *(166)*.

comprehensive correction. Such a definitive approach to severe deformities is associated with acceptable morbidity and eliminates the possibility of recurrence or undercorrection from untreated intrinsic pathology *(3,5, 35,52,70,75,76,78–80,82,83,87,95,98,109,110,121,153,154,168,175–178)*.

When wrist-flexion deformities are severe, release of the wrist flexors is performed. This can be helpful even in a hand with some functional ability. A proximal row carpectomy may be needed to provide additional shortening of the forearm and correct the deformity in persons with severe, longstanding contracture *(52,109,116)*. The wrist is then stabilized with a wrist fusion to eliminate the need for a wrist orthosis after surgery. Splints tend to be lost by these patients and their caretakers. Gravity alone can cause a recurrence of the flexion deformity. Unopposed wrist- or finger-extensor tone can result in a hyperextension deformity. Because the median nerve is

Orthopedic Interventions

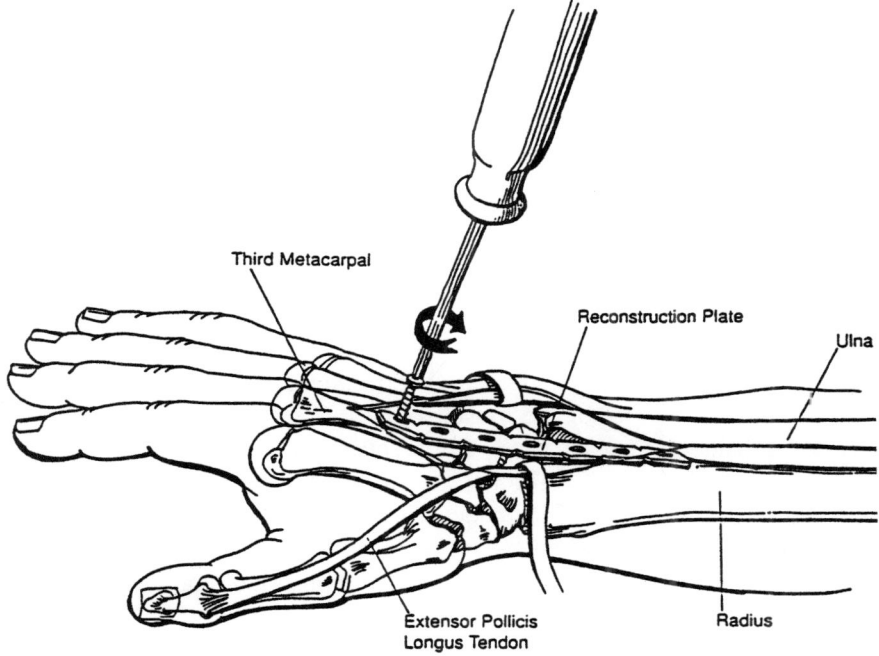

Fig. 2. Wrist arthrodesis using a plate and screws for stabilization. Reprinted with permission from ref. *(166)*.

compressed against the proximal transverse carpal ligament causing a painful neuropathy, a carpal-tunnel release is performed as well.

Spastic Extension

Extension deformity of the wrist causes hygiene problems and may prevent release in patients with poor digital extension. Median-nerve compression may also be caused by prolonged extension. If median-nerve compression is diagnosed, carpal-tunnel release is performed.

When volitional control has been demonstrated in the dyssynergic wrist extensors, myotendinous lengthening of the extensor carpi ulnaris is performed through a short longitudinal incision on the ulnar border of the forearm. The myotendinous junction is identified and the tendinous portion transected, allowing the muscle to stretch. The extensor carpi radialis longus and brevis are then identified in a separate longitudinal incision on the radial side of the forearm. Again, the myotendinous junction is identified and the tendinous portion cut, allowing the muscle to lengthen. The incisions are closed in routine fashion. Active motion is begun immediately after surgery.

When no volitional activity is seen in the wrist-extensor muscle by clinical examination and dynamic EMG, tendon release with wrist fusion with or without proximal row carpectomy is performed. A midline dorsal incision is made. Dissection is carried out medially and laterally exposing the distal extensor carpi radialis longus and brevis and the distal extensor carpi ulnaris. These tendons are transected proximal to their insertions. Wrist fusion with or without proximal row carpectomy is performed as described earlier.

Hand

Functional Procedures vs Hygiene Procedures

Pre-operative evaluation is done to determine which extremities have sufficient volitional control of the muscles to allow surgical procedures aimed at restoring function to the hand. Often severe deformities are present but there is insufficient or no volitional activity in the muscles. In these cases, contracture releases are done to decrease pain, to improve position and cosmesis of the hand, and to ease basic skin care and hygiene. The criteria for determining which procedures are most appropriate are summarized in Table 4 *(75)*.

Spastic Clenched Fist

The spastic clenched-fist deformity is common in spasticity involving the upper extremity. This pattern results from unmasking of the primitive grasp reflex. The fingers are typically clasped into the palm. Fingernails may dig into palmar skin and access to the palm for washing may be compromised. When access is chronically restricted, skin maceration, breakdown, and malodor occurs. Patients may complain of pain with any attempt to pry fingers open in order to gain palmar access. Some relaxation of finger tightness may occur if the wrist is positioned in extreme flexion. The deformity, however, is often accompanied by wrist flexion as well.

The degree of motor control may be masked by the severe amount of tone present in the finger flexors. Passive range of motion should be established first. Following this the patient is asked to open and close the fingers and to flex and extend the wrist. If no active wrist or finger extension is seen, it is still important to assess whether there appears to be active control of finger flexion. In the continuum of neurologic impairment and recovery, control of wrist and finger flexion is seen prior to active control of extension. A finger is placed in the patient's palm and the patient is asked to grasp. Often an increase in the pressure of grasp can be felt, indicating underlying muscle control.

Next an anesthetic block of the median nerve should be performed in the antecubital space to temporarily eliminate flexor tone. A block of the ulnar

Table 4
Criteria for Functional vs Nonfunctional Surgical Procedures

Criteria	Functional	Nonfunctional
Cognition	• Able to obey simple commands. • Able to cooperate with postoperative occupational therapy. • Able to retain what is taught from one session to another. • Able to assimilate newly taught activities into activities of daily living.	• Does not obey commands. • Uncooperative with occupational therapy efforts. • No retention of information from one session to the next. • Unable to use what was taught in daily activities.
Sensation	• Intact pain, light touch, and temperature sensation. • Two-point discrimination less than 10 mm. • Kinesthetic awareness.	• Absent pain, light touch, or temperature sensation. • Two-point discrimination greater than 10 mm. • Unable to reproduce body positions.
Spontaneous use of the Extremity	• Yes	• No
Motor control	• Able to move affected extremity volitionally. • Palpable movement in involved extremity. • EMG shows volitional control during manual muscle testing (Class I, II, or III).	• No volitional movement of extremity. • No movement palpable in involved extremity. • Continuous, stretch response or absent EMG activity during manual muscle testing (Class IV, V, or VI).

Adapted with permission from refs. (5,28,75).

nerve in the cubital canal can supplement relaxation. With the flexor muscles relaxed the activity of the extensor muscles can be more accurately evaluated. When extensor control returns, it is generally seen in the extensor indicis proprius muscle first (75–78,87,98,121).

Muscles that contribute to the clenched fist deformity include FDS and FDP. If the PIP joints flex while the DIP joints remain extended, spasticity of FDS rather than FDP may be suspected. Dynamic EMG studies have shown that the FDS muscles exhibit a marked degree of spasticity while the

FDP muscles are often normal or minimally spastic *(75–78,87,98,121)*. Despite the marked increase in tone, it often has some underlying volitional control. The flexor profundus has less spasticity and better volitional control. Volitional control of the finger extensors is present in 50% of patients with spastic-flexion deformities.

The intrinsics may also be spastic along with the extrinsics but an intrinsic plus posture (i.e., combined metacarpal-phalangeal joint (MCP) flexion and PIP extension) is not seen because spastic extrinsic flexors dominate by flexing the PIP joints. Some degree of contracture of the extrinsics is typical of the chronically clenched fist. From the perspective of active functional potential, some degree of volitional control may also be present in either or both sets of extrinsic finger flexors. Spastic finger flexors may override and mask the patient's potential to extend the fingers. Sometimes a patient presents with spasticity in just one or two muscle slips of either FDP or FDS. For example, we have seen a number of cases of index-finger flexion traced to a spastic FDP muscle slip for that finger alone.

A variety of orthopedic options are available to treat these deformities. When dynamic EMG demonstrates volitional control in the extrinsic flexor muscles, fractional lengthening is indicated. In a hand with skin maceration and malodor from a clenched fist deformity in which no volitional movement is detected, more significant lengthening of the flexor tendons is required. In this situation a STP tendon transfer is performed.

FRACTIONAL LENGTHENING
OF THE FINGER FLEXORS IN A FUNCTIONAL HAND

Fractional lengthening of extrinsic finger flexors is performed through a longitudinal incision on the volar surface of the forearm, commonly at the same sitting with wrist-flexor lengthenings (Fig. 1). The PL tendon is divided if tight. The lengthening of the individual FDS and FDP tendons is performed by sharply incising the tendon fibers as they overly the muscle belly at the musculotendinous junction, allowing the tendon to slide distally. The FPL tendon is lengthened in an identical manner. This technique allows the tendons to lengthen with minimal scarring. By transecting the tendon over the muscle belly, no sutures are needed. This eliminates scarring from foreign-body reaction to suture material. The underlying support and vascularity of the muscle provides an optimal environment for the tendons to heal and reconstitute themselves.

Postoperatively no immobilization is used. The patient is begun on a program of active and active-assisted exercises on the first post-operative day. If the patient has significant pain or spasticity, a short volar splint can be used for comfort. The splint should be removed for exercise. In patients with limited motor control, it is often useful to use the splint to position the wrist while the patient exercises the fingers. This immediate active motion allows the flexor tendons to continue to lengthen in the postoperative period as necessary. Ultimately, the amount of flexor lengthening is determined for each individual muscle by its' underlying tone and control rather than by the surgeon's "educated guess" of tone while the patient is under anesthesia. Using this technique we have had marked improvement in functional results when compared to our previous regimen of postoperative immobilization. In cases where the motor control is very limited, extrinsic finger-flexor lengthening can be combined with wrist fusion.

SUPERFICIALIS TO PROFUNDUS TENDON TRANSFER
IN THE NON-FUNCTIONAL HAND

In a hand with skin maceration and malodor from a clenched fist deformity in which no volitional movement is detected, more significant lengthening of the flexor tendons is required. In this situation, a STP tendon transfer is performed (52,97,179,180). This provides a more cosmetically pleasing hand position, aids in hygiene by getting the fingers out of the palms, and provides, at best, a mass-action grasp pattern, and at least a passive restraint to extension.

The STP tendon transfer is performed through a volar incision that may be extended distally to allow release of the carpal tunnel and access to Guyon's Canal. The PL tendon is identified and transected. The four superficialis tendons are sutured together distally and then transected for the en masse transfer (52,97,179). The profundus tendons are sutured together proximally and then cut. The fingers are extended and the distal end of the superficialis tendons are then sutured en masse to the proximal end of the profundus tendons.

Several other surgical procedures are routinely done in combination with the STP tendon transfer to treat the concurrent deformities. A neurectomy of the motor branch of the ulnar nerve is needed to prevent an intrinsic plus deformity from developing (52,97,179–181). If an intrinsic contracture is seen at the time of surgery following the STP lengthening, then release of the intrinsics is also performed. A carpal-tunnel release is done to decompress the median nerve. To prevent a recurrent wrist-flexion deformity from occurring secondary to passive wrist flexion, the wrist must be stabilized (Fig. 2). Wrist-extensor tenodesis has been attempted but often will stretch out with time. A cock-up wrist splint can be worn but patient compliance is poor. A fusion of the wrist in 15° of extension provides the most reliable means of maintaining hand position and is now routinely performed. A proximal release of the thenar muscles is often needed to correct a thumb-in-palm deformity *(35,52,104,173,182–188)*. Post-operatively, the wrist is immobilized for 3 wk in a short arm splint that includes the fingers and thumb. A volar wrist splint is used until the wrist fusion is healed.

Spastic Thumb-In-Palm Deformity

The thumb-in-palm deformity is heterogeneous in appearance and may be secondary to spasticity of multiple muscles including the FPL muscle and the median and ulnar-innervated thenar muscles *(35,52,104,173,182–188)*. The thumb is held within the palm, the DIP joint of the thumb is commonly flexed, and the thumb is unable to function during key grasp or in three-jaw chuck grasp (i.e., in opposition to the pads of the index and third fingers). In addition, skin maceration and breakdown can occur if proper hygiene is prevented.

Clinically, spasticity of the FPL is indicated by flexion of the interphalangeal joint. Some patients may be able to extend the thumb if the wrist is flexed, suggesting that a spastic flexor pollicis longus (FPL) may be impeding active thumb extension when the wrist is more extended and FPL is tighter. The thumb-in-palm deformity may result from spastic activity in FPL, adductor pollicis (AP), and/or the thenar muscles, particularly flexor pollicis brevis. Adduction of the thumb metacarpal indicates spasticity of the AP muscle and possibly the first dorsal interosseous muscle. A quick stretch of the thumb into abduction will often elicit a clonic response. An anesthetic block of the ulnar nerve in Guyon's Canal at the wrist will temporarily eliminate intrinsic tone. This will demonstrate the presence of any myostatic contractures and will also confirm that the adductor pollicis was an offending muscle in the deformity. Contracture of the skin of the web space and interphalangeal joint contracture of the thumb may also develop over time. If some volitional potential in thumb extensors or thumb abductors is present, lengthening of the spastic FPL and AP will facilitate key grasp. Dynamic EMG and lidocaine blocks are helpful to elucidate the specifics of motor control.

Orthopedic treatment consists of fractional lengthening of the FPL at the myotendinous junction combined with a thenar muscle slide in which the origins of the thenar muscles are detached from the transverse palmar ligament while preserving the neurovascular pedicle. Fractional lengthening of the FPL at the myotendinous junction will improve thumb extension. This is generally performed in conjunction with wrist- or digital-flexor lengthening. In order to provide a functional lateral pinch, it is desirable to stabilize the interphalangeal joint of the thumb.

In those cases with a fixed adduction contracture, surgical lengthening of the thenar muscles is indicated *(35,52,104,173,182–188)*. Generally all of

Orthopedic Interventions

the thenar muscles are spastic or contracted and a proximal myotomy is required to reposition the thumb and decrease the underlying tone in order to improve pinch function. Distal releases are to be avoided as these often result in a hyperextension deformity of the metacarpophalangeal joint of the thumb *(182)*.

If the first dorsal interosseous muscle is contracted, a release is performed through a dorsal incision along the ulnar margin of the thumb metacarpal while protecting the radial sensory nerve. The origin of the first dorsal interosseus is released from its origin on the base of the first metacarpal. In persistent web-space contractures despite appropriate muscle releases, a Z-plasty of the thumb web space is indicated.

Post-operatively, the patient is immobilized in a thumb spica splint for 3 wk. Active therapy is initiated a few days after surgery. The splint is removed for therapy but used at other times to position the thumb.

Deformities from Intrinsic Spasticity

When spasticity of the extrinsic flexors is present, intrinsic muscle spasticity should also be expected *(35,52,97,104,181,190)*. However, intrinsic spasticity and contracture are frequently masked by the presence of extrinsic flexor spasticity or contracture. Extension of the fingers at the metacarpal-phalangeal joints may be blocked by spasticity of the interossei and lumbrical muscles of the hand. Another manifestation of intrinsic spasticity is the tendency to swan-neck or Boutonniere positioning of the fingers. When a release or tendon lengthening of the spastic extrinsic flexor muscles has already been done, an intrinsic positive deformity of the hand will be unmasked. These hand deformities can be painful and disfiguring. Such contractures often lead to maceration of the palmar skin and recurrent nail-bed infections from poor hygiene.

The degree of tension caused by the intrinsic muscles can be demonstrated by comparing the amount of proximal interphalangeal-joint flexion obtained with the metacarpal-phalangeal joints both flexed and extended. If there is less proximal interphalangeal-joint flexion with metacarpal-phalangeal joint extension, then the intrinsic tendons are tight. This test should be performed both before and after a lidocaine block of the ulnar nerve at the wrist in order to distinguish between intrinsic tone and contracture.

Boutonniere deformities are commonly associated with intrinsic spasticity. They result from a combination of intrinsic spasticity combined with FDS tone. Swan-neck deformities may also result from increased intrinsic tone. The central extensor band is relatively shortened relative to the lateral bands because of tension exerted by the intrinsics and long extensor. In both of these cases, care must be taken to distinguish between deformities caused by the intrinsic spasticity, which should improve with treatment and deformities resulting from the more usual mechanisms such as traumatic central-slip injury with lateral band subluxation or traumatic mallet finger, because if not caused by spasticity the deformity will not improve with treatment for spasticity.

Because it is impossible to fully delineate the relative contributions and balance of spasticity and contracture of the intrinsic and extrinsic muscles by clinical assessment alone, we routinely obtain dynamic EMG studies of the intrinsic muscles before embarking on treatment of hand deformities. This is especially important prior to considering any surgical intervention.

Three treatment options are available. The procedure chosen is based on considerations of contracture and the presence or absence of volitional activity in the intrinsic muscles. When no significant intrinsic contracture is present and dynamic EMG indicates that there is no volitional control in the intrinsic muscles, a neurectomy of the motor branches of the ulnar nerve in the palm is performed. The sensory branches are left intact to preserve protective sensation in the hand. When a contracture of the intrinsic muscles is present and the dynamic EMG study shows no volitional activity, a release is performed of the lateral bands of the extensor hood mechanism at the level of the proximal phalanx. In these cases, neurectomy of the motor branches of the ulnar nerve is done simultaneously to prevent recurrence of the intrinsic plus deformity from spasticity of the interosseous muscles. When there is either a dynamic or static intrinsic plus deformity but the EMG demonstrates volitional control, the interossei are released from their proximal origins on the metacarpals and allowed to slide distally *(190,191)*. A static deformity is one in which a myostatic contracture is present. A dynamic deformity is one where the deformity results mostly from increased tone with little or no fixed contracture.

The abductor digiti quinti muscle may contribute to a flexion deformity of the metacarpo-phalangeal joint of the fifth finger. Transecting the tendon within the muscle belly can fractionally lengthen the muscle. This allows lengthening while preserving the function of the muscle.

Intrinsic Minus Deformities

A less common deformity pattern is the intrinsic minus hand. In these patients the intrinsic muscles have normal or weakened tone, but there is spasticity of the extrinsic finger flexors. There may be increased tone in the extrinsic extensors as well. This pattern results in a claw-hand posture, with hyperextension of the metacarpophalangeal joints and flexion of the proximal and distal interphalangeal joints. Ulnar neuropathy must be considered as a possible diagnosis. Hyperextension contracture of the metacarpalphalangeal joint capsule is common. When present the contractures require surgical release. Treatment of this deformity may also require lengthening of the extrinsic digital flexors or STP transfers as described earlier.

Release of the dorsal capsule of the metacarpophalangeal joints from the metacarpal is often needed. Capsulodesis in which the palmar capsule is sutured to create a 40° flexion contracture of the metacarpalphalangeal joints may also be required to place the hand in a more functional and cosmetic position *(173,192)*. Postoperatively, the hand is splinted with the metacarpalphalgeal joints flexed for 3 wk.

Spastic Hip Deformities
Adduction Deformity
OBTURATOR NEURECTOMY

Scissoring of the legs in an ambulatory patient gives the patient a narrow base of support while standing and results in poor balance. A preoperative obturator nerve block will eliminate the adductor spasticity and allow assessment of the adduction contracture *(76,167)*. Alternately the patient can be examined at the time of surgery while under anesthesia to determine if a fixed myostatic contracture is present. When no fixed adduction contracture is present, transection of the anterior branches of the obturator nerve will denervate the adductors and allow the patient with a broader base of support *(1–5,11,32,49,51,57,76,80,84–86,89,105,113,122,125,130–132,134, 136,139,149,153,154,167,193–195,197–199)*. Commonly, a small contracture is found and the adductor longus muscle is released at the time of the obturator neurectomy.

A longitudinal incision is made directly over the adductor longus muscle. The adductor longus muscle is released and retracted. The anterior branch of the obturator nerve is transected over the muscle belly of the adductor brevis. Early gait training with weight bearing as tolerated is instituted in the post-operative period.

HIP-ADDUCTOR TENOTOMY

A hip-adduction contracture that interferes with nursing care and hygiene in a nonambulatory patient or excessive limb scissoring during attempted transfers and ambulation in a patient with active function are indications for surgical release *(1–5,11,32,49,51,57,76,80,84–86,89,105,113,122,125, 130–132,134,136,139,149,153,154,167,193–195,197–199)*.

In a severely spastic patient, a flexion contracture of the hip and knee commonly occurs in conjunction with an adduction contracture. As with any contracture, pre-operative radiographs should be obtained prior to performing soft-tissue releases in order to rule out the presence of heterotopic ossification or an underlying bony deformity that would prevent correction.

With the patient in the supine position, a longitudinal incision is made over the adductor longus muscle. The incision is placed distal to the groin crease to position the incision in a more hygienic location. A longitudinal incision is utilized in order to decrease tension on the wound edges as the leg is brought into a corrected position after surgery. The adductor longus muscle is dissected free and transected using electrocautery. The anterior branches of the obturator nerve are identified and transected. The adductor brevis and gracilis are released close to their origin on the pubis. The wound is closed over a drain.

Daily wound care is essential to prevent infection in this potentially contaminated area. The hips should be kept in abduction for 4 wk using casts or an abduction pillow splint to prevent recurrence of the deformity during wound healing.

Flexion Deformity

FUNCTIONAL RELEASE: PECTINEUS RELEASE WITH ILIOPSOAS RECESSION

Spasticity of the hip flexors can result in a crouched gait with compensatory knee flexion to maintain balance. This is a very costly deformity because it requires constant use of the quadriceps, hip extensor, and calf muscles to maintain upright posture. The energy requirement for the continuous firing of these muscles is extremely high. Few patients are able to remain ambulatory with this deformity.

The hip-flexor muscles are needed to advance the limb during gait *(76,107,114,122,128,130–132,134,139,194,199,200)*. Complete release of the hip flexors should be avoided in any patient with the potential to ambulate. Because the iliopsoas has capsular insertions, release of the iliopsoas tendon from the lesser trochanter of the femur does not provide a complete release. Release of the tendon from the lesser trochanter permits the iliopsoas to recess proximally, thereby diminishing its pull but retaining its function.

A medial approach to the hip is used *(167)*. A longitudinal incision is made overlying the adductor longus tendon beginning 3 cm distal to the pubic tubercle. A plane is bluntly developed between the adductor longus and gracilis muscles. The dissection is continued between the adductor brevis and adductor longus muscles. The anterior division of the obturator nerve is identified and protected. If an adduction deformity is also present, division of the adductor longus muscle is performed. This facilitates exposure of the deeper muscles. The pectineus muscle is identified, as it lies deep to the femoral vessels and medial to the adductor longus. The pectineus muscle is divided using electrocautery. The lesser trochanter of the femur can be palpated in the depth of the wound. The tendon of the iliopsoas is visualized by placing narrow reverse retractors above and below the lesser trochanter. The iliopsoas tendon is divided from the trochanter and allowed to retract proximally. The wound is closed over a drain.

Post operatively, the patient begins range of motion exercises and full weight-bearing gait training as tolerated. Prone lying and electrical stimulation of the gluteus maximus muscle are helpful to correct any residual hip-flexion deformity.

NONFUNCTIONAL RELEASE: COMPLETE HIP RELEASE FOR SEVERE CONTRACTURE

A hip-flexion contracture or severe spasticity in a nonambulatory patient causing poor hygiene or pressure sores that cannot be healed secondary to limited positioning of the patient are indications for surgical release *(1–5,11,32,49,51,57,76,80,84–86,89,105,113,122,125,130–132,134,136, 139,149,153,154,167,193–195,197–199)*.

An adduction contracture of the hip and a flexion deformity of the knee are commonly associated with a hip-flexion contracture in the severely spastic patient. These deformities are common in persons with traumatic brain injury, stroke, cerebral anoxia, and MS. As with any contracture, preoperative radiographs should be obtained prior to performing soft-tissue releases in order to rule out the presence of heterotopic ossification or an underlying bony deformity that would prevent correction.

When a severe adduction contracture of the hip is present, it may be necessary to perform a percutaneous release of the adductor longus tendon in the groin in order to position the patient adequately and prep for further surgery. Any flexion contracture of the knee should be corrected simultaneously to prevent the leg from positioning in flexion and causing a recurrent and more resistant contracture.

With the patient in the supine position, an anterior incision is made beginning 2.5 cm distal to the anterior superior iliac spine and is carried distally following the sartorius muscle for a short distance *(165)*. The incision should not extend over the iliac crest because the patient will be expected to lie in the prone position post-operatively to gain further correction of the deformity. The lateral femoral cutaneous nerve is identified as it passes distal to the anterior superior iliac spine and protected. The sartorius muscle is detached from its origin on the anterior superior iliac spine. The rectus femoris muscle is released from its origin on the anterior inferior spine of the pelvis. The femoral nerve and vessels are gently retracted medially to expose the iliopsoas muscle on the anterior aspect of the hip. The iliopsoas and pectineus muscles are carefully divided over the pelvic brim using the electrocautery to diminish post-operative bleeding. Because the iliopsoas has capsular insertions, release of the iliopsoas tendon from the lesser trochanter of the femur does not provide a complete release. The tensor fascia lata and the anterior portion of the gluteus medius and gluteal aponeurosis may be released from the iliac crest if necessary. The hip-joint capsule is not released.

In a severely contracted patient, care must be taken to identify all structures prior to release because the anatomy is frequently distorted by the long-standing deformity. A large dead space is left after releasing the hip-flexor muscles and a drain should be used. Careful wound closure and a compressive dressing are helpful in preventing post-operative infection.

As with release of other contracted joints, approx 50% of the deformity will be corrected at the time of surgery. Daily wound care will help prevent infection in this area where bacterial contamination is likely and a large dead space remains following surgery. Placing the patient in a prone position three times a day for increasing periods and gentle stretching exercises will assist in correcting any residual hip-flexion deformity. When a release of a knee-flexion contracture has been performed simultaneously, the weight of the long leg cast will also provide a correcting force. Sitting in a wheelchair is allowed for short periods.

On occasion, a patient is seen with chronic hip subluxation or dislocation from severe and very long-standing hip-flexion and adduction spasticity. This is most common with anoxic encephalopathy. The hip joint has advanced osteoarthrosis and is painful. The hip pain increases the spasticity, which in turn causes more pain in a circular fashion. In these cases, it is usually necessary to resect the femoral head at the same time as performing a complete muscle release. It is not advisable to merely resect the femoral head because this will not treat the spasticity and a more severe leg deformity can occur. After this surgery it is very important to maintain the leg in a neutral position for at least 3 mo while soft tissue healing occurs. This can be done with bilateral short leg casts connected with a bar to hold the legs in neutral rotation and slight abduction. If the hip is allowed to position in flexion, abduction, and external rotation while healing occurs, the ability to sit in a chair may be severely compromised.

Extension Deformity

PROXIMAL HAMSTRING RELEASE

Following a severe brainstem injury, spasticity of the extensor muscles of the leg may result in a hip-extension contracture. Although uncommon, an extension contracture will interfere with a person's ability to sit. When good sitting posture cannot be obtained, a release of the proximal origin of the hamstring muscles is indicated *(92,167,201–203)*.

The patient is placed in the prone position for surgery. A longitudinal incision is made over the posterior thigh beginning at the gluteal fold. The posterior femoral cutaneous nerve is identified and protected. The distal edge of the gluteus maximus is lifted proximally to expose the underlying hamstring muscles. The biceps femoris, semimembranosus and semitendinosus muscles are then detached from their origins on the ischial tuberosity and allowed to retract distally. Postoperatively the patient is started on gentle passive range-of-motion exercises to regain hip flexion.

Spastic Knee Deformities
Flexion Deformity
DISTAL HAMSTRING LENGTHENING

A knee-flexion deformity is caused by over-activity of the hamstring muscles *(76,99,108,139,140,204,205)*. When the knee-flexion deformity is less than 60° and the patient has documented volitional activity in the hamstring muscles, then a lengthening procedure is done. This will correct the flexion deformity while preserving the function of the hamstrings.

With the patient in the supine position, a longitudinal incision of approx 8 cm is made on the lateral aspect of the distal thigh just proximal to the knee joint. The peroneal nerve is isolated and protected and the biceps femoris tendon is divided obliquely as it overlies the muscle belly. This allows the tendon to slide distally while still maintaining continuity of the muscle. The portion of the iliotibial band that is posterior to the axis of knee flexion is also divided transversely.

A longitudinal incision is then made on the medial aspect of the distal thigh *(90)*. The tendons of the gracilis and semimembranosus are isolated and fractionally lengthened at the myotendinous junction by making an oblique cut in the tendon as it overlies the muscle belly. The semitendinosus tendon has a very short myotendinous junction, which does not permit fractional lengthening. This tendon is simply transected.

After surgery the extremity is immobilized in a long leg cast. Approximately 50% correction of the knee-flexion deformity can be expected at the time of surgery. Further correction is limited owing to tethering of the neurovascular structures. The extremity is casted in the position of knee extension it assumes while being supported under the heel, without attempting forced extension. Forced knee extension can result in limb ischemia. The long leg cast is changed weekly until full knee extension has been obtained. Splints are used at night for an additional 4 wk to maintain correction.

DISTAL HAMSTRING RELEASE

In a nonambulatory patient with a marked increase in hamstring muscle tone, knee-flexion contractures result *(1,2,49,76,85,99,125,130, 131, 139, 142, 147,149,167,195,199,204–206)*. Spasticity is frequently present. When severe spasticity of the hamstring muscles or a knee-flexion contracture of greater than 60° is present, attempts to correct the knee position with casting or bracing may result in posterior subluxation of the tibia. Distal release of the hamstring tendons does not prevent a patient from becoming ambulatory. If the hip-flexion contracture or spasticity is not corrected at the same time as the hamstring release, a recurrent knee-flexion contracture is likely to develop that is very resistant to surgical correction.

With the patient in the supine position, a longitudinal incision of approx 8 cm is made on the lateral aspect of the distal thigh just proximal to the knee joint. The peroneal nerve is isolated and protected and the biceps femoris muscle and tendon are divided just proximal to its insertion using the electrocautery. The portion of the iliotibial band that is posterior to the axis of knee flexion is also divided transversely.

A longitudinal incision is then made on the medial aspect of the knee and the tendons of the gracilis, semimembranosus, and semitendinosus are isolated and divided. The semitendinosus tendon is usually surrounded by a layer of fat and can closely resemble the posterior tibial nerve. The fatty tissue should be dissected from the tendon to confirm its identity prior to transection. In severe contractures, release of the sartorius muscle is also performed. By using electrocautery, the procedure is easily performed without a tourniquet, which facilitates localization and protection of the posterior tibial artery, vein, and nerve. Following localization of the neurovascular bundle, any remaining restricting bands are divided as required. The posterior fascia at the knee is often thickened, limiting extension, and may require release. The posterior joint capsule may need to be released in long-standing contractures. The joint capsule is stripped from the distal posterior femur using a periosteal elevator. The cruciate ligaments are not divided. If more correction is required, a closing wedge osteotomy can be performed. A closing wedge will allow for some shortening of the femur and release some tension from the neurovascular structures and posterior skin.

Post-op management is the same as for hamstring lengthening.

Extension Deformity

RECTUS FEMORIS TO GRACILIS TRANSFER FOR DYNAMIC STIFF-KNEE GAIT

Patients with a stiff-knee gait are unable to flex the knee during the swing phase of gait. The deformity is a dynamic one meaning that it only occurs during walking. There is no restriction of passive knee motion and the patient does not have difficulty sitting. Usually the knee is maintained in extension throughout the gait cycle. Toe drag, which is likely in the early swing phase, may cause the patient to trip, thus, balance and stability are also affected *(1–3,5,76,91,108,131,138,140,142–146,148,150,152,167, 197,206)*. The limb appears to be functionally longer. Circumduction of the involved limb, hiking of the pelvis, and/or contralateral limb vaulting may occur as compensatory maneuvers.

A gait study with dynamic EMG should be done preoperatively to document the activity of the individual muscles of the quadriceps. Dyssynergic activity is commonly seen in the rectus femoris from pre-swing through terminal swing throughout the gait cycle. Abnormal activity is also common in the rectus intermedius. If knee flexion is improved with a block of the rectus femoris or vastus intermedius, the rationale for surgical intervention is strengthened. Any equinus deformity of the foot should be corrected prior to evaluation of a stiff-knee gait because equinus causes a knee-extension force during stance. Because the amount of knee flexion during swing is directly related to the speed of walking, the patient should be able to ambulate with a reasonable velocity in order to benefit from surgery. Hip-flexion strength is also needed for a good result because it is the forward momentum of the leg that normally provides the inertial force to flex the knee. In the past a selective release of the rectus femoris or rectus and vastus intermedius was done to remove their inhibition of knee flexion. On average, a 15° improvement in peak knee flexion was seen after surgery. Transfer of the rectus femoris to a hamstring tendon not only removes it as a deforming muscle force; it also converts the rectus into a corrective (flexion) force. This procedure provides improved knee flexion over selective release.

A longitudinal incision is made on the anterior thigh from 10 cm above patella to the middle aspect of the patella. The rectus femoris muscle is dissected free from the other vasti muscles both proximally and distally. Dissection is carried distally to the patella where a strip of periosteum is also removed from the patella to gain additional length. If significant spasticity was seen in the vasti muscles on the dynamic EMG study, these muscles are fractionally lengthened by transecting their tendons as they overlay the muscle belly.

A second incision is made over the medial hamstrings just proximal to the knee. The gracilis tendon is identified. A subcutaneous tunnel is then made between the two incisions and through the intermuscular septum. The distal end of the rectus femoris tendon is passed through the tunnel to the medial wound with the knee flexed 90° and the femur externally rotated. The rectus femoris tendon is sewn to the gracilis tendon by means of a Pulvertaft weave. We prefer to use the gracilis as our transfer site because of the strong tendon repair possible as opposed to the sartorius. The gracilis also provides a more posterior attachment of the transfer, which, in turn, increases the flexor moment created. The rectus muscle is transferred under considerable tension. The knee should then be gently extended to be certain that full knee extension could still be obtained. The location of the transfer has not been shown to affect range of motion of the knee *(145)*.

The patient is placed in a knee immobilizer splint for 1 wk after surgery to prevent a knee-flexion deformity from occurring secondary to the tension and discomfort of the transfer. The patient can begin gait training in the immobilizer on the first postoperative day. Because of the good fixation into the gracilis tendon, knee range of motion and ambulation without the splint is started 1 wk later. A marching gait pattern is stressed during therapy to facilitate knee flexion during swing.

QUADRICEPS LENGTHENING

After a brainstem injury, extensor spasticity can cause a knee extension contracture. This is usually seen in combination with a hip-extension contracture. Both deformities result in problems with sitting. The knee-extension deformity can be corrected by lengthening the quadriceps. Quadriceps weakness is not a problem in these patients because they are not ambulatory. In the past a V-Y lengthening of the quadriceps tendon was routinely done *(49,167)*. We have more recently been performing a fractional lengthening of the individual muscles of the quadriceps. This procedure is more easily performed and has less morbidity than the V-Y lengthening. It also does not cause a patella baja deformity. Even severe hyperextension knee deformities can be corrected with this procedure.

A longitudinal incision is made over the anterior thigh at the junction of the middle and distal third of the quadriceps muscle. The rectus femoris tendon is easily dissected free from the vasti at this level. There is a long overlap of the rectus muscle and tendon on the undersurface of the muscle belly. The tendon is sharply transected over the muscle belly leaving the underlying muscle intact. The rectus tends to be the most contracted muscle and two cuts are often made in the tendon. Beneath the rectus femoris muscle the myotendinous junctions of the vastus intermedius, medialis, and lateralis muscles are easily located. Each tendon is individually transected over the muscle belly. The knee is then gently and slowly flexed to at least 120°. The quadriceps muscles can be seen to lengthen as the knee is flexed. The wound is closed in a routine manner. Postoperatively, passive knee flexion is done several times daily to maintain knee flexion. The patient is permitted to sit as much as tolerated. Immobilization is not needed.

Spastic Foot and Ankle Deformities

Equinus

ACHILLES TENDON LENGTHENING

Equinus is the most common spastic deformity causing gait difficulty *(76,93,94,103,105,107,112,117,125,126,128,133–135,137,139,193,207–211)*. Equinus results from over-activity or premature activity of the gastrocnemius and soleus muscles. Surgical lengthening of the Achilles tendon is indicated when the patient foot and ankle position is not adequately controlled by an orthosis or when attempting to make the patient brace-free. Adequate lengthening of the Achilles tendon can be performed using the Hoke triple hemisection technique percutaneously (Fig. 3). With the foot held in maximum dorsiflexion, three percutaneous hemi-transections of the Achilles tendon are made using a #11 knife blade. If a varus deformity of the foot is present, the proximal and distal cuts are made in the medial half of the tendon and the center cut is placed laterally. The foot is then pushed into dorsiflexion, allowing the tendon to lengthen.

Postoperative management requires 6 wk of rigid immobilization. We begin by using a short leg walking cast for 2 wk. We then use a cam walker boot for the next 4 wk. At this time we allow the patient to remove the boot once daily for bathing, provided that they do not stand or walk without the boot. After this the patient uses an ankle foot orthosis (AFO) for an additional 6 wk.

Varus

SPLIT ANTERIOR TIBIAL TENDON TRANSFER (SPLATT)

Varus deformities most commonly occur as the result of increased and inappropriate activity of the tibialis anterior muscle. When dynamic EMG has documented the tibialis anterior to be the cause of varus, the deformity is corrected by a split anterior tibial tendon transfer (SPLATT). The SPLATT maintains the half of the tendon on the medial aspect of the foot and transfers the other half of the tibialis anterior tendon to the lateral side of the foot (Fig. 4) *(3–5,76,80,93,112,115,117,126,127,133,135,137,139,141,147, 152–154,175,193,197)*. Because equinus and toe curling usually accompany the varus deformity, a lengthening of the Achilles tendon should be

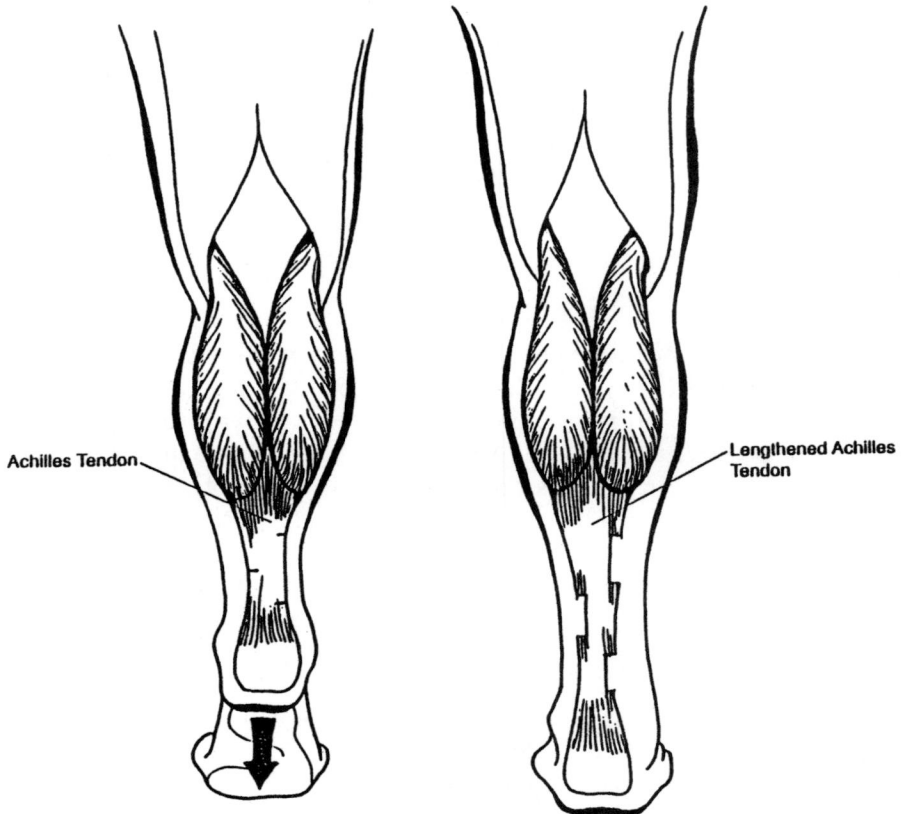

Fig. 3. Diagram of the Hoke technique for Achilles-tendon lengthening. Reprinted with permission from ref. *(166)*.

performed first and the toe-flexor tendons divided. An incision is made over the distal insertion of the tibialis anterior tendon on the medial aspect of the foot. The lateral half of the tendon is sharply divided from its insertion. A nonabsorbable suture is placed in the end of the tendon as a tag for ease of handling. The suture can be used later to help secure the tendon in its new location in the cuboid bone.

A second incision is made approx 10 cm proximal to the ankle joint just lateral to the crest of the tibia over the tibialis anterior muscle. An opening is made in the fascia overlying the tibialis anterior. We use a long twisted wire loop as a tendon passer. The wire loop is passed under the fascia and follows the tibialis anterior tendon to the incision on the medial foot. The suture in the free end of the tendon is passed through the wire loop and is

Orthopedic Interventions

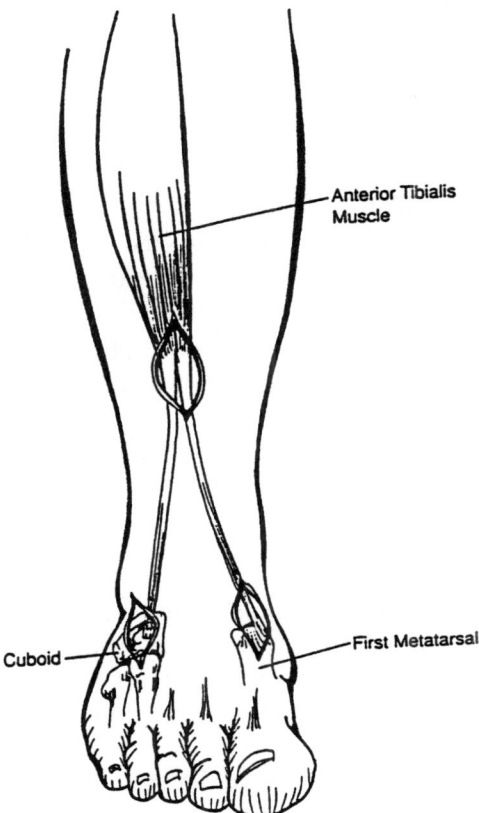

Fig. 4. The split anterior tibialis tendon transfer (SPLATT) for correction of varus caused by overactivity of the tibialis anterior muscle. Reprinted with permission from ref. *(166)*.

pulled into the proximal wound. This suture is used to pull the free end of the tendon into the proximal wound thereby splitting the tibialis anterior tendon and a portion of the muscle belly. The tendon is wrapped in a saline moistened sponge temporarily.

A third incision is then made on the lateral aspect of the foot. The lateral face of the cuboid is subperiosteally exposed. A drill is used to make a tunnel through the cuboid for anchoring of the lateral portion of the tendon. A subcutaneous tunnel is created from the proximal wound to the lateral incision using a long forceps. The lateral arm of the tibialis tendon is passed through this subcutaneous passage to protrude from the lateral incision. The tibialis anterior tendon is secured on the lateral side of the foot through the tunnel in the cuboid bone and sutured to itself to hold the foot in a neutral position. When there is marked osteoporosis the cuboid bone may be too weak to use for the transfer. In this situation the tibialis anterior tendon can be interwoven into the peroneus brevis using a Pulvertaft technique.

Postoperative management is the same as for hamstring lengthening.

TIBIALIS ANTERIOR LENGTHENING

Occasionally a mild varus deformity is seen during walking that is owing to a moderate increase in tibialis anterior activity. In this situation a myotendinous lengthening is sufficient to control the varus deformity. An incision is made over the tibialis anterior muscle approx 10 cm proximal to the ankle joint. The fascial sheath of the tibialis anterior is opened and the tendon is transected over the muscle belly of the tibialis anterior, thereby allowing the muscle to lengthen fractionally. If this is the only procedure performed, no immobilization is needed after surgery. Full weight-bearing ambulation is allowed immediately.

TIBIALIS POSTERIOR LENGTHENING

In approx 10% of stroke and brain-injured patients the tibialis posterior muscle is also spastic and can contributes to the varus deformity *(3,5, 11,76,105,107,126,131,137,141,152–154,193)*. Clinically this is evidenced by the increased heel varus in addition to the forefoot varus caused by the tibialis anterior muscle.

When spasticity of the tibialis posterior muscle is present, a myotendinous lengthening of the tendon is performed posterior and slightly proximal to the medial malleolus. Complete release of the tibialis posterior tendon is not recommended as a planovalgus deformity may occur secondarily.

EXTENSOR HALLUCIS LENGTHENING

With the equinovarus deformity the patient may also have a hitchhiker's great toe secondary to spasticity of the extensor hallucis longus (EHL) tendon *(3,5,122,141,207)*. The EHL also contributes to the varus deformity of the forefoot. Many of these patients complain of shoe wear problems from pressure of the hallux against the shoe. A 3-cm incision is made over the anterior leg beginning 10 cm proximal to the ankle joint. The EHL muscle is identified and fractionally lengthened by transecting the tendon as it overlies the muscle belly. If no other surgical procedures are needed, then no immobilization is used after surgery. Most commonly the EHL is lengthened in combination with a SPLATT procedure. In this situation the postoperative protocol of the SPLATT is followed.

Valgus

Peroneal Lengthening

Spastic valgus foot deformities are less common in the stroke and brain-injured population. The deformity can result from over activity of the peroneus longus, peroneus brevis, or both *(117)*. Dynamic EMG is used to determine which muscles are causing the deformity.

If the deformity is not severe, a myotendinous lengthening can be considered. An incision is made over the lateral leg approx 10 centimeters above the ankle joint. The fascia of the lateral compartment is opened and the offending peroneal muscles are fractionally lengthened. If no other procedures are performed simultaneously, no immobilization is needed after surgery and unrestricted ambulation is allowed.

Peroneus Longus Transfer

A spastic valgus deformity may be seen from over activity of the peroneus longus muscle. This can occur as an isolated deformity but more commonly occurs in combination with spastic equinovarus *(117,167)*. In the "spastic combination foot" deformity, equinovarus is observed during swing phase from premature and prolonged firing of the tibialis anterior and gastroc-soleus muscles. The planovalgus deformity occurs during stance from the inappropriate activity of the peroneus longus muscle. The pronation deformity may be accentuated by a premorbid tendency to flat foot or by the presence of an equinus contracture.

When a severe spastic valgus occurs, the peroneus longus tendon is transferred through the interosseous membrane to the tarsal navicular bone to support the longitudinal arch of the foot during stance (Fig. 5). A small incision is made on the lateral border of the foot just proximal to the base of the fifth metatarsal. The peroneus longus and brevis tendons are identified. The peroneus longus tendon is divided obtaining maximal length. A second incision is made over the lateral leg approx 10 cm above the ankle. The peroneus longus muscle is identified and the distal end of the tendon is pulled proximally into this wound. A third incision is made over the anterior leg 10 cm proximal to the ankle. Dissection is carried down to expose the interosseus membrane. A window is made in the interosseus membrane and the peroneus longus tendon is passed through to the anterior leg wound. A final incision is made over the navicular bone on the medial side of the foot. A drill is used to create a tunnel through the navicular bone. The peroneus longus tendon is then passed subcutaneously to the medial foot using a long forceps. The end of the tendon is passed through the tunnel in the navicular and secured back to itself using nonabsorbable sutures. The tendon is secured to hold the foot in a neutral alignment.

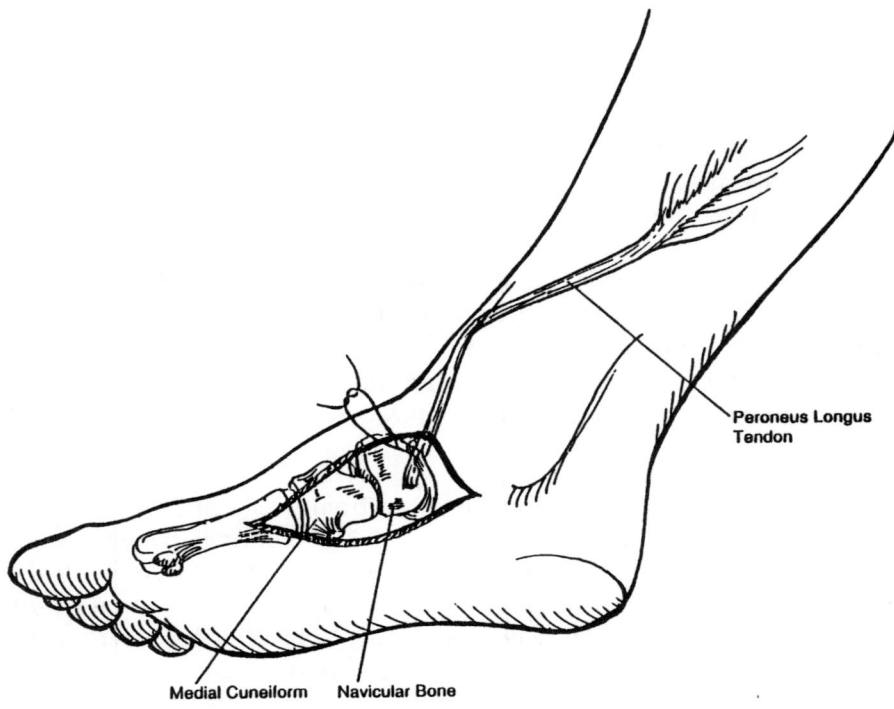

Fig. 5. Transfer of the peroneus longus tendon to the tarsal navicular for correction of a severe spastic valgus foot deformity caused by spasticity of the peroneus longus muscle. Reprinted with permission from ref. *(166)*.

When a combined deformity is present, a SPLATT is performed along with a tendo-Achilles lengthening (TAL) and toe-flexor release (TFR) to correct the swing-phase abnormalities.

Postoperative management is the same as for the SPLATT transfer.

Cavus

STEINDLER STRIPPING (RELEASE OF THE PLANTAR STRUCTURES)

A cavus deformity is defined as an elevated arch that does not flatten with weight bearing. The deformity is probably a result of muscle imbalance of both the intrinsic and extrinsic muscles of the foot *(109)*. If the foot is supple, a soft-tissue procedure can be done; however, if the foot is rigid, a bony fusion must be done.

The plantar fascia is exposed through a medial foot incision. Care is taken to identify and preserve the medial calcaneal nerve branches to the heel pad.

Orthopedic Interventions

The origin of the fascia is released under direct vision. The origin of the abductor hallucis is identified and elevated from the tuberosity of the os calcis. The origin of the flexor brevis and intrinsic muscles of the foot are also released. The foot is then passively corrected and placed into a short leg cast for 2 wk. Weight-bearing can be started on the first postoperative day. Because this procedure is usually done in combination with the SPLATT operation, the SPLATT protocol is generally followed.

Triple Arthrodesis

For severe rigid bony deformities, a triple arthrodesis is done to correct the foot *(212)*. Most commonly this procedure is being done in combination with a planter release and the SPLATT procedure.

An incision is made over the lateral foot from the tip of the fibula to base of the fourth metatarsal. The extensor brevis and fat pad are elevated to expose the calcaneo-cuboid joint and the sinus tarsi. The Superior process of the distal calcaneous is removed using an oscillating saw to facilitate exposure. The bone is saved to use as graft later. A lamina spreader is inserted between the talus and calcaneous to further expose the joint surfaces. The posterior and middle facets of the subtalar joint are denuded of cartilage. The calcaneal cuboid joint is also exposed and the cartilage is removed. The lateral talo-navicular joint is exposed and prepared through the same incision. A small medial incision is made over the talo-navicular joint and the remaining cartilage is removed. At this time the three joints are fixed with three large-diameter cannulated screws confirmed by fluoroscopic guidance. Postoperatively the patient is placed in a short leg walking cast for 6 wk. With the rigid fixation provided by the screw fixation, weight bearing is permissible. If sufficient bony union is seen at 6 wk after surgery, the patient can begin using a rigid, nonarticulated AFO for ambulation. The fusion is protected until full bony healing is seen.

Claw Foot

Toe Flexor Release

Toe clawing or curling is a common accompaniment of over-activity of the gastrocnemius muscles. Toe curling is caused by over-activity of the flexor hallucis longus and flexor digitorum muscle as well as the short toe flexor and occasionally the intrinsic muscles of the foot *(125)*. A longitudinal incision is made on the plantar surface of each toe at the metatarsal phalangeal joint level. The flexor tendons are identified and released under direct vision. This procedure is commonly done in combination with an Achilles tendon lengthening because bringing the foot into a plantigrade position will worsen the toe curling. When an Achilles tendon lengthening has been performed, the foot must be immobilized for 3 mo as described earlier.

Calf Paresis

TRANSFER THE FLEXOR DIGITUROM LONGUS TO OS CALCIS

Muscle paresis (weakness) is an integral part of UMN syndrome. Lengthening the Achilles tendon to correct an equinus deformity weakens the gastrocnemius-soleus muscle group, which was already weak as a consequence of the underlying UMN syndrome. This calf paresis generally results in the need of an AFO during ambulation. Thus transfer of the digitorum longus muscle can be done in order to augment calf strength. With this transfer, more patients eventually achieve brace-free ambulation *(205)*. In prior studies of treatment of a spastic equinovarus foot deformity, 30% of patients were able to walk safely without an AFO *(124)*. When transfer of the FDL to the os calcis augments the gastroc-soleus strength, 70% of patients achieve brace-free ambulation *(205)*.

A 4-cm incision is made on the medial border of the foot dorsal and parallel to the abductor hallucis muscle. The abductor hallucis is reflected plantarward from the base of the first metatarsal and the flexor hallicus longus (FHL) and flexor digitorum longus (FDL) are isolated through the deep fascia at the master knot of Henry. At this level the FDL has not yet split into four tendons and the FHL is easily dissected free. If the flexor brevis tendons are to be released simultaneously to correct toe curling, they are released prior to transecting the FDL tendon. The FHL and FDL are dissected at the knot of Henry.

A 5-cm incision is then made at the medial supramalleolar region where the muscle belly of the FDL is isolated with its tendon and delivered through the medial supramalleolar incision. A 1-cm incision is made over the medial posterior superior oscalcis. A 3/8-inch drill is used to create a tunnel through the posterior superior calcaneous exiting on the lateral side. A small incision is made over the lateral malleolus at the exit site of the drill. A suture ligature is placed in the FDL and the tendon is passed subcutaneously to the medial heel wound. The tendon is then passed through the tunnel created in the calcaneous from medially to laterally. A twisted wire loop is used to first pull the suture ligature through the tunnel. A Sta-tek (Simmer, Warsaw, IN) suture anchor is drilled into the lateral os-calcis and the transferred tendon is securely tied with the foot in maximum dorsiflexion to prevent a recurrent equinus deformity.

Postoperatively the patient is placed in a short leg walking cast at surgery holding the foot in a neutral position. Gait training can be started on the first postoperative day allowing the patient to bear full weight on the foot as tolerated. The cast is kept on the foot for 2 wk. Two weeks after surgery the cast and sutures are removed. The patient is then placed in a cam walker boot for the next 4 wk. With reliable patients we allow the cam boot to be removed once daily for washing and skin care. The foot must be maintained in a neutral position while the boot is off and no weight is allowed on the foot. Six weeks after surgery the patient begins using a nonarticulated, moderately rigid AFO for an additional 6 wk. The patient must sleep wearing AFO during this time to protect the foot from an inadvertent stretch. At 3 mo after surgery, the brace can be removed for sleeping and gait training. The AFO can be discontinued if and when the patient has established sufficient strength in the calf muscles to permit safe walking.

Foot Deformities in the Nonambulatory Patient

Severe deformities of the feet are common in patients with spasticity. Even in the nonambulatory patient, these deformities cause significant problems. The complications include pressure sores, inability to wear shoes or protective footwear, and difficulty positioning the feet on wheelchair supports for improved sitting balance. These deformities should be surgically corrected to maintain a plantigrade foot.

The most common deformity is equinovarus with claw toes. As in the more functional patient, muscle balance must be achieved by performing the SPLATT, an Achilles-tendon lengthening, and release of the toe-flexor tendons and lumbrical insertions. Because the spasticity is often extreme and of long duration, it is commonly necessary to perform a release of the plantar fascia to correct a cavus deformity as well as a triple arthrodesis in conjunction with the tendon transfer.

REFERENCES

1. Keenan, M. A. (1996) Stroke, in *Orthopaedic Knowledge Update 5* (Kasser J.R., ed.), American Academy of Orthopaedic Surgeons, Rosemont, IL p. 689.
2. Keenan, M. A. E. (1996) Rehabilitation of the neurologically disabled patient, in *Neurosurgery,* Vol. (Wilkens, RHaR, S. S, ed.), McGraw-Hill Publishers, New York, NY, p. 445–457.
3. Mayer, N., Esquenazi, A., and Wannstedt, G. (1996) Surgical planning for upper motoneuron dysfunction: the role of motor control evaluation. *J. Head Trauma Rehabil.* **11,** 37–58.
4. Perry, J. and Keenan, M. A. E. (1989) Rehabilitation of the neurologically disabled patient, in *Neurology and General Medicine,* (Aminoff, M. J., ed.), Churchill Livingstone Publishers, New York, p. 747–778.
5. Mayer, N. H., Esquenazi, A., and Keenan, M. A. E. (1996) Analysis and management of spasticity, contracture, and impaired motor control, in *Medical*

Rehabilitation of Traumatic Brain Injury, (Horn L. J. and Zasler N. D., eds.), Hanley & Belfus, Inc., Philadelphia, p. 411–458.
6. Ayers, D. C., Pellegrini, V. D., and Evarts, C.M. (1991) Prevention of heterotopic ossification in high-risk patients by radiation therapy. *Clin. Orthop.* **263,** 87–93.
7. Beck, E. R. and Bell, K.R. (1995) Deep venous thrombosis in the spastic upper limb. *Brain Inj.* **9,** 413–416.
8. Beredjiklian, P. K., Iannotti, J. P., Norris, T. R., and Williams, G.R. (1998) Operative treatment of malunion of a fracture of the proximal aspect of the humerus [In Process Citation]. *J. Bone Joint Surg [Am.]* **80,** 1484–1487.
9. Bidner, S. M., Rubins, I. M., Desjardins, J. V., Zukor, D. J., and Goltzman, D. (1990) Evidence for a humoral mechanism for enhanced osteogenesis after head injury. *J. Bone Joint Surg. [Am.]* **72,** 1144.
10. Bontke, C. F. and Cobble, N. D. (1991) Rehabilitation in brain disorders. Clinical manifestations and medical issues. *Arch Phys Med Rehabil.* **72,** S320–S313.
11. Bontke, C. F. and Cobble, N.D. (1991) Rehabilitation in brain disorders. Clinical manifestations and medical issues. *Arch Phys Med Rehabil.* **72,** S320.
12. Booth, B. J., Doyle, M., and Montgomery, J. (1960,1983) Serial casting for the management of spasticity in the head injured adult. *Phys. Ther.* **63,** 1960–1966.
13. Botte, M. J., Keenan, M. A., Abrams, R. A., von Schroeder, H. P., Gellman, H., and Mooney, V. (1997) Heterotopic ossification in neuromuscular disorders. *Orthopedics* **20,** 335.
14. Botte, M. J., Keenan, M. A. E., and Gelberman, R.H. (1998) Volkmann's ischemic contracture of the upper extremity. *Hand Clin.* **14,** 483–497.
15. Botte, M. J., Nickel, V. L., and Akeson, W. H. (1988) Spasticity and contracture. *Clin. Orthop.* **233,** 7–18.
16. Botte, M. J., Nickel, V. L., and Akeson, W. H. (1988) Spasticity and contracture. *Clin. Orthop.* **233,** 7–18.
17. Braun, R. M., West, F., Mooney, V., Nickel, V. L., Roper, B., and Caldwell, C. (1971) Surgical treatment of the painful shoulder contracture in the stroke patient. *J. Bone Joint Surg [Am].* **53,** 1307–1312.
18. Braun, R. M., West, F., Mooney, V., Nickel, V. L., Roper, B., and Caldwell, C. (1971) Surgical treatment of the painful shoulder contracture in the stroke patient. *J. Bone Joint Surg [Am].* **53,** 1307–1312.
19. Charnley, G., Judet, T., de Loubresse, C. G., and Piriou, P. (1996) Articulated radial head replacement and elbow release for post head-injury heterotopic ossification. *J. Orthop. Trauma* **10,** 68.
20. Chua, H. C., Tan, C. B., and Tjia, H. (1997) A case of bilateral ulnar nerve palsy in a patient with traumatic brain injury and heterotopic ossification. *Singapore Med. J.* **38,** 447, 448.
21. Citta-Pietrolungo, T. J., Alexander, M. A., and Steg, N.L. (1992) Early detection of heterotopic ossification in young patients with traumatic brain injury. *Arch. Phys. Med. Rehabil.* **73,** 258–262.
22. Cosgrove, J. L., Vargo, M., and Reidy, M.E. (1989) A prospective study of peripheral nerve lesions occurring in traumatic brain-injured patients [see comments]. *Am. J. Phys. Med. Rehabil.* **68,** 15–17.

23. Fitzsimmons, A. S., O'Dell, M. W., Guiffra, L. J., and Sandel, M.E. (1993) Radial nerve injury associated with traumatic myositis ossificans in a brain injured patient. *Arch. Phys. Med. Rehabil.* **74,** 770–773.
24. Frischhut, B., Stockhammer, G., Saltuari, L., Kadletz, R., and Bramanti, P. (1993) Early removal of periarticular ossifications in patients with head injury. *Acta Neurol. (Napoli)* **15,** 114–122.
25. Garland, D. E. (1988) Clinical observations on fractures and heterotopic ossification in the spinal cord and traumatic brain injured populations. *Clin. Orthop.* **233,** 86–101.
26. Garland, D. E. (1991) A clinical perspective on common forms of acquired heterotopic ossification. *Clin. Orthop.* 13–29.
27. Garland, D. E. (1991) Surgical approaches for resection of heterotopic ossification in traumatic brain-injured adults. *Clin. Orthop.* 59–70.
28. Garland, D. E. (1992) Evidence for a humoral mechanism for enhanced osteogenesis after head injury [letter; comment]. *J. Bone Joint Surg. [Am].* **74,** 152, 153.
29. Garland, D., Alday, B., and Venos, K. (1984) Heterotopic ossification and HLA antigens. *Arch. Phys. Med. Rehabil.* **65,** 531, 532.
30. Garland, D. E., Blum, C. E., and Waters, R. L. (1980) Periarticular heterotopic ossification in head-injured adults. Incidence and location. *J. Bone Joint Surg. [Am].* **62,** 1143–1146.
31. Garland, D. E., Hanscom, D. A., Keenan, M. A., Smith, C., and Moore, T. (1985) Resection of heterotopic ossification in the adult with head trauma. *J. Bone Joint Surg. [Am].* **67,** 1261–1269.
32. Garland, D. E., Keenan, M. A. (1983) Orthopedic strategies in the management of the adult head-injured patient. *Phys. Ther.* **63,** 2004–2009.
33. Gennarelli, T. A. (1988) Heterotopic ossification. *Brain Inj.* **2,** 175–178.
34. Hurvitz, E. A., Mandac, B. R., Davidoff, G., Johnson, J. H., and Nelson, V.S. (1992) Risk factors for heterotopic ossification in children and adolescents with severe traumatic brain injury. *Arch. Phys. Med. Rehabil.* **73,** 459–462.
35. Keenan, M. A. (1988) Management of the spastic upper extremity in the neurologically impaired adult. *Clin. Orthop.* 116–125.
36. Keenan, M. A. and Haider T. (1996) The formation of heterotopic ossification after traumatic brain injury: a biopsy study with ultrastructural analysis. *J. Head Trauma Rehabil.* **11,** 8–22.
37. Keenan, M. A., Kauffman, D. L., Garland, D. E., and Smith, C. (1988) Late ulnar neuropathy in the brain-injured adult. *J. Hand Surg. [Am].* **13,** 120–124.
38. Keenan, M. E. and Waters, R. L. (1995) Heterotopic ossification, in *Diagnosis and Treatment in Orthopedics,* (Skinner H.B., ed.), Prentice Hall, New Jersey, 580–625.
39. Kolessar, D. J., Katz, S. D., and Keenan, M. E. (1996) Functional outcome following surgical resection of heterotopic ossification in patients with brain injury. *J. Head Trauma Rehabil.* **4,** 78–87.
40. McAuliffe, J. A., and Wolfson, A. H. (1997) Early excision of heterotopic ossification about the elbow followed by radiation therapy. *J. Bone Joint Surg. [Am].* **79,** 749.

41. Meythaler, J. M., Tuel, S. M., Cross, L. L., and Mathew, M. M. (1992) Heterotopic ossification of the extensor tendons in the hand associated with traumatic spinal cord injury. *J. Am. Paraplegia Soc.* **15,** 229.
42. Mital, M. A., Garber, J. E., Stinson, J. T. (1987) Ectopic bone formation in children and adolescents with head injuries: its management. *J. Pediatr. Orthop.* **7,** 83–90.
43. Money, R. A. (1972) Ectopic paraarticular ossification after head injury. *Med J. Aust.* **1,** 125–127.
44. Moore, J. M. (1993) Functional outcome following surgical excision of heterotopic ossification in patients with traumatic brain injury. *J. Orthop. Trauma.* **7,** 11–14.
45. Moore, T. J. (1993) Functional outcome following surgical excision of heterotopic ossification in patients with traumatic brain injury. *J. Orthop. Trauma.* **7,** 11–19.
46. Mysiw, W. J., Tan, J., and Jackson, R. D. (1993) Heterotopic ossification. The utility of osteocalcin in diagnosis and management. *Am. J. Phys. Med. Rehabil.* **72,** 184–187.
47. O'Dwyer, N. J., Ada, L., and Neilson, P. D. (1996) Spasticity and muscle contracture following stroke. *Brain* **119,** 1737.
48. Otfinowski, J. (1993) Heterotopic induction of osteogenesis in the course of neural injury. *Patol. Pol.* **44,** 133–168.
49. Ough, J. L., Garland, D. E., Jordan, C., and Waters, R. L. (1981) Treatment of spastic joint contractures in mentally disabled adults. *Orthop. Clin. North Am.* **12,** 143–151.
50. Ozaki, J. (1996) Pathomechanics and operative management of chronic frozen shoulder. *Ann. Chir. Gynaecol.* **85,** 156–158.
51. Perry, J. (1987) Contractures. A historical perspective. *Clin. Orthop.* **219,** 8–14.
52. Pomerance, J. F., Keenan, M. A. (1996) Correction of severe spastic flexion contractures in the nonfunctional hand. *J. Hand Surg [Am].* **21,** 828–833.
53. Ragone, D. J., Jr., Kellerman, W. C., and Bonner, F. J., Jr. (1986) Heterotopic ossification masquerading as deep venous thrombosis in head-injured adult: complications of anticoagulation. *Arch. Phys. Med. Rehabil.* **67,** 339–341.
55. Ritter, M. A. (1987) Indomethacin: an adjunct to surgical excision of immature heterotopic bone formation in a patient with a severe head injury. A case report. *Orthopedics* **10,** 1379–1381.
56. Rogers, R. C. (1988) Heterotopic calcification in severe head injury: a preventive programme. *Brain Inj.* **2,** 169–173.
57. Roper, B. A. (1987) The orthopaedic management of the stroke patient. *Clin. Orthop.* 78–86.
58. Schaeffer, M. A. and Sosner, J. (1995) Heterotopic ossification: treatment of established bone with radiation therapy. *Arch. Phys. Med. Rehabil.* **76,** 284–286.
59. Sobus, K. M., Alexander, M. A., and Harcke, H. T. (1993) Undetected musculoskeletal trauma in children with traumatic brain injury or spinal cord injury. *Arch. Phys. Med. Rehabil.* **74,** 902–904.

60. Sobus, K. M., Sherman, N., and Alexander, M. A. (1993) Coexistence of deep venous thrombosis and heterotopic ossification in the pediatric patient. *Arch. Phys. Med. Rehabil.* **74**, 547–551.
61. Soren, A. and Fetto, J. F. (1996) Contracture of the shoulder joint. *Arch. Orthop. Trauma Surg.* **115**, 270–292.
62. Spencer, R. F. (1991) Heterotopic ossification in a finger following head injury. *J. Hand Surg.* **16**, 217, 218.
63. Spielman, G., Gennarelli, T. A., and Rogers, C. R. (1983) Disodium etidronate: its role in preventing heterotopic ossification in severe head injury. *Arch. Phys. Med. Rehabil.* **64**, 539–542.
64. Stone, L. and Keenan, M. A. (1988) Peripheral nerve injuries in the adult with traumatic brain injury. *Clin. Orthop.* 136–144.
65. Stone, L. R. and Keenan, M. A. (1992) Deep-venous thrombosis of the upper extremity after traumatic brain injury. *Arch. Phys. Med. Rehabil.* **73**, 486–489.
66. Summerfield, S. L., DiGiovanni, C., and Weiss, A. P. (1997) Heterotopic ossification of the elbow. *J. Shoulder Elbow Surg.* **6**, 321.
67. Swanson, A. B. and de Groot Swanson, G. (1989) Evaluation and treatment of the upper extremity in the stroke patient. *Hand Clin.* **5**, 75–96.
68. Tsur, A., Sazbon, L., and Lotem, M. (1996) Relationship between muscular tone, movement and periarticular new bone formation in postcoma-unaware (PC-U) patients. *Brain Inj.* **10**, 259–262.
69. van der Linden, A. J. (1984) Spontaneous regression of neurogenic heterotopic ossification. *Int. Orthop.* **8**, 25–27.
70. Waters, R. L. (1978) Upper extremity surgery in stroke patients. *Clin. Orthop.* 30–37.
71. Young, S. and Keenan, M. A. E. (1992) Extremity fractures in the brain-injured patient, in *Orthopaedic Rehabilitation*, (Nickel, VL and Botte, MJ, eds.), Churchill Livingstone, New York, p. 401–410.
72. Garland D. E. and Bailey S. (1981) Undetected injuries in head-injured adults. *Clin. Orthop.* **155**, 162–165.
73. Orcutt, S. A., Kramer, W. G. D., Howard, M. W., Keenan, M. A., Stone, L. R., Waters, R. L., and Gellman, H. (1990) Carpal tunnel syndrome secondary to wrist and finger flexor spasticity. *J. Hand Surg. [Am].* **15**, 940–944.
74. Ouellette, E. A. and Kelly, R. (1996) Compartment syndromes of the hand. *J. Bone Joint Surg. [Am.]* **78**, 1515.
75. Hisey, M. S. and Keenan, M. A. E. (1998) Orthopedic management of upper extremity dysfunction following stroke or brain injury, in *Operative Hand Surgery,* vol. 1., (Green D. P., Hotchkiss R. N., and Pederson W. C., eds.), Churchill Livingstone, New York, p. 287–324.
76. Keenan, M. A. (1988) Surgical decision making for residual limb deformities following traumatic brain injury. *Orthop. Rev.* **17**, 1185–1192.
77. Keenan, M. A. and Waters, R. L. (1993) Surgical treatment of the upper extremity after stroke or brain injury, in *Operative Orthopaedics,* (Chapman, M., ed.), Lippincott, Philadelphia, p. 1529–1544.
78. McDaid, P. and Keenan, M. A.: Management of Upper Extremity Dysfunction Following Stroke and Brain Injury. In Chapman's Orthopaedic Surgery,

Chapman, M. W. (ed.), pp. 1809–1854, Lippincott Williams & Wilkins Publishers, Philadelphia, PA, 2001.
79. Kolessar, D. and Keenan, M. A. E. (1993) Surgical management of upper extremity deformities following traumatic brain injury, in *Neurologic and Orthopaedic Sequelae of TBI,* vol. 7, (Stone, L. R., ed.), Hanley & Belfus, Philadelphia, p. 623–636.
80. Kozin, S. H. and Keenan, M. A. E. (1991) Principles of surgery for adult brain injury. *Curr. Orthop.* **5,** 75–83.
81. McCulloch, K. L. and Novack, T. A. (1990) Upper extremity functional assessment in traumatically brain-injured patients. *J. Head Trauma Rehabil.* **4,** 1.
82. Pinzur, M. S. (1993) Dynamic electromyography in functional surgery for upper limb spasticity. *Clin. Orthop.* **288,** 118.
83. Waters, R. L. and Keenan, M. A. (1988) Surgical treatment of the upper extremity after stroke, in *Operative Orthopedics,* vol. 1, (Chapman, M., ed.), Lippincott, Philadelphia, p. 1449–1458.
84. Keenan, M. A., Perry, J., and Jordan, C. (1984) Factors affecting balance and ambulation following stroke. *Clin. Orthop.* 165.
85. Keenan, M. A. (1987) The orthopedic management of spasticity. *J. Head Trauma Rehabil.* **2,** 62–71.
86. Keenan, M. A. and Waters, R. L. (1995) Orthopedic rehabilitation, in *Current Diagnosis and Treatment in Orthopaedics,* (H. B. S., ed.), Appleton & Lange Medical, Norwalk, p. 580–625.
87. Keenan, M. A. E. (1994) Aspekte der orthopadischen behandlung der posttraumaticischen zerebralparese, in *Die Behandlung Der Infantilen Zerebralparese,* (Niethard, F. U. C., and Doderlein, L., ed.), Georg Thieme Verlag, Stuttgart, New York, 119–125.
88. Keenan, M. A. E. and Botte, M. J. (1992) Traumatic brain injury, in *Orthopaedic Rehabilitation* (Nickel, V. L., Botte, M. J., eds.), Churchill Livingstone, New York, p. 361–370.
89. Bauman, J. U., Sutherland, D. H., and Hanggi, A. (1979) Intramuscular pressure during walking: An experimental study using the wick catheter technique. *Clin. Orthop.* **145,** 292–299.
90. Peter, K. S., Hsu, J. D., Keenan, M. A., and Romansky, S.G. (1996) Histology and intramuscular pressure in spastic muscles. *J. Head Trauma Rehabil.* **11,** 1–7.
91. Chambers, H., Lauer, A., Kaufman, K., Cardelia, J. M., and Sutherland, D. (1998) Prediction of outcome after rectus femoris surgery in cerebral palsy: the cocontraction of the rectus femoris and vastus lateralis. *J. Pediatr. Orthop.* **18,** 703–711.
92. Drummond, D. S., Rogala, E., and Templeton, J. (1974) Proximal hamstring release for knee flexion and crouched posture in cerebral palsy. *J. Bone and Joint Surg. [Am.]* **56-A,** 1598–1602.
93. Edwards, P. and Hsu, J. (1993) SPLATT combined with tendo achilles lengthening for spastic equinovarus in adults: results and predictors of surgical outcome. *Foot Ankle* **14,** 335–338.

94. Etnyre, B., Chambers, C. S., Scarborough, N. H., and Cain, T. E. (1993) Preoperative and postoperative assessment of surgical intervention for equinus gait in children with cerebral palsy. *J. Pediatr. Orthop.* **13,** 24.
95. Keenan, M. A., Abrams, R. A., Garland, D. E., and Waters, R. L. (1987) Results of fractional lengthening of the finger flexors in adults with upper extremity spasticity. *J. Hand Surg. [Am.]* **12,** 575–581.
96. Keenan, M. A., Gorai, A. P., Smith, C. W., and Garland, D. E. (1987) Intrinsic toe flexion deformity following correction of spastic equinovarus deformity in adults. *Foot Ankle* **7,** 333–337.
97. Keenan, M. A., Korchek, J. I., Botte, M. J., Smith, C. W., and Garland, D. E. (1987) Results of transfer of the flexor digitorum superficialis tendons to the flexor digitorum profundus tendons in adults with acquired spasticity of the hand. *J. Bone Joint Surg. [Am.]* **69,** 1127–1132.
98. Keenan, M. A., Romanelli, R. R., and Lunsford, B. R. (1989) The use of dynamic electromyography to evaluate motor control in the hands of adults who have spasticity caused by brain injury. *J. Bone Joint Surg. [Am.]* **71,** 120–126.
99. Keenan, M. A., Ure, K., Smith, C. W., and Jordan, C. (1988) Hamstring release for knee flexion contracture in spastic adults. *Clin. Orthop.* 221–226.
100. Koman, L. A., Gelberman, R. H., Toby, E. B., and Poehling, G. G. (1990) Cerebral palsy. Management of the upper extremity. *Clin. Orthop.* 62–74.
101. Kozin, S. H., Keenan, M. A. (1993) Using dynamic electromyography to guide surgical treatment of the spastic upper extremity in the brain-injured patient. *Clin. Orthop.* 109–117.
102. Laroche, M., Ighilahriz, O., Moulinier, L., Constantin, A., Cantagrel, A., and Mazieres, B. (1998) Adhesive capsulitis of the shoulder: an open study of 40 cases treated by joint distention during arthrography followed by an intraarticular corticosteroid injection and immediate physical therapy. *Rev. Rheum. Engl. Ed.* **65,** 313–319.
103. Lawrence, S. J., and Botte, M. J. (1994) Current topic review: management of the adult spastic equinovarus foot deformity. *Foot Ankle Int.* **15,** 340–346.
104. Matev, I. (1991) Surgery of the spastic thumb-in-palm deformity. *J. Hand Surg. [Br.]* **16,** 127–132.
105. Moore, T. (1996) Traumatic brain injury, in *Orthopedic Knowledge Update 5* (Kasser, J. R., ed.), American Academy of Orthopedic Surgeons, Rosemont, IL, p. 695, 696.
106. Ogilvie-Harris, D. J., Biggs, D. J., Fitsialos, D. P., and MacKay, M. (1995) The resistant frozen shoulder. Manipulation versus arthroscopic release. *Clin. Orthop.* 238–248.
107. Piazza, S. J. and Delp, S. L. (1996) The influence of muscles on knee flexion during the swing phase of gait. *J. Biomech.* **29,** 723–733.
108. Perry, J., Waters, R. L., and Perrin, T. (1978) Electromyographic analysis of equinovarus following stroke. *Clin. Orthop.* 47.
109. Pinzur, M. S. (1996) Carpectomy and fusion in adult-acquired hand spasticity. *Orthopedics* **19,** 675.
110. Pomerance, J. and Keenan, M. A. (1975) Management of the spastic elbow and forearm, in *Disorders of the Upper Extremity,* (Herndon, J., ed.), in press.

111. American Academy of Orthopedic Surgeons Instructional Course Lectures (1975) Upper extremity management and surgery, vol. 24. C. V. Mosby, St. Louis, MO, p. 51.
112. Vogt, J. C. (1998) Split anterior tibial transfer for spastic equinovarus foot deformity: retrospective study of 73 operated feet. *J. Foot Ankle Surg.* **37,** 2.
113. Waters, R. and Montgomery, J. (1974) Lower extremity management of hemiparesis. *Clin. Orthop.* **0,** 133.
114. Waters, R. L., Hislop, H. J., Perry, J., and Antonelli, D. (1978) Energetics: application to the study and management of locomotor disabilities. Energy cost of normal and pathologic gait. *Orthop. Clin. North. Am.* **9,** 351.
115. Waters, R. L., McNeal, D. R., and Clifford, B. (1984) Correction of footdrop in stroke patients via surgically implanted peroneal nerve stimulator. *Acta. Orthop. Belg.* **50,** 285.
116. Weiss, A. -P. C., Wiedeman, G. P., Jr., Quenzer, D., Hanington, K. R., Hastings, H. I., and Strickland, J. W. (1995) Upper extremity function after wrist arthrodesis. *J. Hand Surg.* **20A,** 818.
117. Young, S., Keenan, M. A., and Stone, L. R. (1990) The treatment of spastic planovalgus foot deformity in the neurologically impaired adult. *Foot Ankle* **10,** 317.
118. Zorowitz, R. D., Idank, D., Ikai, T., Hughes, M. B., and Johnston, M. V. (1995) Shoulder subluxation after stroke: a comparison of four supports. *Arch. Phys. Med. Rehabil.* **76,** 763.
119. Hendricks, H. T., Hageman, G., and van Limbeek, J. (1997) Prediction of recovery from upper extremity paralysis after stroke by measuring evoked potentials. *Scand. J. Rehabil. Med.* **29,** 155.
120. Keenan, M. A., Haider, T. T., and Stone, L. R. (1990) Dynamic electromyography to assess elbow spasticity. *J. Hand Surg. [Am.]* **15,** 607.
121. Keenan, M. A. E. and Perry, J. (1992) Motion analysis: Upper extremity, in, *Orthopedic Rehabilitation,* (Nickel, V. L., and Botte, M. J., ed.), Churchill Livingstone, New York, p. 243.
122. Keenan, M. A., R., A., Lazarus, M., and Perry, J. (1996) Selective release of spastic elbow flexors in the patient with brain injury. *J. Head Trauma Rehabil.* **11,** 57.
123. Esquenazi, A. and Keenan, M. A. (1993) Gait Analysis, in *Rehabilitation Medicine: Principles and Practice,* (DeLisa, J. A., ed.), Lippincott, Philadelphia, p. 122.
124. Hoffer, M. M., Barakat, G., and Koffman, M. (1985) 10-year follow-up of split anterior tibial tendon transfer in cerebral palsied patients with spastic equinovarus deformity. *J. Pediatr. Orthop.* **5,** 432.
125. Jordan, C. (1988) Current status of functional lower extremity surgery in adult spastic patients. *Clin. Orthop.* 102.
126. Keenan, M. A., Creighton, J., Garland, D. E., and Moore, T. (1984) Surgical correction of spastic equinovarus deformity in the adult head trauma patient. *Foot Ankle* **5,** 35.
127. Keenan, M. A., Gorai, A. P., Smith, C.W., and D. E., G. (1987) Intrinsic toe flexion deformity following correction of spastic equinovarus deformity in adults. *Foot & Ankle* **7,** 333.

128. Kerrigan, D. C. and Glenn, M. B. (1994) An illustration of clinical gait laboratory use to improve rehabilitation management. *Am. J. Phys. Med. Rehabil.* **73**, 421.
129. Lawrence, S. J. and Botte, M. J. (1994) Management of the adult, spastic, equinovarus foot deformity. *Foot Ankle Int.* **15**, 340.
130. Perry, J. (1992) *Gait Analysis. Normal and Pathological Function,* Slack Inc., Thorofare.
131. Perry, J. (1993) Determinants of muscle function in the spastic lower extremity. *Clin Orthop.* 10.
132. Perry, J., Giovan, P., Harris, L. J., Montgomery, J., and Azaria, M. (1978) The determinants of muscle action in the hemipareitc lower extremity. *Clin. Orthop.* **131**, 71.
133. Piccioni, L. and Keenan, M. A. (1992) Surgical management of the spastic equinovarus foot deformity. *Operative Tech. Orthop.* **2**, 146.
134. Pinzur, M. S., Sherman, R., DiMonte-Levine, P., Kett, N., and Trimble, J. (1986) Adult-onset hemiplegia: changes in gait after muscle-balancing procedures to correct the equinus deformity. *J. Bone Joint Surg. [Am.]* **68**, 1249.
135. Roper, B. A., Willaims, A., and King, J. B. (1978) The surgical treatrment of equinovarus deformity in adults with spasticity. *J. Bone Joint Surg. [Br.]* **60-B**, 533.
136. Waters, R., Rhoades, M., and Montgomery, J. (1975) Improvement of physical function after stroke: surgical and orthotic management. *J. Am. Geriatr. Soc.* **23**, 248.
137. Waters, R. L., Frazier, J., Garland, D. E., Jordan, C., and Perry, J. (1982) Electromyographic gait analysis before and after operative treatment for hemiplegic equinus and equinovarus deformity. *J. Bone Joint Surg. [Am.]* **64**, 284.
138. Waters, R. L., Garland, D. E., Perry, J., Habig, T., and Slabaugh, P. (1979) Stiff-legged gait in hemiplegia: surgical correction. *J. Bone Joint Surg. [Am.]* **61**, 927.
139. Waters, R. L., Perry, J., and Garland, D. (1978) Surgical correction of gait abnormalities following stroke. *Clin. Orthop.* 54.
140. Damron, T. A., Breed, A. L., and Cook, T. (1993) Diminished knee flexion after hamstring surgery in cerebral palsy patients: prevalence and severity. *J. Pediatr. Orthop.* **13**, 188.
141. Esquenazi, A., Keenan, M. A., and Mayer, N. (1995) Evaluacion y manejo de espasticidad, contracturas y disfuncion del control motor. *Kinesiologia* **42**, 60.
142. Gage, J. R. (1990) Surgical treatment of knee dysfunction in cerebral palsy. *Clin. Orthop.* 45.
143. Mazurkiewicz, S. (1974) Evaluation of some elements of gait in patients with a stiff knee. *Chir. Narzadow Ruchu. Ortop. Pol.* **39**, 627.
144. Miller, F., Cardoso Dias, R., Lipton, G. E., Albarracin, J. P., Dabney, K. W., and Castagno, P. (1997) The effect of rectus EMG patterns on the outcome of rectus femoris transfers. *J. Pediatr. Orthop.* **17**, 603.
145. Ounpuu, M. S., Muik, E., Davis III, R. B., Gage, J. R., and DeLuca, P. A. (1993) Rectus femoris surgery in children with cerebral palsy. Part II: A comparison between the effect of transfer and release of the distal rectus femoris on knee motion. *J. Pediatr. Orthop.* **13**, 331.

146. Perry, J. (1987) Distal rectus femoris transfer. *Dev. Med. Child. Neurol.* **29,** 153.
147. Pinzur, M. S. (1996) Surgical correction of lower extremity problems in patients with brain injury. *J. Head Trauma Rehabil.* **44,** 69.
148. Riley, P. O. and Kerrigan, D. C. (1998) Torque action of two-joint muscles in the swing period of stiff-legged gait: a forward dynamic model analysis [In Process Citation]. *J. Biomech.* **31,** 835.
149. Smith, C. W. and Levanthal, L. (1987) Surgical management of lower extremity deformities in adult head injured patients. *J. Head Trauma Rehabil.* **2,** 53.
150. Botte, M. J., Keenan, M. A. E., and Jordan, C. (1992) Stroke, in *Orthopedic Rehabilitation,* (Nickel, V. L., and Botte, M. J., eds.), Churchill Livingstone, New York, p. 337.
151. Botte, M. J. and Keenan, M. A. E. (1991) Brain injury and stroke, in *Operative Nerve Repair and Reconstruction,* (Gelberman, R. H., ed.), Lippincott, Philadelphia, p. 1413.
150. Sutherland, D. H. and Davids, J. R. (1993) Common gait abnormalities of the knee in cerebral palsy. *Clin. Orthop.* 139.
152. Sutherland, D. H., Santi, M., and Abel, M. F. (1990) Treatment of stiff-knee gait in cerebral palsy: a comparison by gait analysis of distal rectus femoris transfer versus proximal rectus release. *J. Pediatr. Orthop.* **10,** 433.
153. Botte, M. J., Waters, R. L., Keenan, M. A. E., Jordan, C., and Garland, D. E. (1988) Orthopaedic management of the stroke patient: Part I: Pathophysiology, limb deformity, and patient evaluation. *Orthop. Rev.* **27,** 637.
154. Botte, M. J., Waters, R. L., Keenan, M. A. E., Jordan, C., and Garland, D. E. (1988) Orthopaedic mangement of the stroke patient: Part II: Treating deformities of the upper and lower extremities. *Orthop. Rev.* **27,** 891.
155. Andersen, N. H., Sojbjerg, J. O., Johannsen, H. V., and Sneppen, O. (1998) Frozen shoulder: arthroscopy and manipulation under general anesthesia and early passive motion. *J. Shoulder Elbow Surg.* **7,** 218.
156. Gellman, H., Keenan, M. A., Stone, L., Hardy, S. E., Waters, R. L., and Stewart, C. (1992) Reflex sympathetic dystrophy in brain-injured patients. *Pain* **51,** 307.
157. Grubbs, N. (1993) Frozen shoulder syndrome: a review of literature. *J. Orthop. Sports Phys. Ther.* **18,** 479.
158. Ikai, T., Tei, K., Yoshida, K., Miyano, S., and Yonemoto, K. (1998) Evaluation and treatment of shoulder subluxation in hemiplegia: relationship between subluxation and pain. *Am. J. Phys. Med. Rehabil.* **77,** 421.
159. Murninghan, J. P. (1988) Adhesive capsulitis of the shoulder: current concepts and treatment. *Orthopedics* **2,** 152.
160. Raj, P., Caloodney, A., Janisse, T., and Cannella, J. (1992) Reflex sympathetic dystrophy, in *Skeletal Trauma: Fractures, Dislocations, Ligamentous Injuries,* vol. 1. (Browner, B. D., J. J., Levine, A. M., and Trafton, P. G., eds.), W. B. Saunders, Philadelphia, p. 471.
161. Shaffer, B. (1992) Frozen shoulder: a long term follow-up. *J. Bone Joint Surg. [Am.]* **74,** 738.
162. Shaffer, B. (1992) Frozen shoulder: a long term follow-up. *J. Bone Joint Surg. [Am.]* **74,** 738.
163. Kumar, R., Metter, E. J., Mehta, A. J., and Chew, T. (1990) Shoulder pain in hemiplegia. The role of exercise. *Am. J. Phys. Med. Rehabil.* **69,** 205.

164. Poulin de Courval, L., Barsauskas, A., Berenbaum, B., Dehaut, F., Dussault, R., Fontaine, F. S., et al. (1990) Painful shoulder in the hemiplegic and unilateral neglect. *Arch. Phys. Med. Rehabil.* **71,** 673.
165. Zorowitz, R. D., Hughes, M. B., Idank, D., Ikai, T., and Johnston, M. V. (1996) Shoulder pain and subluxation after stroke: correlation or coincidence? *Am. J. Occup. Ther.* **50,** 194.
166. Keenan, M. A. E., Kozin, S. H., and Berlet, A. C. (1993) *Manual of Orthopedic Surgery for Spasticity,* Raven Press, New York.
167. Gellman, H., Keenan, M. A., and Botte, M. J. (1996) Recognition and management of upper extremity pain syndromes in the patient with brain injury. *J. Head Trauma Rehabil.* **11,** 23.
168. Keenan, M. A. E. and Perry, J. (1990) Evaluation of upper extremity motor control in spastic brain-injured patients using dynamic electromyography. *J. Head Trauma Rehabil.* **5,** 13.
169. Meals, R. A. (1988) Denervation for the treatment of acquired spasticity of the brachioradialis. *J. Bone Joint Surg. [Am.]* **70,** 1081.
170. Caldwell, C. and Braun, R. M. (1974) Spasticity in the upper extremity. *Clin. Orthop.* **0,** 80.
171. Keenan, M. A., Tomas, E. S., Stone, L., and Gersten, L. M. (1990) Percutaneous phenol block of the musculocutaneous nerve to control elbow flexor spasticity. *J. Hand Surg [Am.]* **15,** 340.
172. Stotz, S. and Heimkes, B. (1992) Surgical treatment concepts of deformities of the upper extremities in infantile cerebral palsy. *Orthopade.* **21,** 301.
173. Suso, S., Vicente, P., and Angles, F. (1985) Surgical treatment of the nonfunctional spastic hand. *J. Hand Surg. [Br.]* **10,** 54.
174. Pinzur, M. S., Sherman, R. S., and Dimonte-Levine, P. (1977) Triceps spasticity in traumatic hemiplegia: diagnosis and treatment. *Arch. Phys. Med. Rehabil.* **68,** 446.
175. Botte, M. J., Abrams, R. A., Keenan, M. A. E., and Mooney, V. (1992) Limb rehabilitation in stroke patients. *J. Musculoskeletal Med.* **9,** 66.
176. Botte, M. J. and Keenan, M. A. (1987) Reconstructive surgery of the upper extremity in the patient with head trauma. *J. Head Trauma Rehabil.* **2,** 34.
177. Pinzur, M. S. (1991) Flexor origin release and functional prehension in adult spastic hand deformity. *J. Hand Surg. [Br.]* **16,** 133.
178. Pinzur, M. S., Wehner, J., Kett, N., and Trilla, M. (1988) Brachioradialis to finger extensor tendon transfer to achieve hand opening in acquired spasticity. *J. Hand Surg. [Am.]* **13,** 549.
179. Botte, M. J., Keenan, M. A., Korchek, J. I., and Waters, R. L. (1987) Modified technique for the superficialis-to-profundus transfer in the treatment of adults with spastic clenched fist deformity. *J. Hand Surg. [Am.]* **12,** 639.
180. Braun, R. M. and Vise, G. T. (1973) Sublimis-to-profundus tendon transfers in the hemiplegic upper extremity. *J. Bone Joint Surg. [Am.]* **55,** 873.
181. Keenan, M. A., Todderud, E. P., Henderson, R., and Botte, M. (1987) Management of intrinsic spasticity in the hand with phenol injection or neurectomy of the motor branch of the ulnar nerve. *J. Hand Surg. [Am.]* **12,** 743.

182. Botte, M. J., Keenan, M. A., Gellman, H., Garland, D. E., and Waters, R. L. (1989) Surgical management of spastic thumb-in-palm deformity in adults with brain injury. *J. Hand Surg. [Am.]* **14,** 174.
183. Dahlin, L. B., Komoto-Tufvesson, Y., and Salgeback, S. (1998) Surgery of the spastic hand in cerebral palsy. Improvement in stereognosis and hand function after surgery. *J. Hand Surg. [Br.]* **23,** 334.
184. Matev, I. (1963) Surgical treatment of spastic "thumb-in-palm" deformity. *J. Bone Joint Surg. [Br.]* **45,** 703.
185. Matev, I. (1991) Surgery of the spastic thumb-in-palm deformity [see comments]. *J. Hand Surg. [Br.]* **16,** 127.
186. Rayan, G. M. and Saccone, P. G. (1996) Treatment of spastic thumb-in-palm deformity: a modified extensor pollicis longus tendon rerouting. *J. Hand Surg. [Am.]* **21,** 834.
187. Sakellarides, H. T., Mital, M. A., Matza, R. A., and Dimakopoulus, P. (1995) Classification and surgical treatment of the thumb-in-palm deformity in cerebral palsy and spastic paralysis. *J. Hand Surg. [Am.]* **20,** 428.
188. Silver, C. M., Litchman, H. M., Simon, S. D., and Motamed, M. (1976) Surgical correction of spastic thumb-in-palm deformity. *Dev. Med. Child. Neurol.* **18,** 632.
189. House, J. H., Gwathmey, F. W., Fidler, M. O. (1981) A dynamic approach to the thumb-in palm deformity in cerebral palsy. *J. Bone Joint Surg. [Am.]* **63,** 216.
190. Smith, R. J (1975) Intrinsic muscles of the fingers: function, dysfunction, and surgical reconstruction, in *Instructional Course Lectures,* vol. 24. (AAOS, ed.), C. V. Mosby, St Louis, p. 200.
191. Smith, R. J. (1975) Surgical treatment of the claw hand, in *Symposium on Tendon Surgery in the Hand* (AAOS, ed.), C.V. Mosby, St. Louis, p. 181.
192. Zancolli, E. A., and Zancolli, E. R. (1983) The infantile spastic hand. Surgical indications and management. *J. Hand Surg. [Am.]* **5,** 766.
193. Anmuth, C., Esquenazi, A., and Keenan, M. A. E. (1994) Lower extremity surgery for the spastic patient, in: *Spasticity,* vol. 8. (Katz, R., ed.), Hanley & Belfus, Philadelphia, p. 547.
194. De Quervain, I. A., Simon, S. R., Leurgans, S., Pease, W. S., and McAllister, D. (1996) Gait pattern in the early recovery period after stroke. *J. Bone and Joint Surg. [Am.]* **64-A,** 1506.
195. Guanche, C., and Keenan, M. A. E. (1992) Principles of orthopaedic rehabilitation. *Phys. Med. and Rehab. Clin. North A.* **3,** 417.
196. Keenan, M. A., Botte, M. J., Hsu, J., Liebenberg, R., and Moore, T. J. (1993) Symposium: orthopaedic management of patients with traumatic brain injuries. *Contemp. Orthop.* **27,** 357.
197. Lee, G. A. and Keenan, M. A. Management of lower extremity deformities following stroke and brain injury, in *Operative Orthopedics,* (Chapman, M., ed.), Lippincott, Philadelphia, in press.
198. Perry, J. and Waters, R. L. Orthopedic evaluation and treatment of the stroke patient. Part
199. Waters, R. L., Clifford, B., and Jordan, C. (1984) Surgical correction of spastic lower extremity deformities. *Acta. Orthop. Belg.* **50,** 172.

200. Kerrigan, D. C. and Annaswamy, T. M. (1997) The functional significance of spasticity as assessed by gait analysis. *J. Head Trauma Rehabil.* **12,** 29.
201. Seymour, N., and Sharrard, W. J. W. (1968) Bilateral proximal release of the hamstrings in cerebral palsy. *J. Bone Joint Surg. [Br.]* **50-B,** 274.
202. Sharps, C. H., Clancy, M., and Steele, H. H. (1984) A long term retrospective study of proximal hamsting release for hamstring contracture in cerebral palsy. *J. Pediatr. Orthop.* **4,** 443.
203. Waters, R. L., Perry, J., McDaniels, J. M., and House, K. (1974) The relative strength of the hamstrings during hip extension. *J. Bone Joint Surg. [Am.]* **56,** 1592.
204. Bauman, J. U., Ruetsch, H., and Shurman, K. (1980) Distal hamstring lengthening in cerebral palsy. *Int.Orthop.* **3,** 305.
205. Grujic, H., and Asparisi, T. (1982) Distal hamstring release in knee flexion deformity. *Int. Orthop.* **6,** 103.
206. Keenan, M. A. E. and Waters, R. L. (1993) Surgical treatment of the lower extremity after stroke, in *Operative Orthopedics,* (Chapman, M., ed.), Lippincott, Philadelphia, p. 3449.
207. Keenan, M. A. E., Lee, G. A., Tuckman, A. S., and Esquenazi, A. Improving calf muscle strength in patients with spastic equinovarus deformity by transfer of the long toe flexors to the os calcis. *J. Head Trauma Rehabil.,* in press.
208. Morita, S., Yamamoto, H., and Furuya, K. (1994) Anterior transfer of the toe flexors for equinovarus deformity due to hemiplegia. *J. Bone and Joint Surg. [Br.]* **76-B,** 447.
209. Morita, S., Yamamoto, H., and Furuya, K. (1994) Anterior transfer of the toe flexors for equinovarus deformity due to hemiplegia. *J. Bone and Joint Surg. [Br.]* **76-B,** 447.
210. O'Byrne, J. M., Kennedy, A., Jenkinson, A., and O'Brien, T. M. (1997) Split tibialis posterior tendon transfer in the treatment of spastic equinovarus foot. *J. Pediatr. Orthop.* **17,** 481.
211. Synder, M., Kumar, S. J., and Stecyk, M. D. (1993) Split tibialis posterior tendon transfer and tendo-Achillis lengthening for spastic equinovarus feet. *J. Pediatr. Orthop.* **13,** 20.
212. Mann, R. A. (1993) Pes Cavus, in *Surgery of the Foot and Ankle* (Mann, R. A. and Coughlin, M., eds.), Mosby, St. Louis, p. 785.

16
Neurosurgical Management

Jose A. Espinosa

INTRODUCTION

Over the years, a number of surgical procedures have been developed to treat spasticity. Sophistication in surgical techniques has led to the maximal preservation of sensation and useful motor function. Increased experience with these surgical procedures and progress in monitoring techniques has drastically decreased the number of postoperative complications that had been seen earlier, leading to improved outcomes. Despite all of these advances, spasticity is still a significant problem affecting patients with a wide variety of underlying pathologies.

Fortunately, a variety of noninvasive interventions are generally effective in the treatment of spasticity, including medications, nerve blocks, botulinum toxin, and intrathecal pumps. However, for patients with refractory spasticity, surgical interventions can be considered. This chapter reviews some of the ablative procedures used to treat intractable spasticity (see Table 1). Nonablative procedures are described elsewhere in this book.

PERCUTANEOUS NEUROTOMY

The pioneering work of Walshe in which procaine was injected into the muscles of spastic patients producing a transitory decrease in tone led to the technique known as percutaneous neurotomy (1). Today, intramuscular neurolysis is usually accomplished by injection of an sclerosing agent, either ethanol or phenol, into the region of the targeted nerve. Because both agents have systemic side effects, the number of branches lesioned per procedure are limited (2). Phenol has been used extensively as a neurolytic agent in various settings and it is usually the agent of choice. Five mL of 5% phenol in sterile water can be used safely in a single sitting. When injected in the proximity of a nerve, it results in selective denervation and produces focal reduction of muscle tone and weakness.

From: *Current Clinical Neurology: Clinical Evaluation and Management of Spasticity*
Edited by: D. A. Gelber and D. R. Jeffery © Humana Press, Inc., Totowa, NJ

Table 1
Neuroablative Procedures for Spasticity

With partial preservation of function	Without preservation of function
Motor-point block	Intrathecal injection
Phenol nerve block	Selective anterior rhizotomy
Selective neurectomies	Cordectomy
Percutaneous radiofrequency foraminal rhizotomy	Cordotomy
Myelotomies	
Selective dorsal rhizotomy	
Stereotaxic thalamotomy or dentatotomy	

The motor branches of the nerve selected for neurolysis are localized by electrical stimulation using an insulated 22-gauge needle and then, a maximum of 0.5 mL of phenol is injected into each targeted branch *(3,4)*. The procedure partially preserves motor and sensory function. A greater reduction in tone with better maintenance of useful muscle strength can be obtained by injecting the nerve at a more proximal location.

Unfortunately, almost all patients undergoing percutaneous neurotomies for spasticity do not obtain long-lasting relief of their symptoms. Muscle tone invariably returns to preoperative status in few months to months *(5)*.

The main advantages of the procedure is that it is safe, simple, and does not require a complex operating room setting. Because the effects of percutaneous neurotomy are often transitory, the procedure is sometimes performed prior to an open neurotomy to asses the effects of a specific muscle group on overall limb spasticity and useful motor function.

SELECTIVE OPEN NEUROTOMY

This technique has the advantage over percutaneous neurotomy in that there is direct exposure of the nerve to be treated. The nerve is exposed at the known anatomical region where it branches. Electrical stimulation of the different branches helps in tailoring the degree and extension of the lesion to be created.

The obturator, sciatic, tibial, ulnar, and pudendal are among the nerves that are frequently selected for open neurotomies. Selective section of the anterior branch of the obturator nerve is the procedure more commonly performed and is considered for intractable hip-adductor spasticity. The motor fibers are partially sectioned and the sensory supply is spared. Complete transection of the nerve is avoided as contracture of the unopposed hip abductors can develop *(6)*. Approximately 80% of patients obtain relief from the procedure *(7)*.

A major drawback from the procedure is that open neurectomy can cause permanent flaccid paralysis with muscle atrophy and weakness in the myotomes inervated by the nerve sectioned. Permanent hypoesthesia arises after sectioning mixed nerves.

ANTERIOR RHIZOTOMY

In 1945, Munro reported a series of 42 patients with severe lower-extremity spasticity that underwent anterior rhizotomies (sectioning of ventral nerve roots) *(8)*. In his series, all of the roots from T_{11} to S_1 were sectioned. Improvement of spasticity was noted in 92% of the patients. His results were later duplicated by Freeman *(9)*.

Anterior rhizotomy is an effective treatment of severe spasticity producing long-lasting results. The drawback of the procedure is that it requires extensive, multiple-level laminectomies with obvious sacrifice of any potential for future functional motor recovery. Permanent flaccid paralysis with muscle atrophy are the end result of complete sectioning of the anterior nerve roots.

PERCUTANEOUS RADIOFREQUENCY FORAMINAL RHIZOTOMY

Percutaneous radiofrequency foraminal rhizotomy is based on the principle that small, unmyelinated fibers are more sensitive to heat lesions than larger, myelinated A-alpha fibers. This technique was first published by Kenmore in 1983. He achieved excellent results in a series that included patients with spasticity secondary to brain and spinal-cord injury *(10)*. Similar results were reported in two separate series *(11,12)*. In the Kasdon series, most of the prospectively identified goals were met in 24 of 25 surgically treated patients. Despite the fact that his patients had severe pre-operative spasticity, improvement persisted for an average follow-up period of 12 months *(11)*.

The procedure is performed under fluoroscopic control and with the patient under general anesthesia. Patients with spasticity of the lower extremities generally have rhizotomies from L_1 to S_1 bilaterally. The position of the needle is confirmed by fluoroscopy and by electrical motor stimulation in order to obtain an appropriate response in the desired muscle group. The tip of the needle should be extradural. Heat lesions then are made at 90°C for 2 min at S_1 and at 70°C for 2 min from T_{12} to L_5. Herz reported that the needle angulation necessary to perform the rhizotomies at L_5 and

S_1 was difficult to negotiate and made the procedure technically more demanding. He complemented the radiofrequency rhizotomies with a percutaneous radiofrequency sciatic neurectomy in 32 out of 77 patients treated. With the aid of fluoroscopy, he localized the sciatic nerve just below the gluteal crease. The needle position was corroborated by application of a motor-stimulation current until either hamstrings or gastrosoleus muscle activity was observed. Then the lesion was made with the heated probe at 90°C for 90 s. Herz obtained satisfactory results in 95% of his cases with a complication rate of only 5% *(12)*, although one of his earlier publications showed a high recurrence rate of spasticity after surgery *(4)*.

MYELOTOMY

The theory of myelotomy is that spasticity can be reduced by interruption of the spinal-reflex arc by sectioning tracts in the cord. Over the years, several techniques for myelotomy have been proposed. In 1951, Bischof introduced a posterolateral approach dividing the anterior and posterior horns, between the spinothalamic and corticospinal tracts, using a laterally placed incision. In essence, the spinal cord was divided into two halves from L_1 to S_1 *(13)*. The procedure led to elimination of the spasticity; however, there was also lost of voluntary motor activity below the level of the lesion.

The surgical technique was later on modified in order to prevent the mandatory loss of motor function in those patients with useful limb motility. In 1960, Pourpre reported his technique of "T" myelotomy. He described opening the posterior median sulcus and incising the spinal cord from L_1 to S_1. Then, using a knife at a depth of 3 mm, he cut the intermediate gray matter with bilateral horizontal incisions separating anterior from posterior horns. Unilateral extension to the conus increases bladder capacity before reflex emptying occurs. A modification of the procedure allows for preservation of the lateral column with results similar to selective functional rhizotomies *(14,15)*.

More recently, Padovani utilized a bilateral triangular griseotomy (sectioning of gray matter) in three patients with severe spasticity that resulted in some degree of preservation of motor function. His technique is a modification of Ivan and Wiley's circular griseotomy, which at that time had been performed only experimentally *(16,17)*.

In summary, myelotomies are extensive surgical procedures requiring multilevel laminectomies. Patients usually experience motor deficits after surgery and often have associated bladder and sensory disturbances.

SELECTIVE SPINAL CORDECTOMY

Spinal cordectomy, an extensive and radical surgical procedure, was first introduced in 1948 by MacCarty when he treated a patient with spasticity secondary to a malignant spinal-cord tumor. Later he treated four patients with spastic paraplegia secondary to trauma with this procedure *(18)*. Segments of the thoracic spinal cord were removed "in block" in these patients with the hope of maintaining abdominal muscle tone in order to improve urinary evacuation. After surgery, all patients showed markedly decreased tone of the lower extremities with loss of benefits from mild spasticity; however, his patients were able to handle a wheelchair and occasionally perform transfers without assistance.

ABLATIVE INTRATHECAL SCLEROSING AGENTS

Sclerosing agents administered intrathecally destroy neurons and interrupt reflex arcs, thereby alleviating symptoms related to spasticity. Ethanol is superior to phenol; however, the agent is hypobaric and therefore more difficult to manage.

Intrathecal administration of chemical agents like ethanol, phenol, or a mixture of phenol and glycerin with metrizamide has been used to treat refractory spasms in paraplegic patients *(19,20)*. Scott used 4 mL of a solution containing phenol, glycerin, and metrizamide, with a concentration of 6% phenol, and instilled it into the thecal sac via lumbar puncture at the L_2-L_3 interspace. The patient was kept in the lateral decubitus position for 20 min and then rolled to the other side for further administration of 3 mL of the solution. His patient experienced recurrent spasticity 48 h after treatment that required similar treatment 1 wk later. The result was complete obliteration of the symptoms. Others have had similar results *(21)*.

The procedure is simple and does not require sophisticated monitoring. The main disadvantage is the high risk of voluntary motor weakness as well as bowel and bladder dysfunction.

STEREOTAXIC ABLATIVE PROCEDURES

Cerebral and cerebellar lesioning have been used by several investigators to treat spasticity in patients with cerebral palsy (CP). In the brain, multiple targets have been lesioned sterotactically. Cooper used a pulvinectomy to treat spasticity in patients with cerebrovascular accidents or traumatic head injuries *(22)*. Seven of his 10 patients showed improvement after the procedure. However, his results were not duplicated by subsequent investigators *(23)*. Gornall reported satisfactory results after ventrolateral thalamotomies *(24)*. Mundinger reported similar findings *(25)*; however, Narabayschi concluded that this procedure was useful in treating rigidity but had no effect on spasticity *(25,26)*.

Stereotaxic ablation of the dentate nucleus was introduced by Heimburger and Whitlock in 1965 *(27)*; however, the procedure only relieved spasticity to a moderate degree. Bilateral dentatotomies improved spasticity in only 30% of the cases and when the procedure was performed only unilaterally, no functional improvement was seen *(28,29)*. Conversely, Gornall found that all his patients treated with unilateral or bilateral dentatotomies had improvement in upper- and lower-extremity spasticity to some degree and suggested that the procedure should be performed as early as possible in order to obtain maximal benefits *(24)*.

Overall, the results of stereotaxic ablative procedures for spasticity are conflicting and in the cases of stereotaxic thalamotomies, the variety of different targets chosen and the limited number of patients studied does not allow for a meaningful interpretation of results.

DORSAL RHIZOTOMIES

The theory behind selective dorsal rhizotomy is that in patients with spasticity, certain dorsal rootlets are involved in abnormal overactive spinal-reflex circuits. By ablating these specific rootlets (usually at levels L2-S2), muscle tone is reduced. The current surgical procedures used for dorsal rhizotomies for the treatment of spasticity represent an evolution of techniques over almost a century *(30)*. In 1913, Foerster introduced a technique characterized by complete division of the lumbosacral dorsal roots with preservation of the motor roots in order to maintain stength and some tone in the lower extremities *(31)*. Gros modified the Foerster technique by partially sectioning dorsal spinal roots in an attempt to preserve at least some sensory function and afferent input from muscles *(32)*. Sindou changed the surgical target from the dorsal roots to the dorsal-root entry zone were he found that afferent fibers segregate and enter the cord in a specific location according to fiber type. By making a continuous lesion ventral to the dorsal-root entry zone, he reported excellent results in 75% of his patients *(33)*.

Further modifications and refinements to Foerster's technique were made originally by Fasano and later by Peacock, Deletis, and others *(34–36)*. Fasano's surgical technique involved sectioning dorsal rootlets based on their electrophysiological responses. Abnormal responses to intraoperative electrical stimulation of individual dorsal rootlets consisted of sustained muscle contraction, diffusion to other myotomes and a high stimulation threshold to elicit the response *(34)*. Peacock changed the operative target from the conus medularis to the cauda equina in an attempt to limit bowel and bladder complications *(35)*. Deletis actively monitored action potentials from S1 to S3 dorsal rootlets. His technique spared rootlets that carried afferent signals effectively, thus avoiding bladder complications *(36)*.

Functional posterior rhizotomy is a common modality used to treat lower extremely spasticity in children with CP. A number of studies have demonstrated improvement in lower-extremity spasticity, standing, sitting, and ambulation, with benefits persisting for over 10 yr *(37–40)*. One randomized clinical trial has shown that selective dorsal rhizotomy followed by physiotherapy is superior to physiotherapy alone *(41)*. Several studies have also reported improvement in upper-extremity function and speech following this procedure *(42,43)*. Because dorsal-root neurons have collateral fibers that ascend to the cervical spinal cord and brainstem nuclei, it is thought that sectioning lumbar dorsal rootlets could reduce facilitatory influences at rostral levels. Complications after surgery are usually transient *(38,40,44)*; however, the effects of multilevel laminectomies in children and the possibility of deformity will require further assessment.

REFERENCES

1. Walshe, A. E. (1924) Observations on the nature of the muscular rigidity of paralysis agitans, and on its relationship to tremor. *Brain* **47**, 159–177.
2. Easton, J. K. M., Ozel, T., and Halpern, D. (1979) Intramuscular neurolysis for spasticity in children. *Arch. Phys. Med. Rehabil.* **60**, 155–158.
3. Garland, D. E., Lucie, R. S., and Waters, R. L. (1982) Current uses of phenol nerve block for adult acquired spasticity. *Clin. Orthop.* **165**, 217–222.
4. Herz, D. A., Looman, J. E., Tiberio, A., et al. (1990) The management of paralytic spasticity. *Neurosurgery* **26**, 300–306.
5. Khalil, A. A. and Betts, H. B. (1967) Peripheral nerve block with phenol in the management of spasticity. *JAMA* **200**, 1155–1157.
6. Wheeler, M. E. and Weinstein, S. I. (1984) Adductor tenotomy-obturator neurectomy. *J. Pediatr. Orthop.* **4**, 48–51.
7. Silver, C. M., Simon, S. D., and Litchman, H. M. (1966) The use and abuse of obturator neurectomy. *Dev. Med. Child. Neurol.* **8**, 203–205.
8. Munro, D. (1945) The rehabilitation of patients totally paralyzed below the waist: with special reference to making them ambulatory and capable of earning their living. *N. Engl. J. Med.* **223**, 453–461.
9. Freeman, L. W. and Heimburger, R.F. (1947) The surgical relief of spasticity in paraplegic patients. *J. Neurosurg.* **4**, 435–443.
10. Kenmore, D. (1983) Radiofrequency neurotomy for peripheral pain and spasticity syndromes. *Contemp. Neurosurg.* **5**, 1–6.
11. Kasdon, D. L. and Lathi, E. S. (1984) A prospective study of radiofrequency rhizotomy in the treatment of posttraumatic spasticity. *Neurosurgery* **15**, 526–529.
12. Herz, D. A., Parsons, K. C., and Pearl, L. (1983) Percutaneous radiofrequency foraminal rhizotomies. *Spine* **8**, 729–732.
13. Bischof, W. (1951) Die longitudinale myelotomy. *Zbl. Neurochir.* **2**, 79–88.
14. Laitinen, L. and Singounas, E. (1971) Longitudinal myelotomy in the treatment of spasticity of the legs. *J. Neurosurg.* **35**, 536–540.
15. Laitinen, L. (1991) Longitudinal myelotomy for spasticity, in *Neurosurgery for Spasticity: A Multidisciplinary Approach* (Sindou, M., Abbott, R., and Keravel, Y., eds.), Springer-Verlag, Wien, Austria, pp. 183–186.

16. Padovani, R., Tognetti, F., Pozzati, E., et al. (1982) The treatment of spasticity by means of dorsal longitudinal myelotomy and lozenge-shaped griseotomy. *Spine* **7,** 103–109.
17. Ivan, L. P. and Wiley, J. J. (1975) Myelotomy in the management of spasticity. *Clin. Orthop.* **108,** 52–56.
18. MacCarthy, C. S. (1954) The treatment of spastic paraplegia by selective spinal cordectomy. *J. Neurosurg.* **11,** 539–545.
19. Scott, B. A., Weinstein, Z., Chiteman, R., Polliam, W. M. (1985) Intrathecal phenol and glycerin in metrizamide for treatment of intractable spasms in paraplegia. *J. Neurosurg.* **63,** 125–127.
20. Kelly, R. E. and Gauthier-Smith, P. C. (1959) Intrathecal administration of phenol in the treatment of reflex spasms and spasticity. *Lancet* **2,** 1102–1105.
21. Lourie, H. and Vanasupa, P. (1963) Comments on the use of intrathecal phenol-pantopaque for relief of pain and spasticity. *J. Neurosurg.* **20,** 60–63.
22. Cooper, I.S., Waltz, J.M., Amin, I., Fujita, S. (1971) Pulvinectomy: a preliminary report. *J. Am. Geriatr. Soc.* **19,** 553–554.
23. Guidetti, B. and Fraioli, B. (1977) Neurosurgical treatment of spasticity and dyskinesias. *Acta. Neurochir. Suppl. (Wein)* **24,** 27–39.
24. Gornall, P., Hitchcock, E., and Kirkland, I. S. (1975) Stereotaxic neurosurgery in the management of cerebral palsy. *Dev. Med. Child Neurol.* **17,** 279–286.
25. Mundinger, F. and Ostertag, C. (1977) Multilocular lesions in the therapy of cerebral palsy. *Acta. Neurochir. Suppl. (Wein)* **24,** 11–14.
26. Narabaysahi, H. (1977) Experiences of stereotaxic surgery on cerebral palsy patients. *Acta. Neurochir. Suppl. (Wein)* **24,** 3–10.
27. Heimburger, R. F. and Whitlock, C. C. (1965) Stereotaxic destruction of the human dentate nucleous. *Neurology* **26,** 346–358.
28. Sigfried, J. and Verdie, J. C. (1977) Long-term assessment of stereotactic dentatotomy for spasticity and other disorders. *Acta. Neurochir. Suppl. (Wein)* **24,** 41–48.
29. Zervas, N. (1977) Long-term review of dentatectomy in dystonia musculorun deformans and cerebral palsy. *Acta. Neurochir. Suppl. (Wein)* **24,** 49–51.
30. Abbott, I. R. (1996) Management of congenital spasticity in children, in *The Practice of Neurosurgery* (Tindall, G. T., Cooper, P. R., and Barrow, D.L., eds.), Williams & Wilkins, Baltimore, pp. 2805–2818.
31. Foerster, O. (1913) On the indications and results of the excision of posterior spinal nerve roots in men. *Surg. Gynecol. Obstet.* **16,** 463–475.
32. Gros, C. (1979) Spasticity: clinical classification and surgical management. *Adv. Tech. Stand Neurosurg.* **6,** 55–97.
33. Sindou, M. and Jeanmonod, D. (1991) Surgery in the dorsal root entry zone: microsurgical DREZ-otomy for the treatment of spasticity, in *Neurosurgery for Spasticity: A Multidisciplinary Approach* (Sindou, M., Abbott, R., and Keravel, Y., eds.), Springer-Verlag, Wein, pp. 165–182.
34. Fasano, V. A., Barolat-Romana, G., Zeme, S., Squazzi, A. (1979) Electrophysiological assessment of spinal circuits in spasticity by direct dorsal root stimulation. *Neurosurgery* **4,** 146–151.
35. Peacock, W. J. and Arens, L. J. (1982) Selective posterior rhizotomy for the relief of spasticity in cerebral palsy. *S. Afr. Med. J.* **62,** 119–124.

36. Deletis, V., Vodusek, D., Abbott, R., et al. (1992) Intraoperative monitoring of dorsal sacral roots. Minimizing the risk of iatrogenic micturation disorders. *Neurosurgery* **30,** 72–75.
37. Peter, J. C. and Arens, L. J. (1993) Selective posterior lumbosacral rhizotomy for the management of cerebral palsy spasticity. *S. Afr. Med. J.* **83,** 745–747.
38. Steinbok, P., Reiner, A., Beauchamp, R. E., et al. (1992) Selective functional posterior rhizotomy for treatment of spastic cerebral palsy in children. *Pediatr. Neurosurg.* **18,** 34–42.
39. Peacock, W. J., Arens, A. J., and Berman, B. (1987) Cerebral palsy spasticity. Selective posterior rhizotomy. *Pediatr. Neurosci.* **13,** 61–66.
40. Nishida, T., Thatcher, S. W., and Marty, G. R. (1995) Selective posterior rhizotomy for children with cerebral palsy: a 7-year experience. *Child. Nerv. Sys.* **11,** 374–380.
41. Steinbock, P., Reiner, A., Beuchamp, R., et al. (1997) A randomized clinical trial to compare selective posterior rhizotomy plus physiotherapy with physiotherapy alone in children with spastic diplegic cerebral palsy. *Dev. Med. Child. Neurol.* **39,** 179–184.
42. Albright, A. L., Barry, M. J., Fasick, M. P., and Janosky, J. (1995) Effects of continuous intrathecal baclofen infusion and selective posterior rhizotomy on upper extremity spasticity. *Pediatr. Neurosurg.* **23,** 82–85.
43. Beck, A. J., Gaskill, S. J., and Marlin, A. E. (1993) Improvement in upper extremity function and trunk control after selective posterior rhizotomy. *Am. J. Occup. Ther.* **47,** 704–707.
44. Peacock, W. J. and Staudt, L. A. (1990) Management of spasticity by ablative techniques, in *Neurological Surgery* 4th ed. (Youmans, J. R., ed.), Saunders, Philadelphia, pp. 3671–3686.

III
A Coordinated Approach to the Treatment of Spasticity in Neurologic Diseases

17
Management of Spasticity in Children with Cerebral Palsy

Carol Green, Daniel R. Cooperman, Susan E. Gara, and Carrie Proch

INTRODUCTION

Cerebral palsy (CP) refers to a disorder of motor function resulting from a nonprogressive brain lesion occurring before the brain is fully mature. CP refers exclusively to the motor dysfunction, although affected individuals may also have other symptoms of a static encephalopathy, such as cognitive dysfunction or seizures. Although the lesion is static, the symptoms often change with time. Examples include the transformation of hypotonia to hypertonia in the first years of life, increasing dystonia with age, as well as the appearance of complications, such as contractures and bony deformities. The classification of CP is based on the motor deficit rather than the underlying etiology. It is defined by the limbs involved, e.g., monoplegia, triplegia, hemiplegia, or quadriplegia; type of tone abnormality, e.g., hypotonia or spasticity; and associated movement disorders, such as dystonia, chorea and athetosis, or ataxia.

EDUCATIONAL PLANNING

As with all childhood illnesses, an important role of the medical caregivers is the education of families. When introducing the diagnosis to them, it is important to keep in mind that many individuals often have a preconception of what CP means; this may represent a much more disturbing picture than the clinician intends to convey. In helping patients and families meet current needs and anticipate future needs, it is useful to consider the physical and developmental impact of CP at a variety of ages, including infancy, the toddler/preschool years, elementary school years, adolescence, and adulthood.

From: *Current Clinical Neurology: Clinical Evaluation and Management of Spasticity*
Edited by: D. A. Gelber and D. R. Jeffery © Humana Press, Inc., Totowa, NJ

During infancy and preschool, a major goal of intervention should be to educate the family about the diagnosis and to discuss services available to individuals with CP. These include local (county) services, public-school services, and referral to organizations such as the United Cerebral Palsy Association. Overall, the diagnosis of CP should be made with caution in infants. During early years, motor delays and abnormal tone may actually improve with age. In others, spasticity may not appear until the end of the first year, as anti-gravity skills develop. Increased problems with spasticity often occur during growth spurts in the 4–5 yr age range, when physical progress may plateau or even decline.

For grade-school children with CP, the focus turns to the development of an appropriate educational plan with adaptive devices and services provided to meet each child's ability level, in an environment that is the least restrictive. Health-care providers should be familiar with public-school services, which are often available as early as preschool.

Adolescence is a time of physical growth, social maturation, and preparation for the workplace. Children and teenagers with physical disabilities often have less opportunity to develop appropriate social interactions than their typical peers do. In addition to the emotional stress of isolation during the teenage years, poor social interactions may be one of the key obstacles to successful employment in adulthood. As such, adolescents can benefit from directed social-skill training, a service that has become more available in the past few years *(1)*. Depending on the level of functioning, the focus of training may vary from hygiene issues to that of maintaining friendships and dating. In addition, teenagers with hemiplegia may discover a newfound interest in improving their posture and use of a dysfunctional limb, or in improving their gait. Such interest should be anticipated, and good motor patterning should be encouraged in younger children despite their frequent disinterest (and even resistance!).

Young adults often see their physicians because of worsening complications of spasticity, often resulting from relative immobility; symptoms include generalized early-morning stiffness, increasing contractures, or tightness in hamstrings and Achilles tendons. At this point, medical or surgical interventions are often needed to enhance a return to a physical therapy or exercise program. Attention should be given to accommodations in the workplace, such as making architectural adjustments to allow for wheelchair accessibility.

The treatment of spasticity in CP is similar to that of traumatic brain injury and spinal-cord disorders, although associated clinical features may differ. For example, many individuals with CP and spasticity also have concurrent movement disorders, such as dystonia and choreoathetosis. As well, it is well-recognized that individuals with CP are at risk for poor growth owing a combination of factors, including sustained muscle contraction and, at times, impaired or inefficient eating (2). For those patients with oromotor dysfunction, careful attention should be paid not only to nutrition and growth, but also to pulmonary function, as these individuals are often at risk of aspiration injury or infection. Also, as for individuals with any type of disability, health in areas of normal function, such as vision and hearing, should be promoted.

Many individuals with CP will need assistance with educational and job planning, not only because of physical disability, but also because of associated learning disabilities or mental retardation. Great care should be taken that the educational assessment does not underestimate an individual's ability, as might happen when standard tests that depend on specific verbal or motor skills are used. It should be kept in mind that most sports can be adapted to physical disabilities. Many career opportunities can be made available with appropriate planning. Families might need assistance with supportive and anticipatory guidance regarding emotional and financial aspects of a motor disability. Patients and their families should know their legal rights when negotiating education and employment opportunities.

ASSESSMENT AND TREATMENT OF SPASTICITY

Medical treatment of CP involves multiple disciplines. Setting appropriate goals is key in developing an intervention program. The goals must be realistic to avoid repeated disappointments, and sufficiently challenging to allow a child or adult to realize their full potential. Patients and families are often hoping to improve their level of function, such as progressing from requiring assistance with transfers to ambulating independently. Such expectations should be openly discussed so that appropriate education and planning can take place. Treatment should also include management and prevention of complications of spasticity and immobility, such as constipation, muscular pain with positioning or sleep, joint contractures, and hip dislocation.

Assessment of spasticity in patients with CP includes evaluation by physical and occupational therapists, and gait analysis. Primary-care physicians and rehabilitation specialists may choose to involve speech therapists, neurologists, orthopedists, and neurosurgeons. The assessment includes evaluation not only of muscle tone and range of motion, but also should quantify the contribution of associated movement disorders, such as dystonia. In addition, careful consideration should be given to areas in which spasticity may be disguising an underlying weakness, and, in these cases, actually improving function. For example, some individuals depend on lower-limb spasticity to support their weight and will be further disabled when their spasticity is relieved. Finally, because some surgical and medical interventions require a commitment from the patient to participate in an intensive physical-therapy (PT) program and be diligent in keeping follow-up medical appointments, there may be a need for a formal psychosocial assessment.

Physical and Occupational Therapy

Physical and occupational therapy (PT/OT) have long been the cornerstone of spasticity treatment in patients with CP. PT intervention is typically indicated to maximize gross motor skills. OT addresses upper-limb function, fine motor skills, and self-cares. Oromotor incoordination that affects sucking and feeding can be addressed by experienced speech and occupational therapists. Therapists can suggest devices and adaptive equipment, which may allow independent functioning in many areas, including gross and fine motor skills, mobility, and communication.

Occupational and physical therapists assess children with CP by utilizing a combination of standard evaluations, clinical observations, and handling techniques to establish rehabilitation goals and a treatment plan. A working knowledge base of developmental milestones, muscle tone, and classifications of CP are needed for an appropriate evaluation. Therapists work with patients and families to maximize development of normal functional movement patterns, minimize bony and muscular deformities, minimize or prevent sequela to abnormal skeletal alignment, and to maximize functional independence in activities of daily living, such as self-cares, work, play, and leisure *(3)*. A brief review of some of the standard therapy approaches are presented below.

Children with spastic cerebral palsy respond to PT and OT with a focus on passive range of motion (PROM) and active range of motion (AROM) of the limbs, increasing spinal mobility, use of varied and differential movement patterns incorporating varied speed and directions, use of adaptive equipment to aid with weight bearing, movement, and position transitions promoting muscle elongation as well as joint mobility and stability. Children with athetoid CP respond to PT/OT with focus on balance and postural tone, promoting midline and symmetrical muscle control and small graded movements *(3)*. Children with hypotonic CP respond to PT/OT with focus on antigravity positioning of the head, trunk control, promoting automatic reactions, and stabilization of the joints.

The therapeutic needs change with age. During infancy and toddler years, the therapy focus is to instruct caregivers in promoting optimal movement patterns and postures during daily-care activities such as feeding, playing, carrying, toileting, and movement. Generally, families are introduced to adaptive equipment such as special strollers, bath chairs and feeding equipment, and fist, hand or limb splints. During preschool, therapists continue to work with families to promote skill acquisition for independent function. Therapy promotes strength, endurance, and movement patterns. Mobility issues, such as use of wheelchairs, crutches, walkers, strollers, car seats, school chairs, splints, and orthotics are addressed.

During grade school, the occupational or physical therapist may function on a more consultative basis, advising on architecture adaptations such as widening doorways, making home modifications, and installing wheelchair lifts. Classroom accommodations may involve use of an aide, computer, and adjustable tabletop, and adaptation of recreational activities. In high school, therapists continue to address classroom modifications to enhance mobility and fine motor skills, evaluate new areas such as driving or use of public transportation, and address self-image issues including puberty and sexuality. In addition, preparation for the work place or college provides new issues for therapists to explore with students. In adulthood, therapists often deal with medical concerns, including overuse syndromes, lack of joint integrity, contractures, osteoporosis, weakness, and poor endurance, which may be complicated by poor nutrition habits, employment and housing limitations, pregnancy, and child care.

Formal Evaluation Tools

Formal evaluation tools include, but are not restricted to, the following:

MODIFIED ASHWORTH SCALE (4)

This assessment offers a way to measure resistance to passive movement in upper/lower joints.

GONIOMETER MEASUREMENTS (5)

Measurements of PROM/AROM for children with CP employ the same universal measurement procedures as those used for adults. The standard bony landmarks for axis of movement are the same for adults and children. Measurements may be unreliable owing to postural-tone changes, and abnormal reflexes, and therefore clinical observations may be recorded as well.

GROSS MOTOR FUNCTIONAL MEASURE (GMFM) (6)

GMFM is a standardized test designed to evaluate change in gross motor function of children with CP. The GMFM also describes a child's current level of function and provides goals for treatment. It is intended for use in both clinical and research settings.

PEDIATRIC EVALUATIONS OF DISABILITY INVENTORY (PEDI) *(7)*

One hundred ninety-seven items are completed by interview with parents/caregivers to quantify functional skills in the areas of mobility, self-care, and social function in children ages 6 mo to 7.5 years. Scores are compared with norms for typical performance in the same age groups.

PEABODY DEVELOPMENTAL MOTOR SCALES *(8)*

These scales assess gross and fine motor skills from 0–7 yr of age. This is a good assessment tool for children with hemiparesis to document change in skills.

BERMAN MOVEMENT SCALE *(9)*

This scale quantifies functional movement in a variety of standard positions.

ERHARDT PREHENSION/HAND ASSESSMENT *(10)*

This is an assessment that analyzes hand function from birth to 6 yr of age. This evaluates involuntary arm and hand patterns, voluntary movements, and pre-writing skills.

STRENGTH MEASUREMENTS *(11)*

Strength measurements may be performed using the Dynamometer and Pinch meter to measure grip and pinch strength. Standardized scores begin at 5 yr of age.

Useful clinical measurements include videotaping functional tasks such as seating (positioning in or out of wheelchair), movement transitions, gait, and fine motor tasks. This technique offers qualitative evidence of change when numerical scores do not reflect change or progress. In addition, timed tests of activities of daily living (ADL) and gait may demonstrate progress in a controlled setting using consecutive times recorded before and after a given treatment. Strength may be assessed using manual tests as well as observations of movement transition in graded antigravity positions, such as sit to stand for quadriceps, one leg standing for hip extensors, and assessment of trunk control with bench sitting and stooping or reaching to the floor.

Facilitation of movement patterns

The following techniques are described in the literature, but are not necessarily considered standard treatment. They are intended to facilitate movement patterns:

NEURODEVELOPMENTAL TRAINING (NDT)/BOBATH *(12)*T

The basic concept involves inhibiting abnormal muscle tone and primitive reflexes and to facilitate normal movement patterns via positioning and handling techniques that promote sensation of normal movement. Emphasis is placed on acquiring functional skills. The main treatment principles are weight bearing, weight shifting, and normalizing tone to facilitate quality of movement. Results can be difficult to quantify because they deal with efficiency of movement.

ELECTRICAL STIMULATION

Research is ongoing regarding the effects of the therapeutic electrical stimulation (TES) and functional electrical stimulation (FES), which is used during functional activities such as hand grasp/release or ambulation. Electrical stimulation can assist with improvement in AROM/PROM; however, it must be used in conjunction with other therapies to provide maximal results.

Other therapies to provide maximal results

STRENGTHENING/STRETCHING

Strengthening of specific muscles and muscle groups focuses on grading or timing of movement in activities such as sitting to standing, standing to sitting, ambulation, and weight shifting through the upper limbs.

SERIAL CASTING

Serial casting is used for upper and lower limbs with very spastic muscles to provide prolonged stretch of the muscles in a lengthened state. This results in permanently increased muscle length by addition of sarcomeres. Casts are reapplied every few weeks, gradually increasing the range of motion.

TONE REDUCTION AND TONE FACILITATION
BY INHIBITION CASTING AND TAPING

This uses the principles of positioning and of pressure application. The exact mechanism of spasticity reduction in casting is not known, but might be the result of neutral warmth and constant pressure. Taping of muscles may be performed with materials like Coban or Hypafix tape. The taping is along the muscle fibers for stimulation to encourage muscle-fiber generation.

FUNCTIONAL ACTIVITIES

Functional activities can be encouraged with a dynamic (motor learning) approach that takes into consideration all systems (including sensory, biomechanical, and proprioception). Treatment is geared toward repetition of activities by the patient, with a "hands off" approach by the therapist.

ADAPTIVE EQUIPMENT

Equipment includes seating systems that may be used in a wheelchair, stroller, or car seat to allow for improved postural control and improvement in movement patterns (upper-limb use, respiration, head control, and oromotor control). Adaptive equipment such as walkers, canes, built-up spoon handles, pencil grips, sock aides, and so on allow a child to explore and gain independence at home and school.

SPLINTING *(13)*

Splinting uses low-temperature thermoplastics, such as aquaplast, to fabricate upper- and lower-limb splints as a precursor in obtaining braces fabricated the orthotist. Splints made by the therapists are done so in an attempt to minimize the cost of bracing in rapidly growing infants and children. Examples of splints include: heel splints to provide optimal foot alignment; knee hyperextension splints to prevent "back kneeing;" elbow splints to limit range of hypermobile joints; wrist and thumb splints for functional grasp and for preservation of joint integrity; air splints for upper- and lower-limb joints; and neoprene thumb, wrist, forearm, elbow, and knee splints to allow for dynamic function.

Oral Pharmacotherapy

In general, results of oral medication for the treatment of spasticity of cerebral origin are limited at best. However, it is important to thoughtfully and systematically complete reasonable trials of medications prior to considering surgical interventions. As with any therapy, it is important to clearly identify the goals of treatment, the specific symptoms that seem to be limiting achievement of that goal, and to carefully follow up on the effects of treatment. While a patient may gain significant improvement in spasticity from a medication, if goals are not clearly discussed then success may be confused with failure, e.g., an individual who is more comfortable during sleep and makes gains in physical therapy but fails to achieve a new skill such as walking.

Oral medications may be used to reduce spasticity and perhaps lessen some of the associated movements such as dystonia. Medications may be effective at the level of the central nervous system (CNS), e.g., the benzodiazepines, tizanidine, and baclofen, or at the level of the muscle, such as dantrolene. Benefits are often limited by side effects. Pharmacologic details of these medications have been previously reviewed *(14,15)*. Some general comments follow:

The benzodiazepines (such as diazepam, clonazepam, and lorazepam) are thought to work via effects of the inhibitory neurotransmitter gamma-aminobuytric acid (GABA) in the spinal cord. Benefits include prompt relief of painful muscular spasm often with resultant improvement in sleep, and a long-term decrease in muscle tone. These medications also have anticonvulsant properties. Side effects include habituation, sedation, increased secretions, and possible rebound seizures with abrupt withdrawal. In addition, with higher doses, downregulation of receptors is thought to occur, resulting in waning clinical benefits (tachyphylaxis).

Baclofen has been demonstrated to have actions at the GABA receptor in the spinal cord *(16–18)*. However, side effects such as fatigue also suggest a cortical effect. Baclofen is generally well-tolerated by patients over the long term, and is effective in reducing both active and passive tone *(19)*, but use is limited by side effects including sedation, truncal hypotonia, and change in bladder habits. As such, some patients respond better to baclofen delivered intrathecally; this allows application more directly to the spinal cord and a more delicate control of dosing.

Clonidine, quanfacine, and tizanidine, have alpha$_2$ adrenergic effects *(20,21)*. These medications have antihypertensive effects, are used in the treatment of movement disorders, such as tics, and are effective in the treatment of spasticity. Side effects include fatigue and disturbed sleep as well as a risk of rebound hypertension if stopped suddenly. Improvement in spasticity has been reported in the settings of multiple sclerosis (MS) *(22)* and spinal-cord injury *(23)*, but extensive experience in the treatment of CP is lacking at the present time.

Dantrolene works directly on the sarcoplasmic reticulum of muscle, and, as such, is effective in reducing muscle tone *(14)*. Individual reports vary in extent of benefits for patients with CP *(24)*. Side effects include muscle weakness, gastrointestinal upset, and fatigue. In addition, serum liver enzymes should be monitored because of potential hepatotoxicity.

Anticholinergic medications have been reported to be of benefit in pediatric movement disorders. Specifically, trihexyphenidyl was reported to be beneficial in children who have dystonia as a clinical feature of their CP *(25)*. In addition, dopamine-blocking drugs, such as reserpine, may be a reasonable choice of treatment for hyperkinetic movements. In extreme and urgent situations, antipsychotic medications such as haloperidol can be beneficial for hyperkinetic movements such as choreoathetosis, but pose the recognized concern for significant and potentially long-lasting side effects such as tardive dyskinesia. Tetrabenazine is a dopamine-depleting drug not currently available in the US, but is reported to improve dystonia without the·significant concern for tardive dyskinesia as seen with psychotropic medications *(26)*.

With experience, it is possible to determine to what extent an individual might benefit from medications within a few months of systematic trials. Not all the medications above need to be tried in every situation, but the care provider should have a consistent sequence of medication options. If therapy and oral medications fail to provide satisfactory results, then alternative modes of medication administration or surgical options should be considered.

The use of intrathecal baclofen (ITB) in patients with spasticity of cerebral origin has received great attention in recent years, and has been recently approved for such use. Originally approved by the Food and Drug Administration (FDA) in 1992 for treatment of populations with spasticity attributed to a spinal origin, such as spine injury and MS, ITB has a very promising role in CP *(27)*. This system delivers a continuous infusion of baclofen into the intrathecal space, and allows for individual titration *(28)*. As with all other interventions mentioned, clarification of treatment goals is key for this intervention. Appropriate goals include a decrease of spasticity to improve function and alleviate spasm pain *(29)*. Disadvantages of treatment include the physical presence of the pump and catheter, as well as the need for frequent medical visits for medication refills. Candidates include those with moderate and more severe spasticity who have failed oral medications because of ineffectiveness or side effects, and individuals with dystonia. Candidates must be able to return each 2–3 mo for a pump refill.

While there are no published guidelines, our team has found the baclofen pump to be helpful in individuals who would normally be candidates for selective dorsal rhizotomy (SDR), but in whom there are specific concerns such as underlying weakness and dystonia. ITB dosing can be varied throughout the day to address specific needs, such as increasing the dose at night for comfortable sleep, and decreasing the daytime dose if tone is helpful for weight support. Side effects can include decline of truncal tone, bladder dysfunction, and daytime sleepiness. Complications of surgery, unintended overdose, or sudden infusion discontinuation are less likely as each generation of pump is improved, but these issues must be discussed openly with potential candidates.

Interventions such as SDR and ITB are directed at lessening spasticity long-term. In comparison, shorter-acting medications such as phenol and botulinum toxin injected at the site of muscle and neuromuscular junction selectively weaken spastic muscles to provide a "window of opportunity" to address specific problems. Injections address only a few muscle groups at a time, and are temporary. These agents should be considered when there are specific goals that can be met within a finite time, such as during a period when more intensive physical and occupational therapy can be performed, more aggressive bracing or casting is being considered, or to "buy time" until surgical management can be considered. Because the effects of nerve blocks and botulinum toxin are temporary, additional interventions must be adequate to maintain the therapeutic advantage even after spasticity returns.

In essence, the premise is that linear growth of muscle occurs by addition to sarcomeres *(30)*, a process that can be facilitated by injections and muscle stretching, such that even when the spasticity returns to the targeted muscle, the muscle is now longer and thus the skeletal effects of spasticity are lessened.

Until the recent introduction of botulinum toxin, nerve blocks with alcohol or phenol, or shorter-acting anesthetics, such as lidocaine, were commonly performed to focally weaken specific muscle groups and decrease muscle tone. The limiting factor with these agents is the need for general anesthesia for administration in children, because of significant pain with injection. However, these agents still have a role in treatment of spasticity when administered by a skilled individual.

Botulinum toxin was approved by the FDA for treatment of blepharospasm and strabismus in 1989. Since that time, a number of studies have evaluated the use of botulinum toxin for the treatment of spasticity *(2,31)*, including its use in children *(32,33)*. The toxin is injected into spastic muscle where it diffuses in the neuromuscular junction and is taken up by presynaptic nerve terminals and interrupts the release of acetylcholine *(34)*. Muscle weakening and a reduction of tone, owing to this chemical denervation, develops within 1–2 wk, and lasts 3–4 mo until new nerve terminals sprout.

Orthopedic Surgery

In addition to physical and occupational therapies, orthopedic surgery has been a mainstay of treatment for complications of spasticity. The details of orthopedic interventions have been recently reviewed by Renshaw et al. *(2)* and is discussed in detail in Chapter 7. Briefly, the orthopedic surgeon's focus is to maintain the mobility and stability of joints. Children with mobile, stable joints tend to have the best function and least amount of pain.

The youngest children with CP seldom need orthopedic surgery, as they tend to be hypotonic and have good range of motion at major joints. As hypertonicity subsequently develops, patients may lose range of motion in the spine and extremities in spite of aggressive nonoperative efforts, such as oral and injected medications; active and passive range-of-motion exercises; and uses of braces, splints, and casts. As children lose range of motion at joints, they are at risk for developing permanent contractures of soft tissues and bony deformities. Whether these will adversely effect function or lead to pain needs to be addressed by the treatment team.

Assessment of function and comfort is guided by the child's overall condition. Some children are neurologically devastated such that they cannot communicate, have no head control, cannot feed themselves, roll, or sit. Our primary goal for them is comfort. Scoliosis is generally well-tolerated in this group. Although knee and ankle contractures seldom cause problems with positioning, hygiene, or pain, hip contractures can, and these patients may benefit from soft tissue and/or bony procedures if these problems develop.

Children with the potential for sitting and either assisted or independent transfers benefit from having a balanced spine, located hips, and plantargrade feet. Spinal balance can be achieved with bracing, chair modifications, or surgery to support the functional goal of sitting. Located hips are important to prevent pain deformation *(35,36)*. Studies by Cooperman et al. suggest that hip dislocations are painful in 50% of adults with CP *(37)*. The surgical and medical options for treating a painful dislocated hip in CP are not always successful; consequently, it is best to try to maintain the hips in the proper position preventively and to monitor closely for suggestions of hip pain. Hip and knee-flexion contractures are seldom an obstacle to sitting or transfers, although they can interfere with ambulation. In patients who do not have the potential to walk, hip and knee-flexion contractures are usually well-tolerated. Neutral-positioned ankles help to comfortably place the feet on wheelchair leg rests or to weight bear for standing transfers. Consequently, soft-tissue and/or bony procedures can be useful in maintaining neutral ankle alignment *(37,38)*.

Similarly, children with the potential to stand and walk (with or without aids) benefit from a balanced spine, stable hips, as well as reasonable hip extension, knee extension, and ankle dorsiflexion. Spinal balance can be maintained orthotically or with a spinal fusion. Hip, knee, and ankle position and range of motion can be balanced with soft-tissue and bony procedures followed by bracing, when nonsurgical interventions are unsuccessful.

Soft-tissue and bony procedures are generally used to return normal range of motion to joints. Physical and occupational therapy and bracing are important in the postoperative period, to maintain the gains of surgery. The earlier that soft-tissue surgery is performed the more likely it will need repeating. We seldom do heel cord or hamstring surgery in children younger than 5 yr of age because they are often difficult to treat with therapy and orthoses. Bony deformities seldom develop at the knees and ankles as a result of soft-tissue contractures in children this young. Conversely, we recommend surgery at the first sign of hip subluxation or when abduction is less than 30°. Because hip-joint deformities develop quickly following subluxation, this must be treated aggressively.

Bracing is used extensively in the treatment of spasticity. There are several indications. Bracing is used to improve function, to prevent worsening of contractures, and to prevent the recurrence of deformities that have been corrected by surgery. We do not prescribe braces for children with normal range of motion who do not have functional goals that can be achieved with bracing. For instance, a child with a developmental age of 5 mo and no contractures does not require bracing, as there is no independent functional goal this child can achieve. However, a child with a developmental age of 5 mo with evolving equinus contractures would benefit from bracing to prevent the worsening of contractures.

Each type of brace has a prerequisite for its use as well as limitations. A spinal orthosis does little to retard progression of scoiliosis in patients with curves over 40°. At this point, the forces required to straighten the back are too great to be placed on the skin and ribs of the patient by a brace. Instead, surgery is preferred.

A long leg brace is seldom useful in correcting a knee flexion contracture over 15°. When force is applied to the flexed knee, the knee tends to internally or externally rotate within the orthosis rather than extend, as desired. This rotation defeats the purpose of the brace. If knee extension is necessary for function, surgery is often useful.

A patient who cannot dorsiflex their ankle by at least 15° will have difficulty wearing a solid ankle or free dorsiflexion ankle foot orthosis. As patients walk, their body weight rolls over their feet; if they have a tight Achilles tendon the forward rotation of the tibia is inhibited. When this pattern occurs, children either externally rotate their foot or "pop out" of their brace. In these individuals, other interventions, such as serial casting or surgery would be needed before they could benefit from bracing *(39)*.

Nighttime braces are frequently worn following surgical procedures on the lower limbs. The vast majority of hip surgery is occasioned by decreasing abduction and increasing flexion, leading to hip subluxation. Postoperatively, most children are braced into abduction and extension at night for 6–12 mo. Most knee and ankle surgery is done to correct knee-flexion ankle equinus contractures. Similarly, night braces are frequently prescribed for 6–12 mo following these procedures.

The upper limb is less often treated orthopedically than the lower limb. However, in some children with CP, the upper limb can become quite deformed. The major difficulty with the upper limb in children with CP is the lack of fine motor control and perceptual distortions. In individuals who have demonstrated a potential to use their upper limbs more effectively, coordinated treatment with an occupational therapist and hand surgeon can have positive results. At times a trial of botulinum toxin to lessen the overpowering muscle groups can unmask potential in other muscle groups, and thereby identify a candidate for tendon surgery.

As children approach skeletal maturity, soft-tissue surgery is less often done to improve function. When tight tendons are lengthened to increase range of motion, there is a change in the length-tension relationship of the muscle unit. Gains in range of motion may be accompanied by a loss of strength. In growing children, this loss of strength is more easily tolerated than in the adult because their body mass is relatively small compared to their muscle strength. The strength of muscle is related to its cross sectional area (length × length) while the mass the muscle supports is related to its volume (length × length × length). As we get bigger, our mass increases faster than our strength (as the parent of any 5-yr-old will attest to). As such, surgery should be approached with caution in individuals who have reached full growth, because adults do not compensate as readily as children do to change in muscle dynamics.

Selective Dorsal Rhizotomy

SDR is a neurosurgical procedure in which the dorsal nerve roots are partially transected to diminish sensory afferent input to the spinal reflex arc. Then lessens excessive muscle tone and movement resulting from decreased descending spinal inhibition caused by brain injury. In brief, SDR involves exposing the dorsal-nerve roots from L2 to S1 or S2, avoiding the innervation to bowel and bladder. Selectivity is provided by EMG technique, where the individual dorsal rootlets are isolated by the surgeon and stimulated electrically, with measurement of the muscular response. Based on the electrical responses, the most abnormal of the rootlets are transected. The most effective extent of surgical intervention and benefit of electromyography (EMG) selectivity remain areas of debate. The history of SDR was recently reviewed by Peacock *(40)* and details the controversy regarding its long-term benefit. Another review of this procedure was recently provided by Rekate *(41)*.

Presurgical assessment and postsurgical rehabilitation are key to a successful surgery. Selection criteria are currently a developing area, worthy of continued discussion *(42,43)*. One key concern is the underlying muscular strength in the lower limbs, because many weak patients may actually be depending on spasticity to support their weight for transfers and ambulation. Also key is the individual and family's ability to access and cooperate with aggressive therapy after surgery, and the patients chronological and developmental age. Associated movement disorders that would not be affected by SDR, such as dystonia, can make assessment of the effect of spasticity on the patients' disability difficult to isolate, and therefore obscure the clear benefit of surgery. Children with poor spatial awareness and apraxia may also be limited in their progress even with a reduction in spasticity. Presurgical evaluation includes thorough medical as well as physical- and occupational-therapy assessments. Care should be taken to establish whether the individual and families goals can be reasonably be met by surgery. Surgical goals can include comfort and ease of care for severely affected individuals with spastic quadriplegia, where risk of functional loss from surgery is low.

A more complicated decision arises in patients who are functioning well with spastic diplegia, where goals relate more to independence and ease of ambulation and self-care. Gait analysis and associated EMG evaluations are used in many institutions for preoperative evaluation, although currently no clear guidelines are available for use of these assessments. Many multidisciplinary groups, including our own, have recognized improvement in upper-limb use and speech after SDR *(44)* and therefore must consider whether surgical goals should include these areas of function as well. Details on the role of physical and occupational therapies in SDR have been detailed by Stern and Webb *(45,46)*.

FUTURE DIRECTIONS

The effects of CP are dramatically different from one individual to the next. These effects are life-long and their impact varies with age, growth, life-style, and personal goals. Spasticity, hypotonia, weakness, and associated movement disorders such as dystonia can impact significantly on an individual ability to reach their physical, social, and intellectual potential. Physical and occupational therapies remain the mainstay of treatment; however, new surgical and medical interventions are becoming available for treatment.

The future of treatment for CP will focus on prevention of CP as well as effective and permanent treatments for disordered movement at the level of the brain. Until such solutions are achieved, treatment occurs most effectively with a multidisciplinary approach to assessment and treatment. The task at hand for the medical community must include thoughtful establishment of criteria for patient selection in the use of the treatments currently available.

REFERENCES

1. Mooney, J. F., Koman, L. A., and Smith, B. P. (1993) Neuromuscular blockade in the management of cerebral palsy. *Adv. Oper. Orthop.* **1,** 337–343.
2. Koman, L. A., Mooney III, J. F., Smith, B., Goodman, A., and Mulvaney, T. (1993) Management of cerebral palsy with botulinum-A toxin: Preliminary investigation. *J. Pediat. Orthop.* **13,** 489-495.
3. Pauls, J. and Reed, K. (1996) *Quick Reference to Physical Therapy Pediatric Disorders.* Aspen Publishers, Inc., Gaithersburg, MD, pp.421–432.
4. Bohanan, R. W. and Smith, M. B. (1987) Interaction reliability of modified Ashworth scale of muscle spasticity. *Phys. Ther.* **67,** 206–207.

5. Trombly, C. A. and Scott, A. (1977) Occupational therapy for physical dysfunction. Williams and Wilkins, Baltimore.
6. Russel, D., Rosenbaum, P., Gowland, C., et al. (1993) *Gross Motor Function Measure Manual,* 2nd ed. McMaster University, Hamilton, Ontario, Canada.
7. Haley, S. M., Coster, W. J., Ludlow, L. H., et al. (1992) *Pediatric Evaluation of Disability Inventory (PEDI): Development, Standardization and Administration Manual.* PEDI Research Group, New England Medical Center Hospitals, Boston.
8. Folio, M. R., Fewell. (1983) *Peabody Developmental Scales Manual.* DLM Teaching Recourse, Allen, TX.
9. Berman, B. (1989) Selective posterior rhizotomy: does it do any good? *Neurosurg. State Art Rev.* **4(2),** 431–444.
10. Erhardt, R. P. (1982) *Developmental hand dysfunction: Theory, Assessment, Treatment.* RAMSC.
11. Ager, C., Olinett, B., and Johnson, C. (1985) Grasp and pinch strength in children 5 to 12 years old. *Am. J. Occup. Ther.* **38(2),**107–112.
12. Bobath, K. and Bobath, B. (1984) The neuro-developmental treatment, in *Management of Motor Disorders of Children with Cerebral Palsy* (Scrutton, D., ed.), JB Lippencott, Philadelphia, pp.6–18.
13. Cusick, B. (1988) Splints and casts: managing foot deformity in children with neuromuscular disorder. *Phys. Ther.* **68,** 903–912.
14. Davidoff, R. A. (1985) Antispasticity drugs: mechanisms of action. *Ann. Neurol.* **17,** 107–116.
15. Pranzatelli, M. R. (1996) Oral pharmacotherapy for the movement disorders of cerebral palsy. *J. Child Neurol.* **11(S1),** S13–S22.
16. Curtis, D. R., Game, C. J. A., Johnston, G. A. R., et al. (1974) Central effects of B-p-chlorophenyl-gamma-aminobutyric acid. *Brain Res.* **70,** 493–499.
17. Davidoff, R. A. and Sears, E. S. (1974) The effects of lioresal on synaptic activity in the isolated spinal cord. *Neurology* **24,** 957–963.
18. Pedersen, E., Arlien-Soborg, P., and Mai, J. (1974) The mode of action of the GABA derivative baclofen in human spasticity. *Acta Neurol. Scand.* **50,** 665–680.
19. Milla, P. J. and Jackson, A. D. M. (1977) A controlled trial of baclofen in children with cerebral palsy. *J. Int. Med. Res.* **5,** 398–404.
20. Pranzatelli, M. R. (1996) Antidyskinetic drug therapy for pediatric movement disorders. *J. Child Neurol.* **Sept 11(5),** 355–369.
21. Coward, D. M. (1994) Tizanidine: neuropharmacology and mechanisms of action. *Neurology* **Nov. (Suppl. 9),** S6–S11.
22. Smith, C., Birnbaum, G., Carter, J. L., Greenstein, J., and Lublin, F. D. (1994) Tizanidine Study Group. Tizanidine treatment of spasticity caused by multiple sclerosis: results of a double-blind, placebo-controlled trial. *Neurology* **Nov. (Suppl. 9),** S34–S43.
23. Nance, P. W., Bugaresti, J., Shellenberger, K., Sheremata, W., Martinez-Arizala, A. and North American Tizanidine Study Group. (1994) Efficacy and safety of tizanidine in the treatment of spasticity in-patients with spinal cord injury. *Neurology* **Nov. (Suppl. 9),** S44–S52.

24. Joynt, R. L. and Leonard Jr., J. A. (1980) Dantrolene sodium suspension in treatment of spastic cerebral palsy. *Dev. Med. Child Neurol.* **22,** 755–767.
25. Burke, R. E., Fahn, S., and Marsden, C. D. (1986) Torsion dystonia: a double-blind prospective trial of high-dosage trihexyphenidal. *Neurology* **36,** 160–164.
26. Jankovic, J. and Orman, J. (1988) Tetrabenazine therapy of dystonia, chorea, tics, and other dyskinesias. *Neurology* **38,** 391–394.
27. Rawlins, P. (1995) Intrathecal baclofen for spasticity of cerebral palsy: Project coordination and nursing care. *J. Neurosci. Nurs.* **27(3),** 157–163.
28. Campbell, S. K., Almeida, G. L., Penn, R. D., and Corcos, D. M. (1995) The effects of intrathecally administered baclofen on function in patients with spasticity. *Phys. Ther.* **75(5),** 21–31.
29. Broseta, J., Garcia-March, G., Sanchez-Ledesma, M. J., Anaya, J., and Silva, I. (1990) Chronic intrathecal administration of severe spasticity. *Stereotact. Funct. Neurosurg.* **54–55** 147–153.
30. Simpson, D. M., Alexander, D. N., O'Brien, C. F., et. al. (1996) Botulinum toxin type A in the treatment of upper extremity spasticity. A randomized, double-blind placebo-controlled trial. *Neurology* **46(1),** 1306–1310.
31. Cosgrov, A. P., Corry, I. S., and Graham, H. K. (1994) Botulinum toxin in the management of the lower limb in cerebral palsy. *Dev. Med. Child Neurol.* **36,** 386–396.
32. Chutoran, A. M. and Root, L. (1994) Management of spasticity in children with botulinum-A toxin. *Int. Ped.* **9 (Suppl. 1),** 35–43.
33. Koman, L. A., Mooney III, J. F., and Smith, B. P. (1993) The use of botulinum toxin in the management of cerebral palsy in pediatric patients, in *Botulinum and Tetanus Neurotoxins* (DasGupta, ed.), Plenus Press, New York, pp. 581–587.
34. Calderon-Gonzalez, R. and Canderon-Sepulveda, R. F. (1994) Pathophysiology of spasticity and the role of botulinum toxin in its treatment. *Acta Neuropediatr.* **1(1),** 45–57.
35. Beals, R. K. (1969) Developmental changes in the femur and acetabulum in spastic paraplegia and diplegia. *Dev. Med. Child Neurol.* **11,** 303–313.
36. Sharrard, W. J. W. (1961) The mechanism of deformity in cerebral palsy. *Proc. R. Soc. Med.* **54,** 1016.
37. Cooperman, D. R., Bartucci, E., Dietrick, E., and Millar, E. A. (1987) Hip dislocation in spastic cerebral palsy: long term consequences. *J. Pediatr. Orthop.* **7,** 268–276.
38. Gould, S. J. (1980) *The Panda's Thumb.* W.W. Norton and Co., New York, p. 300.
39. Root, L. and Spero, C. R. (1981) Hip adductor transfer compared with adductor tenotomy in cerebral palsy. *J. Bone Joint Surg.* **63A,** 767–772.
40. Peacock, W. J. and Staudt, L. A. (1991-92) Selective posterior rhizotomy: evolution of theory and practice. *Ped. Neurosurg.* **17,** 128–134.
41. Rekate, H. L. (1995) Neurosurgical management of spasticity in cerebral palsy. *BNI Q.* **11(1),** 2–10.
42. Hendricks-Ferguson, V. L. and Ortman, M. R. (1995) Selective dorsal rhizotomy to decrease spasticity in cerebral palsy. *AORN J.* **61(3),** 514–525.

43. Gregg, S. A. (1995) Criteria for selective dorsal rhizotomy. *BNI Q.* **11(1),** 11–13.
44. Albright, A. L., Barry, M. J., Fasick, M. P., and Janosky, J. (1995) Effects of continuous intrathecal baclofen infusion and selective posterior rhizotomy on upper extremity spasticity. *Pediat. Neurosurg.* **23,** 82–85.
45. Stern, L. (1995) The role of physical therapy in selective dorsal rhizotomy. *BNI Q.* **11(1),** 19–24.
46. Webb, S. J. (1995) The role of occupational therapy in selective dorsal rhizotomy. *BNI Q.* **11(1),** 25–26.

18
The Evaluation and Treatment of Spasticity in Patients with Multiple Sclerosis

Douglas R. Jeffery

INTRODUCTION

Spasticity is defined as a motor disorder characterized by a velocity-dependent increase in muscle tone associated with an increase in deep tendon reflexes, which occurs in the context of an upper motor neuron syndrome (see Table 1) (1). In patients suffering from multiple sclerosis (MS), spasticity is quite common and constitutes an important clinical problem. Its clinical manifestations and its effect on day to day function and quality of life vary considerably between patients. In its mildest form, patients may only suffer from muscle stiffness and occasional cramps. In its more severe form, spasticity may have severe consequences including contractures, spontaneous spasms, impairment in the ability to carry out activities of daily living, and impairment of mobility. The severity of spasticity may also vary over time and even within the course of a day. It is not a static phenomena and its severity and impact in MS may vary over time. In addition, numerous medications used in symptom management as well as immunomodulating therapy can further increase tone in a spastic limb or muscle group (2,3). The implications for the management of spasticity in the clinical setting are clear. Flexibility in the regimen employed is essential and treatment must be tailored to both the timing and severity of symptoms.

Clinical manifestations of spasticity include increased deep tendon reflexes, increased muscle tone, painful cramps, increased nociceptive flexor reflexes, clonus, and decreased dexterity. The functional consequences of spasticity create the need for effective therapy. This has an important consequence for management. Treatments should be directed not at the phenomena of spasticity but at improving the functional consequences of the increased muscle tone.

From: *Current Clinical Neurology: Clinical Evaluation and Management of Spasticity*
Edited by: D. A. Gelber and D. R. Jeffery © Humana Press, Inc., Totowa, NJ

Table 1
Symptoms Associated with Spasticity (Upper Motor Neuron Syndrome)

1. Exaggerated cutaneous reflex including nociceptive and flexor withdrawal reflexes
2. Autonomic hyperreflexia
3. Paresis
4. Fatiguability
5. Lack of dexterity
6. Cramps
7. Spasms

Approximately 60–80% of patients with MS suffer from spasticity as a result of demyelinating lesions in the brain and spinal cord *(4)*. In 26% of these patients, spasticity is severe enough to interfere with the activities of daily living *(5)*. Consequently the treatment of spasticity in the patient with MS becomes a critical aspect of symptom management. This is especially important when considered in light of the fact that disease-modifying therapies such as interferons may transiently worsen spasticity. This chapter will review the functional consequences of spasticity in patients with MS and discuss treatment strategies and therapeutic modalities available for MS patients.

ORIGINS OF SPASTICITY IN MS

Spasticity may result from lesions of the central nervous system (CNS), which occur in a variety of locations including the cerebrum, brainstem, and spinal cord. Multiple lesions occurring in the deep white matter may give rise to increased muscle tone and deficits in motor control resulting in impaired ambulation. This has been well-documented in multi-infarct states *(6)*. In patients with MS, a more common source of spasticity is that which results from lesions within the spinal cord. Demyelinating lesions in the cervical and thoracic spinal cord give rise to the clinical syndrome of spastic paraparesis. Patients with advanced disability owing to MS often exhibit increased tone, especially in the lower extremities accompanied by weakness, increased deep tendon reflexes, and decreased control of movement. The pathophysiology of spasticity is quite complex and is discussed in Chapter 1.

The most basic and simply stated mechanism at play in spasticity is the result of a blockade of inhibitory inputs from higher centers *(6)*. In MS this is owing to structural lesions in the form of demyelinating lesions. The final common pathway for both voluntary and involuntary movement is the anterior horn cell (AHC). A portion of the input into the AHC pool is derived from spinal interneurons that are located within the dorsal and intermediate gray matter of the spinal cord and use gamma-amino butryic acid (GABA) as their transmitter. These interneurons mediate presynaptic inhibitory inputs, which result in the modification of excitatory inputs from primary afferents and from higher centers. They are under the control of descending pathways and under normal circumstances there is a tonic level of presynaptic inhibition. The loss of this inhibitory input as a result of interruption of descending fiber tracts results in increased excitation by 1a afferents and results in increased muscle tone.

Descending pathways are also involved in the pathophysiology of spasticity. Corticospinal-tract fibers synapse directly on AHCs and allow, in part, for the voluntary control of movement and the inhibition of tone in antigravity muscles. Their interruption leads to a decrease in the control of movement and impaired dexterity. In a similar fashion, the pontine reticulospinal tract is excitatory to AHCs and its interruption may lead to similar impairments of motor control. The medullary reticulospinal tract is inhibitory in nature and its interruption leads to increased excitatory tone. There is a complex balance between inhibitory and excitatory inputs involved in motor conrol and some evidence suggests that tendon hyperreflexia and increased muscle tone may be caused by different mechanism *(7,8)*.

In summary, in the absence of a clearer understanding the neurophysiologic underpinning of motor control, spasticity can best be conceptualized as the result of increased excitatory input to AHCs, which results from an interruption of higher pathways. As with any demyelinating lesion of the spinal cord, several descending pathways are probably involved and the result is impaired control of movement, simultaneous contraction of agonist and antagonist muscles, increased deep tendon reflexes, and increased muscle tone.

FUNCTIONAL CONSEQUENCES OF SPASTICITY

The functional consequences of spasticity are outlined in Table 2. In its mildest form, spasticity manifests itself as a sensation of tightness in the muscles. This is particularly true of the lower extremities. It tends to be more bothersome to the patient after they have been on their feet for several hours, at which point the muscles become stiff and sore. Mild gait changes may be noted later in the day and the energy cost of walking increases slightly. Often patients with a mild increase in muscle tone will experience painful cramps and occasional spontaneous spasms in the evening. Usually this will occur when the patient gets into bed. This is an important consideration for treatment. Therapy should be directed at relieving the symptom and timed appropriately so as not to produce unwanted side effects. Hence patients with nighttime muscle cramps and spasms should be treated only in

Table 2
Functional Consequences of Spasticity in Multiple Sclerosis

Mild	Moderate	Severe
Increased energy expenditure in ambulation.	Increased energy cost of walking may be as much as two-fold	Gait impaired to the point that ambulation becomes very difficult with high energy expenditure.
Sensation of stiffness in the affected limb.	Impaired gait. Stresses joints and tendons in affected limbs.	Spontaneous spasms are easily brought on by attempted active or passive movements.
Fatiguability in affected limbs.	Cramps and spontaneous spasms throughtout the day.	Cramps become severe.
	Sensation of stiffness may become painful.	Risk of orthopedic injuries as a result of stresses placed on joints and tendons.
	Spasms of the affected limb with attempted use.	Contracture and pressure soars may result from limitation of movement.

the evening. A daytime dose of an agent that carries with it side effects such as fatigue and lightheadedness is not warranted. Tizanidine may be of particular benefit in patients whose spasticity becomes symptomatic at night. One side effect is sedation and this can be used to advantage to help induce sleep.

As muscle tone increases, the consequences increase on a functional level. Patients may experience stiffness that becomes painful and impairs movement. In addition, the energy cost of walking is increased two-fold in those with moderate spasticity (9). Consequently, mobility is limited owing to pain and increased energy expenditure. One factor that may contribute to pain in patients with moderate spasticity is the stress placed on tendons and joints as a result of increased tone. Nonsteroidal antiinflammatory agents may be of help in treating this type of pain. Other consequences of increased tone in patients with moderate spasticity include the presence of spontaneous spasms which occur throughout the day. This can further impair mobility and may give rise to falls when a patient develops clonus upon rising to upright posture. Clearly, the presence of moderate spasticity brings about functional consequences that may limit the patients motivation to remain active. Effective therapy is required for patients with this degree of spasticity.

When spasticity becomes severe the resulting impairment in functional ability increases exponentially. This is usually seen in patients with advanced disability. If they remain ambulatory, gait is severely impaired and bilateral assistance is required for ambulation. In such patients, it is important to consider the side effects of pharmacotherapy. Agents that bring about an increase in weakness will predispose those with pre-existing decrease in muscle strength to falls. This can be particularly important in middle-aged women whose bone density may be decreased, increasing the susceptibility to bone fractures.

In those with severe spasticity attempted active or passive movement of a limb may bring about spontaneous clonus. Often these patients will have advanced disability and may be bed-bound. When tone is increased to the point where it prevents movement of the limb, a pressure point is created and this can give rise to decubitus ulcer formation. Another consequence is the development of fixed contractures at the joints that exacerbate pressure points already established by the inability to move the limbs. Those points that are most susceptible include the heels and the hips. The ankles tend to be plantar-flexed and immobile while increased tone in the hamstrings and weakness in the iliopsoas muscles create pressure points at the hips. It is important to note that decreasing the spasticity will shift, but not relieve, the pressure points. These patients will remain susceptible to decubitus ulcer formation.

APPROACH TO THE TREATMENT OF SPASTICITY IN MS

There are several important principles of treatment worthy of statement prior to discussion of treatment modalities. The first principle is that the goal of spasticity treatment is to improve quality of life. More clearly stated, it is not the phenomena of spasticity that requires treatment, but the consequences of spasticity and the associated deficits brought about by increased muscle tone, which are the targets of therapy. The presence of spasticity alone is not a reason for treatment. Treatment of spasticity should be undertaken when it interferes with function or when it becomes painful or exacerbates other painful syndromes seen in MS.

The second principle of treatment calls for flexibility in the treatment regimen. Treatment should be targeted to the timing of the symptoms. For example, many patients complain of nighttime cramps and spasms and have almost no noticeable difficulty with increased tone during daylight hours. In this group of patients, the use of antispasticity agents during the day will only bring about unwanted side effects without particular benefit. A single evening dose of antispasmodic agent may be of considerable benefit in this group of patients. The point to be made is that the timing of the symptoms is an important consideration in the schedule of drug administration.

Dosage is also an important issue. Often in clinical practice doses are not titrated to effect and the flexibility is not brought into the regimen. For effective treatment, the dose must be titrated to maximize functional ability. Doses above that level may produce increased weakness or sedation. Doses below the desired level are subtherapeutic. As pointed out earlier, the severity of spasticity may vary over time and even within the course of the day. As a result, it is sometimes useful to use additional doses on an as needed basis. This allows the patient more control over their symptoms and can be useful when spasticity is exacerbated as a result of interferon side effects or other environmental factors.

SPECIFIC AGENTS USEFUL IN SPASTICITY IN THE MS PATIENT

A host of treatment modalities are available for MS patients suffering from spasticity. A partial list of the agents that have found widespread use are listed in Table 3. First-line agents include tizanidine and baclofen. Other agents have proven useful as either primary or adjunctive treatments. These include diazepam, dantrium, gabapentin, clonidine, botulinum toxin, phenol blocks, and physical treatments *(10–18)*.

Tizanidine

Tizanidine is an imidazoline derivative that acts both as an alpha$_2$-adrenergic agonist and as an imidazoline agonist *(19,20)*. Its mechanisms of action are complex and its activity may result from pharmacologic effects at several different sites. It decreases polysynaptic spinal cord-reflex activity and has been shown to block the release of excitatory neurotransmitters and substance P from nociceptive afferents *(20)*. It also decreases the firing rate of neurons within the locus correleus. The half-life of the compound is short (2.5 h) but may be increased in patients with renal insufficiency and in women taking oral contraceptives. One of the major advantages of tizanidine is that it has little or no effect on muscle strength at doses that bring about significant relief from painful spasms and cramps *(22–25)*. It is the only oral agent available that has been shown to improve independence in the activities of daily living *(22)*.

Tizanidine has proven efficacy in spasticity resulting from spinal-cord injury and MS *(26)*. The pathophysiology of spasticity in these two disease states are quite similar, in part, because much of the spasticity seen in MS arises from lesions in the spinal cord. Tizanidine has been studied in both spinal-cord injury and in MS. In large, multi-center, double-blind trials, tizanidine reduced the frequency of daytime spasms and clonus in both groups of patients *(25,27)*. In combined analysis of these studies tizanidine reduced

Table 3
Treatment Modalities

1. Stretching
2. Tizanidine
3. Baclofen
4. Diazepam
5. Dantrium
6. Gabapentin
7. Botulinum toxin
8. Baclofen pump
9. Clonidine
10. Klonapin
11. Phenol block
12. Orthopedic procedures

scores on the Ashworth scale and showed dramatic effects on spasticity as measured by the pendulum test *(28)*. The pendulum test is an objective measure of spasticity in which a patients legs are extended over the edge of an examining table. On release, the legs of a patient with normal tone will swing freely back and forth until they come to rest. In a patient with moderate to severe spasticity the legs tend to remain suspended and slowly, in a ratcheting, step-like fashion become flexed at the knees (Fig. 1). When knee angle is plotted against velocity, a sinusoidal pattern is seen in the normal individual. In the patient with moderate to severe spasticity, this pattern is severely disrupted (Fig. 2A). Following tizanidine administration, the pattern returned to near normal (Fig. 2B). This illustrates a dramatic reduction in muscle tone and is far more objective measure than the Ashworth scale. Nevertheless, it is a measure of muscle tone in an isolated muscle group and may not always reflect the drugs effect on functional abilities.

Tizanidine has several advantages over baclofen and the benzodiazepines and has been compared to baclofen in several trials *(22,23,29–31)*. Most have reported equal efficacy in the reduction of spasms and clonus and a similar incidence of side effects. Tizanidine was superior to baclofen in that activities of daily living were improved to a greater extent on tizanidine *(23)*. Hoogstraten et al. *(22)* reported equal efficacy but patients treated with baclofen experienced greater muscle weakness, resulting in ambulatory difficulties and trouble with standing in some patients. Bass et al. *(29)* also reported similar efficacy but weakness was more evident with baclofen. In another trial comparing the two agents the efficacy of tizanidine improved after 8 wk of therapy whereas that of baclofen decreased *(31)*.

The most important advantage of tizanidine is that it has little or no effect on muscle strength in doses that significantly reduce muscle tone. Baclofen, diazepam, and dantrium all cause muscle weakness at doses that are effective in relieving spasticity. This is of considerable importance for those MS patients with moderate disability who require unilateral or bilateral support for ambulation. The weakening of postural-support muscles by pharmacologic agents in this group of patients will predispose them to falls. That may have a significant impact on future function and could result in injury in the form of hip fractures. Other important advantages of tizanidine include its lack of a withdrawal syndrome such as those seen with baclofen and the benzodiazepines. It can be discontinued at any time without the need for a taper. In addition, the therapeutic efficacy of tizanidine may increase with time on drug whereas other agents may lose efficacy. Further, it has no abuse potential, which is typically encountered with benzodiazepines. Its ease of dosing and mild side-effect profile contribute to its advantages as a first-line agent.

The most frequently encountered side effects in clinical trials include fatigue and dry mouth *(32)*. However, in clinical practice the only limiting side effect encountered is fatigue with daytime administration. The fatigue can be avoided by using a dose-titration schedule in which 2-mg increments are added as tolerated (*see* Table 4). In clinical trials, tizanidine was dosed on a t.i.d. schedule but in clinical practice q.i.d. dosing may be more appropriate given its short half-life. In patients who suffer from spasms only at night it can be administered in a single h.s. dose and used to advantage in inducing sleep and controlling evening spasms and cramps.

In clinical trials, 5% of patients showed a rise in liver-function tests, which returned to normal levels with a decrease in dose or with discontinuation of the agent. There was no significant effect on blood pressure despite its mechanistic similarity to clonidine. Nevertheless, a rare patient may exhibit a drop in blood pressure, particularly in the presence of co-administered antihypertensive medications.

Baclofen

Baclofen has been a mainstay of antispasticity therapeutics since its introduction in the late 1970s. Despite several disadvantages when compared to newer agents, it remains in widespread clinical use and is still a first-line agent for spasticity of spinal-cord origin. Baclofen acts primarily at GABA-B receptors and inhibits monosynaptic extensor and polysynaptic flexor reflexes *(33)*. Its primary action is presynaptic, where it reduces the release of excitatory neurotransmitters in the corticospinal tract, directly antagonizing one mechanism of spasticity. This same mechanism may be responsible for the weakness induced by baclofen at higher doses because it also decreases the release of excitatory transmitters inhibiting the activation of motor neurons in the anterior horns.

Baclofen is effective for spasticity of both spinal-cord and cerebral origin *(32)*. In MS patients, baclofen reduced the frequency of painful spasms and cramps and enhanced passive range of motion. When compared to diazepam in double-blind trials, the two drugs were equally effective in reducing clonus and flexor spasms but diazepam caused more sedation *(10)*. Despite its beneficial effect on reducing muscle tone, baclofen has not been effective in improving independence in the activities of daily living or in improving ambulation *(34)*. In one study, ambulation and strength actually deteriorated owing to baclofen *(34)*. This is likely attributable to its effect on muscle strength. Nevertheless, baclofen can significantly improve quality of life as a result of its ability to reduce spasms and clonus.

In clinical use, baclofen is best started at a dose of 5 mg three times daily. Initial doses higher than this may not be well-tolerated owing to sedation. The dose can be titrated upward to either a t.id. or q.i.d. schedule and doses higher than 200 mg/d have been used but are not well tolerated. In general, with any of the agents used to treat spasticity, it is useful to start at a low dose and move up slowly. In patients with moderately severe spasticity, dose ranges of 80 mg/d are generally needed before any significant beneficial effect is observed.

Baclofen can produce a variety of adverse effects including central depression, sedation, drowsiness, fatigue, muscle weakness, and confusion. In elderly patients and probably in those with significant hemispheric disease, baclofen can impair memory and concentration. While driving ability remains a sensitive issue in patients with MS, those on baclofen should be cautioned against driving while under the influence of this agent because of decreased alertness and increased muscle weakness, which may impair motor control. One of the major disadvantages of baclofen is the withdrawal syndrome, which can accompany abrupt cessation of the agent. Abrupt discontinuation has been associated with seizures, confusion, hallucinations, and rebound muscle over activity *(35,36)*. Aside from these major side effects, baclofen has a good safety record with long-term use and has not been associated with major toxicity.

Benzodiazepines

Benzodiazepines have proven useful in treatment of spasticity of spinal-cord and cerebral origin *(37)*. The prototype agent is diazepam, which has been in use since the 1960s for treatment of spasticity of spinal-cord origin. Other agents such as clonezepam are acceptable alternatives. The benzodiazepines act pre- and postsynaptically to enhance the affinity of GABA receptors for their endogenous ligand. Diazepam is effective in the treatment of spasticity in MS but suffers from several important drawbacks compared to newer agents. It increases weakness at doses that relieve painful spasms. As pointed out earlier, this is important for those patients requiring unilateral or bilateral assistance for ambulation. Increasing weakness in that group of patients will predispose them to falls, which can result in serious injury. In addition, it suffers from abuse potential and is associated with a withdrawal syndrome, which may involve anxiety, agitation, irritability, and seizures. Finally, it clouds consciousness and may bring about significant confusion. Since 45–60% of MS patients suffer from cognitive dysfunction, it can further impair the day to day function.

In rare instances when patients are unable to tolerate first-line agents such as tizanidine or baclofen, diazepam may be a useful alternative. In such instances it should be introduced at doses of 2 mg b.i.d. or t.i.d. and titrated to effect. It may also be dosed in the evening for patients suffering from nocturnal spasms. It suffers from the same drawback as seen with baclofen in that strength is adversely effected and gait may be more impaired as a result.

Dantrium

Dantrium has also been shown effective in the treatment of spasticity. Its mechanism differs from other agents in that it acts directly on muscle. Dantrium blocks the release of calcium from the sarcoplasmic reticulum and effectively interferes with excitation-contraction coupling (16). As a result, it decreases spasticity by interfering with muscle contraction. In disease states such as MS where weakness is owing to demyelinating lesions, dantrium will significantly increase weakness. Its use in MS is not often recommended because of this effect. Dantrium suffers from other major drawbacks the most important of which is hepatotoxicity. The overall risk of hepatotoxicity is 1.8% and fatal reactions occur in 0.3%. Those at the greatest risk are women over the age of 30 taking more than 300 mg/d for over 2 mo. Those patients taking other agents that are metabolized by the liver are also at higher risk. Given the variety of agents that have proven efficacy in spasticity in MS patients, the risk associated with dantrium and its deleterious effect on muscle strength outweigh the potential benefit in the majority of cases.

ALTERNATIVE AND ADJUNCT THERAPIES FOR SPASTICITY IN MS

A wide variety of adjunctive agents have a useful role in the treatment of spasticity in MS. These include gabapentin, clonidine, clonezepam, cyclobenzaprine, cannabinoids, and opiates, which have been shown in smaller studies to reduce muscle tone and decrease the frequency of painful spasms and clonus *(39–46)*. Alternative and adjunct therapies are discussed in detail in this volume (*see* Chapter 14). Each of these agents may prove useful as adjuct therapy but none has the efficacy required of a first-line agent. Gabapentin deserves mention because of its beneficial effect on central pain syndromes seen in MS patients. Pain syndromes characterized by dysthesthetic burning sensations in the extremities may worsen spasticity and increased muscle tone may exacerbate pain. Gabapentin is effective in the treatment for chronic pain syndromes in MS and in doses greater than 900 mg daily it may bring about relief from painful spasms and clonus *(13)*. The other agents mentioned earlier find use as adjuncts when first-line agents are not tolerated at fully therapeutic doses or when first-line agents fail to bring the manifestations of spasticity under sufficient control.

Intrathecal Baclofen

When patients with MS develop spasticity that cannot be controlled with oral medication at maximal doses, the baclofen pump becomes a possible therapeutic alternative. Refractory spasticity tends to occur only in those individuals with advanced disability and whose spasticity is intractable. It should not be considered in those with spasticity of only moderate severity. In those with advanced disability, it can be a very effective alternative. The intrathecal baclofen pump is discussed in detail in this volume (*see* Chapter 15). Briefly, when a patient with intractable spasticity has failed oral medication, a test dose of intrathecal baclofen (ITB) is administered. A baseline measure of tone is obtained and a test dose of 50–100 μg is administered intrathecally over a period of 5 min. The patient is then observed for 8–12 h and measurements of spasticity are made periodically. The Ashworth scale is the recommended measure. The effect of ITB is usually quite impressive and brings about a dramatic reduction in muscle tone within an hour. In patients who do not show a reduction in tone or in those who develop increased weakness, the baclofen pump may not be appropriate. If the test dose is successful, pump implantation can proceed.

A variety of reports have confirmed the efficacy of ITB in spasticity of cerebral and spinal origin *(47–55)*. Significant reductions in the Ashworth score as well as decreases in the frequency of spasms and clonus have been confirmed. In spinal-cord injury patients, functional independence measures were also improved with ITB *(52)*. In patients with advanced disability, it can also improve quality of life and ease the burden care for caretakers as well as nursing staff. Following pump implantation, an inpatient stay in a rehabilitation facility is appropriate to adjust the dose and to facilitate adjustment to the decrease in tone so that functional independence is maintained or improved. During the first year after implantation, some tolerance occurs and the dose of baclofen must be adjusted upward to maintain therapeutic effect in the desired range. After the first year there is little additional tolerance that takes place.

While the ITB pump has proven to be an invaluable aid in the treatment of severe spasticity, several words of caution are in order. First, the baclofen pump is only appropriate for those patients with intractable spasticity whose quality of life and functional abilities are severely impaired owing to spasticity. A majority of patients can be adequately treated with available oral medication. There are a number of other potential problems and pitfalls. Overdosage can occur quite easily and this may be seen in the early stages after pump implantation. Mechanical failure of the pump and catheter kinks and dislodgment may also be problematic and can precipitate baclofen-withdrawal syndromes. This can result in hallucinations, psychosis, and seizures. Further, it may be difficult to distinguish between overdose and withdrawl. A test dose of physostigmine may be helpful in this regard because it will block some of the toxic effects of overdose. Nevertheless, the problem of abrupt withdrawl necessitates the availability of personnel familiar with pump operation 24 h a day. In addition, patients who are not reliable are poor candidates for the baclofen pump because they are more likely to miss refill appointments and run the risk of abrupt withdrawl. It is useful for patients to have oral baclofen to prevent withdrawl should a pump malfunction or catheter kink occur. Despite its potential pitfalls, in patients with intractable generalized spasticity there is no better therapeutic option.

Botulinum Toxin and Nerve Blocks

In patients with focal spasticity, the use of botulinum toxin may be of benefit when used in conjunction with other approaches. The use of botulinum toxin is discussed in greater detail in Chapter 9. The best clinical example of a potential botulinum toxin candidate is that of a patient with severe hip-adductor spasms that interfere with hygiene. Isolated spasticity rarely occurs in MS but some muscle groups may exhibit an increase in tone out of proportion to other muscle groups. It is in these instances where botulinum toxin may be useful. It acts directly on muscle and results in the inhibition of acetylcholine release from presynaptic terminals. The major drawback of botulinum toxin is that it weakens the muscle and is not rapidly reversible. Although functional abilities of the involved limbs do not usually improve, it may have beneficial effects on pain and ease of care.

Nerve blocks are another alternative in the treatment of focal spasticity. The same indications and limitations that apply with botulinum toxin are also applicable to nerve blocks. They are discussed in detail in Chapter 8.

The most commonly used agent is phenol. Alternative agents include ethanol and lidocaine. Phenol is a neurolytic agent that destroys axons and myelin but leaves the endoneurial sheath intact. Muscle weakness brought about by phenol block has a duration of 1–12 mo. Phenol blocks have the ability to reduce focal spasticity and may be beneficial in targeting muscle groups whose tone is increased out of proportion to the rest of the body. They produce muscle weakness and would not be expected to improve function but may improve comfort and ease of care. When compared with botulinum toxin, there is no specific advantage of phenol block over toxin injection. In fact, botulinum toxin injection is less complicated and does not require surgical intervention as does open motor-point blocks. Again, both botulinum toxin and nerve blocks have limited use in the treatment of spasticity owing to MS. This is primarily because the development of focal spasticity in MS is relatively uncommon and when present, is usually accompanied by more generalized increase in muscle tone. As a result, the baclofen pump is also a reasonable alternative in patients with this pattern of involvement.

Orthopedic Procedures

Patients with advanced disability owing to MS are prone to develop contractures, which may impair range of motion and predispose to decubitus-ulcer formation. This occurs when a contracture produces a pressure point. For example, a patient with a severe flexion contracture at the ankle would be highly susceptible to decubitus-ulcer formation on the heel. Similarly, a patient with flexion contractures at the hip is susceptible to decubitus-ulcer formation on the posterior aspects of the hips and at the heels. In these patients with advanced disability and fixed contractures, orthopedic procedures may be used to advantage to achieve normal position and to allow for improved range of motion. Used alone, they are of little benefit, but when used in conjunction with a coordinated plan to treat severe spasticity they may have significant benefit in the treatment of severe spasticity in advanced MS. Orthopedic procedures are discussed in Chapter 15. Briefly, tenotomies and tendon lengthenings are among the most commonly employed procedures. These are generally performed on muscles in which there is no voluntary movement. Examples include Achilles-tendon lengthening to allow for extension of the ankle and release of the hamstrings tendon to correct flexion contracture at the knee. These procedures are usually employed to prevent tertiary complication of advanced disability including the prevention of decubitus ulcers and to ease nursing care. Occasionally they can be employed in patients with less-advanced disability to improve function. An example can be found in an Achilles tendon-lengthening procedure, which would allow for the use of an ankle foot orthotic (AFO) to improve ambulation.

SUMMARY

A wide array of treatment options are now available for MS patients with spasticity of nearly any degree. In recent years, the availability of new options has truly improved the ability of physicians to manage disabling symptoms of MS. With regard to spasticity, it is important to recognize that it is not the phenomena of spasticity which requires treatment. It is the functional consequence of that spasticity that is the target of pharmacologic intervention. It should be remembered that spasticity is not fixed in time and varies considerably over months and even within a day. As a result, treatment regimens must be flexible and tailored to individual patient needs. Each of the treatment modalities available for spasticity should be viewed as a tool to diminish the functional consequence of spasticity and improve quality of life.

REFERENCES

1. Lance, J. W. (1980) Symposium synopsis, in *Spasticity: Disordered Motor Control* (Feldman, R. G., Young, R. R., and Koella, W. P., eds.), Yearbook Medical, Chicago, pp. 485–494.
2. Stolp-Smith, K. A. and Wainberg, M. C. (1999) Antidepressant exacerbation of spasticity. *Arch. Phys. Med. Rehabil.* **80,** 339–342.
3. Gelbert, D. A. and Jozefczk, P. B. (1999) Management of spasticity in multiple sclerosis. In press.
4. Paty, D. W. and Ebers, G. C. (1998) Clinical features, in *Multiple Sclerosis* (Paty, D. W. and Ebers, G. C., eds.), F.A. Davis Company, Philadelphia, pp. 135–191.
5. Freal, J. E., Kraft, G. H., and Coryell, J. K. (1984) Symptomatic fatigue in multiple sclerosis. *Arch. Phys. Med. Rehabil.* **65,** 135–138.
6. Young, R. R. (1994) Spasticity: a review. *Neurology* **44(Suppl. 9),** S12–S20.
7. Katz, R. T. and Reymer, W. Z. (1999) Spastic hypertonia: mechanisms and measurement. *Arch. Phys. Med. Rehabil.* **70,** 144–155.
8. Mayer, N. H. (1997) Clinicophysiologic concepts of spasticity and motor dysfunction in adults with an upper motoneuron lesion. *Muscle Nerve* **6(Suppl. 6)** S1–S13.
9. Chiara, D., Carlos, J., Martin, D., Miller, R., and Nadeau, S. (1998) Cold effect on oxygen uptake, perceived exertion, and spasticity in patients with multiple sclerosis. *Arch. Phys. Med. Rehabil.* **79,** 523–528.
10. From, A. and Heltberg, A. (1975) A double-blind rial with baclofen (lioresal®) and diazepam in spasticity due to multiple sclerosis. *Acta. Neurol. Scand.* **51,** 158–166.
11. Gelenberg, A. J. and Poskanzer, D. C. (1973) The effect of dantrolene sodium on spasticity in multiple sclerosis. *Neurology* **23,** 1313–1315.
12. Levine, A. M. (1985) Management of multiple sclerosis: how to improve the quality of life. *Multiple Sclerosis* **77(5),** 121–127.

13. Mueller, M. E., Gruenthal, M., and Olson, W. L. (1997) Gabapentin for relief of upper motor neuron symptoms in multiple sclerosis. *Arch. Phys. Med. Rehabil.* **78**, 521–524.
14. Gracies, J. M., Elovic, E., McGuire, J., and Simpson, D. (1997) Traditional pharmacological treatments for spasticity part I: local treatments. *Muscle Nerve* **20(Suppl. 6)**, S61–91.
15. Donovan, W. H., Carter, R. E., Rossi, C. D., and Wilkerson, M. A. (1988) Clonidine effect on spasticity: a clinical trial. *Arch. Phys. Med. Rehabil.* **69**, 193–194.
16. Pinder, R. M., Brogden, R. J. N., Speight, T. M., and Avery, G. S. (1997) Dantrolene sodium: A review of its pharmacological properties and therapeutic efficacy in spasticity. *Drugs* **13**, 3-23.
17. Khalil, A. A. and Betts, H. B. (1967) Peripheral nerve block with phenol in the management of spasticity. *JAMA* **200**, 1155–1157.
18. Snow, B. J., Tsui, J. K., Bhatt, B. H., Varelas, M., Hashimoto, S. A., and Calne, D. B. (1990) Treatment of spasticity with botulinum toxin: a double blind study. *Ann Neurol* **28**, 512–515.
19. Wagstaff, A. J. and Bryson, H. M. (1997) Tizanidine: a review of its pharmacology, clinical efficacy and tolerability in the management of spasticity associated with cerebral and spinal disorders. *Drugs* **53**, 435–452.
20. Georgiev, M. I. (1994) Mechanisms of tizanidine action on spasticity. *Acta. Neurol. Scand.* **89**, 274–279.
21. Wallace, J. D. (1994) Summary of combined clinical analysis of controlled clinical trials with tizanidine. *Neurology* **44(Suppl. 9)**, S60–S69.
22. Smolenski, Ch., Muff, S., and Smolenski-Kautz, S. (1981) A double-blind comparative trial of a new muscle relaxant, tizanidine (DS 103-282), and baclofen in the treatment of chronic spasticity in multiple sclerosis. *Curr. Med. Res. Opin.* **7(6)**, 374–383.
23. Hoogstraten, M. C., van der Ploeg, R. J. O., Burg, Wvd., van Marie, S., and Minderhoud, J. M. (1988) Tizanidine versus baclofen in the treatment of spasticity in multiple sclerosis patients. *Acta. Neurol. Scand.* **77**, 224–230.
24. Smith, C., Birnbaum, G., Carter, J. L., Greenstein, J., Lublin, F. D., and the US Tizanidine Study Group. (1994) Tizanidine treatment of spasticity caused by multiple sclerosis: results of a double-blind, placebo-controlled trial. *Neurology* **44 (Suppl. 9)**, S34–S43.
25. The United Kingdom Tizanidine Trial Group. (1994) A double-blind, placebo-controlled trial of tizanidine in the treatment of spasticity caused by multiple sclerosis. *Neurology* **44(Suppl. 9)**, S70–S78.
27. Nance, P. W., Bugaresti, J., Shellenberger, K., Sheramata, W., Martinez-Arizala, A., and the North American Tizanidine Study Group. (1994) Efficacy and safety of tizanidine in the treatment of spasticity in patients with spinal cord injury. *Neurology* **44 (Suppl. 9)**, S44–52.
28. He, J., Norling, W. R., and Wang, Y. (1997) A dynamic neuromuscular model for describing the pendulum test of spasticity. *Biomed. Eng. J.* **44(3)**, 175–184.

29. Bass, B., Weinshenker, B., Rice, G. P. A., Noseworthy, J. H., Cameron, M. G. P., Hader, W., et al. (1988) Tizanidine versus baclofen in the treatment of spasticity in patients with multiple sclerosis. *Can. J. Neurol. Sci.* **15,** 15–19.
30. Stien, R., Nordal, H. J., Oftedal, S. I., and Slettebo, M. (1987) The treatment of spasticity in multiple sclerosis: a double-blind clinical trial of a new anti-spastic drug tizanidine compared with baclofen. *Acta. Neurol. Scand.* **75,** 190–194.
31. Eyssette, M., Rohmer, F., Serratrice, G., Warter, J. M., and Boisson, D. (1988) Multi-centre, double-blind trial of a novel antispastic agent, tizanidine, in spasticity associated with multiple sclerosis. *Curr. Med. Res. Opin.* **10(10),** 699–708.
32. Nance, P. W. (1997) Tizanidine: An alpha$_2$-agonist imidazoline with antispasticity effects. *Today's Therapeut. Trends* **15,** 11–25.
33. Davidoff, R. A. (1985) Antispasticity drugs: mechanisms of action. *Ann. Neurol.* **17,** 107–116.
34. Pedersen, E., Arlien-Soborg, P., Grynderup, V., and Henriksen, O. (1970) GABA derivative in spasticity. *Acta. Neurol. Scand.* **46,** 257–266.
35. Rivas, D. A., Chancellor, M. B., Hill, K., and Freedman, M. K. (1993) Neurological manifestations of baclofen withdrawal. *J. Urol.* **150,** 1903–1905.
36. Khorasani, A. and Peruzzi, W.T. (1995) Dantrolene treatment for abrupt intrathecal baclofen withdrawal. *Anesth. Analg.* **80,** 1054–1056.
37. Reeves, R. K., Stolp-Smith, K. A., and Christopherson, M. W. (1998) Hyperthermia, rhabdomyolysis, and disseminated intravascular coagulation associated with baclofen pump catheter failure. *Arch. Phys. Med. Rehabil.* **79,** 353–356.
38. Gracies, J. M., Nance, P., Elovic, E., McGuire, J., and Simpson, D. (1997) Traditional pharmacological treatments for spasticity part II: general and regional treatments. *Muscle Nerve* **(Suppl. 6),** S92–S121.
39. Gruenthal, M., Mueller, M., Olson, W. L., Priebe, M. M., Sherwood, A. M., and Olson, W. H. (1997) Gabapentin for the treatment of spasticity in patients with spinal cord injury. *Spinal Cord* **35,** 868–869.
40. Priebe, M. M., Sherwood, A. M., Graves, D. E., Mueller, M., and Olson, W. H. (1997) Effectiveness of gabapentin in controlling spasticity: a quantitative study. *Spinal Cord* **35,** 171–175.
41. Barbeau, H., Richards, C. L, and Bedard, B. J. (1982) Action of cyproheptadine in spastic paraparetic patients. *J. Neurol. Neurosurg. Psychiatry* **45,** 923–926.
42. Nance, P. (1994) A comparison of clonidine, cyroheptadine and baclofen in spastic spinal cord injured patients. *J. Am. Paraplegia Soc.* **17,** 151–157.
43. Weingarden, S. I. and Belen, J. G. (1992) Clonidine transdermal system for treatment of spasticity in spinal cord injury. *Arch. Phys. Med. Rehabil.* **73,** 876–877.
44. Erickson, D. L., Blacklock, J. B., Michaelson, M., Sperling, K. B., and Lo, J. N. (1985) Control of spasticity by implantable continuous flow morphine pump. *Neurology* **16,** 215–217.
45. Donovan, W. H., Carter, R. E., Rossi, C. D., and Wilkerson, M. A. (1988) Clonidine effect on spasticity: a clinical trial. *Arch. Phys. Med. Rehabil.* **69,** 193–194.

46. Meinck, H. M., Schönle, P. W., and Conrad, B. (1989) Effect of cannabinoids on spasticity and ataxia in multiple sclerosis. *J. Neurol.* **236,** 120–122.
47. Coffey, R. J., Cahill, D., Steers, W., and Park, T. S. (1993) Intrathecal baclofen for intractable spasticity of spinal origin: results of long-term multicenter study. *J. Neurosurg* **78,** 226–232.
48. Nance, P., Schryvers, O., Schmidt, B., Dubo, H., Loveridge, B., and Fewer, D. (1995) Intrathecal baclofen therapy for adults with spinal spasticity: therapeutic efficacy and effect on hospital admissions. *Can. J. Neurol. Sci.* **22,** 22–29.
49. Lazorthes, Y., Sallerin-Caute, B., Verdie, J., Bastide, R., and Carillo, J. (1990) Chronic intrathecal baclofen administration for control of severe spasticity. *J. Neurosurg.* **72,** 393–402.
50. Rifici, C., Kofler, M., Kronenberg, M., Kofler, A., Bramanti, P., and Saltuari, L. (1994) Intrathecal baclofen application in patients with supraspinal spasticity secondary to severe traumatic brain injury. *Funct. Neurol.* **9,** 29–34.
51. Penn, R. D., Savoy, S. M., Corcos, D., Latash, M., Gottlieb, G., Parke, B., and Kroin, J. S. (1989) Intrathecal baclofen for severe spinal spasticity. *N. Engl. J. Med.* **320,** 517–521.
52. Latash, M. L., Penn, R. D., Corcos, D. M., and Gottlieb, G. L. (1990) Effects of intrathecal baclofen on voluntary motor control in spastic paresis. *J. Neurosurg.* **72,** 388–392.
53. Loubser, P. G., Narayan, R. K., Sandin, K. J., Donovan, W. H., and Russell, K. D. (1991) Continuous infusion of intrathecal baclofen: long-term effects on spasticity in spinal cord injury. *Paraplegia* **29,** 48–52.
54. Ochs, G., Struppler, A., Meyerson, B. A., Linderoth, B., and Gybels, J. (1989) Intrathecal baclofen for long-term treatment of spasticity; a multicentre study. *J. Neurol. Neurosurg. Psychiatry* **52,** 933–939.
55. Meythaler, J. M., DeVivo, M. J., and Hadley, M. (1996) Prospective study on the use of bolus intrathecal baclofen for spastic hypertonia due to acquired brain injury. *Arch. Phys. Med. Rehabil.* **77,** 461–466.

19
The Development and Management of Spasticity Following Traumatic Brain Injury

Patricia B. Jozefczyk

INTRODUCTION

Traumatic brain injury (TBI) results from either a penetrating skull injury or closed trauma to the head, and is a major health problem in the United States and worldwide. Penetrating head injuries account for approx 10% of all traumatic injuries and closed head trauma for the other 90%. These injuries tend to occur more commonly in males. There is a bimodal peak of incidence, with males between 16 and 25 yr of age and people over the age of 65 yr tending to have more TBIs (1). Motor-vehicle accidents account for at least 50% of all TBIs with falls, assaults and violence, and sports and recreational accidents following. Approximately fifty to seventy-five thousand people per year in the United States suffer a severe TBI and approx one-third to one-half of those die (2). The remaining survive with varying degrees of cognitive and neurologic damage.

The Glasgow Coma Scale (GCS) provides a standardized measure of the patient's response to eye opening, motor response, and verbal response, upon presentation to the hospital after a TBI (see Table 1). This scale serves to classify the degree of TBI and to help project outcome. The patient's long-term outcome is highly variable, and residual impairments, which may include spasticity, depend on the pattern and severity of the head injury.

The vast majority of TBIs within the United States are mild, with the patient suffering no loss of consciousness or only a brief period of altered consciousness. These patients present with a GCS of 13–15, loss of consciousness for less than 20 min, and post-traumatic amnesia (PTA) of less than 24 h. These patients may suffer a post-traumatic syndrome that can include imbalance, headaches, vertigo, memory, cognitive, or concentration problems. Patients with admission GCS of less than 9, a duration of coma

From: *Current Clinical Neurology: Clinical Evaluation and Management of Spasticity*
Edited by: D. A. Gelber and D. R. Jeffery © Humana Press, Inc., Totowa, NJ

Table 1
Glasgow Coma Scale

Test	Patient's response	Score
Eye opening	Spontaneous eye opening	4
	Opens eyes to voice	3
	Opens eyes to pain	2
	Does not open eyes	1
Best motor response	Follows commands	6
	Localizes to painful stimulus	5
	Withdraws from painful stimulus	4
	Decorticate posturing	3
	Decerebrate posturing	2
	No motor response	1
Best verbal response	Oriented	5
	Confused or disoriented	4
	Speaks with inappropriate words	3
	Incomprehensible sounds	2
	No speech or sounds	1

greater than 8 h, or PTA of greater than 24 h are classified as having a severe TBI, whereas those with an admission GSC of 9–12 are considered to have a moderate TBI. Patients with severe TBI represent only 5% of all TBI yet they require the most intense rehabilitative efforts. Ten percent of all TBI are considered moderate and the rest minor in nature (3).

Patients with mild TBI typically do not develop focal neurologic deficits or spasticity. Those with moderate or severe TBI frequently have spasticity and their management will be the focus of the discussion in this chapter. For discussion and management purposes, these patients are divided into acute, subacute, and chronic stages of TBI. In the acute phase, the patient may be comatose, have PTA, or be agitated. Depending on the type of injury sustained, focal motor or sensory signs may or may not be present. If a motor deficit does exist, motor recovery may be expected. It is impossible to predict at this stage the degree of recovery that may ultimately occur. Therefore, all patients should be aggressively treated. In the subacute (3-6 mo) or chronic (greater than 6–12 mo) stages after TBI, rehabilitative goals may shift. Treatment of the patient's motor deficit or spasticity will depend on the functional goals to be achieved. In most cases of moderate to severe TBI, patients are left with the combination of physical and cognitive impairments.

PATHOPHYSIOLOGY OF TRAUMATIC BRAIN INJURY

The neurologic deficits that may result from TBI are varied. They depend on the primary type of injury, location of the head trauma, and a series of secondary injuries that may occur (*see* Table 2). Primary injuries to the central nervous system (CNS) may be focal or diffuse. Focal injuries may occur both in open and closed head injuries. With penetrating head injuries, the location of the injury and velocity of the projectile determines the neurologic sequelae. With closed head injuries, hematomas or contusions are most typical. These occur as a result of coup and contra-coup mechanisms and are typically seen in the frontal, orbital, temporal, and occipital poles of the brain. Contusions or frank intracerebral hemorrhage may result.

Diffuse primary injuries include diffuse axonal injury (DAI) or hypoxic ischemic injury (HII). DAI is most typically found after an acceleration-deceleration injury typical of motor-vehicle accidents. This type of injury results in multiple petechial hemorrhages, axonal swelling, and retraction followed by microglial infiltration and later axonal degeneration. This axonal disruption may occur over a course of more than 12 h (*4*). DAI tends to occur in the midline structures of the brain with the areas of primary involvement in the upper brainstem, cerebellum, and corpus callosum. This results in deafferentation and dysfunction in many areas including the thalamic nuclei and prefrontal cortex. Owing to this pathology, DAI does not typically cause focal motor deficits or spasticity, unless also combined with focal cortical or subcortical lesions. HII occurs as a result of microvascular injury, arterial occlusion or dissection, or may be related to local vasospasm, generalized hypotension, or hypoxemia. Pathologically this results in cortical laminar necrosis especially noted in the hippocampus, cerebellum, and basal ganglia.

Primary injuries to the brain after a TBI typically lead to varying degrees of secondary injury. Both closed head injuries and penetrating head injuries may result in a series of cellular events, which include the release of excitotoxins, free radicals, the development of lactic acidosis, calcium and other ion fluxes, glutamate neurotoxicity, and toxic cytokine production (*5*). In addition, there is a secondary increase in intracranial pressure. This may be secondary to neurogenic or vasogenic edema. Depending on the location and the extent of the increased intracranial pressure, herniation may follow. Communicating hydrocephalus may also evolve especially if subarachnoid blood is present. Hypothalamic-pituitary dysfunction can occur with an increase in catecholamines and aldosterone, a drop in thyroid hormone release, diabetes insipidus, or inappropriate antidiuretic hormone secretion.

Table 2
Pathophysiology of Traumatic Brain Injury

Primary Injury	Focal	Intracerebral hemorrhage
		Contusion
		Hematoma
		Focal hypoxic-ischemic injury
	Diffuse	Diffuse axonal injury
		Diffuse hypoxic-ischemic injury
Secondary Injury		Cascade of toxic cellular events
		Hydrocephalus
		Increased intracranial pressure
		Metabolic/endocrine dysfunction

INDICATORS OF OUTCOME AFTER TBI

Epidemiological observations of TBI patients have helped identify some predictors of functional outcome. The GCS has become the most widely used acute predictor. However, the accuracy may be limited by the presence of alcohol, drugs, or other acute surgical or medical complications at the time of the head injury. It is also difficult to administer to young children or patients with language impairments, those intubated, or sedated.

The duration of coma is also a predictor of functional outcome and does have a linear relationship in patients with DAI (6). The duration of PTA also correlates with outcome, with PTA of more than 14 d associated with a higher incidence of moderate-to-severe disability (7). Reactive pupils are also associated with better outcomes than nonreactive pupils. Age also plays a factor. Children and young adults typically have a better outcome than older adults do, although children less that 5 yr old and adults older than 65 yr have the highest degree of mortality. In addition, pre-injury substance abuse (8) and medical or psychological factors also may affect the recovery process.

It appears from outcome statistics, that the majority of neurological recovery from acute brain injury occurs within the first 6 mo. In addition, some impairments recover more quickly than others. Physical disabilities and functional skills such as mobility can show improvement within 3 mo after injury, and the same is generally true for recovery of speech and language functions, which typically plateau by 6 mo after injury. Perceptual-motor skills, however, do not typically plateau until 12 mo after injury. It is unclear, however, what the maximal duration of the recovery period is in these patients. Some suggest that neurologic recovery is virtually complete within one year whereas others feel that recovery can continue two or more years postinjury (9).

PATTERNS OF RECOVERY AFTER TBI

In the acute stage, the patient who suffers a moderate to severe TBI is typically cared for in an intensive-care setting. In addition to the brain injury, many of these patients suffer from multiple fractures, soft-tissue injuries, and abdominal or thoracic problems that may require surgical intervention. These patients are typically comatose and acute care should include careful monitoring for prevention of complications such as contractures, decubitus ulcers, the development of heterotopic ossification, and bowel and bladder function. In addition, maintaining adequate nutrition and monitoring the metabolic and endocrine status are important factors in the care of these patients. Next, the patient may clinically emerge from the comatose stage and their medical and surgical problems stabilize. This phase of care may last several months. These patients will require continued in-patient care until their medical problems stabilize. Neurologic complications during this period can include seizures, the development of hydrocephalus, or infections. The more severely brain injured patient however, may remain in a persistent vegetative state (PVS). PVS follows severe TBI in 1–14% of 1-mo survivors (10). Prognosis for recovery, regaining consciousness, and return of function in patients in a PVS is poor. Many die, remain vegetative, or have severe disability even if they do regain consciousness. These patients typically require continued management in a nursing home environment.

As the brain-injured patient emerges from coma, they typically progress through a confusional state with PTA, agitation, and behavioral disturbances. It is during this time that their physical mobility will begin to improve. Management in an acute rehabilitation facility or an extended-care facility will depend on the patient's ability to tolerate intensive rehabilitation. If the patient has primarily cognitive or behavioral problems with little or no physical impairments, management focuses on cognitive retraining. If the patient can be managed at home, a day-care program can be an acceptable option. If not, a behavioral-management program leading to transitional living situations and community reintegration is commonly advocated for the cognitively impaired TBI patient.

The majority of patients who survive TBI and recover from a comatose state typically suffer from cognitive and neurobehavioral problems. In the mid-1970s, focus on the rehabilitation of memory, behavior, and psychosocial reintegration was emphasized (11). Unfortunately, this resulted in a relative de-emphasis on physical rehabilitation such as treatment of motor paresis or limb spasticity. When a brain injury produces an upper motor neuron syndrome, the degree of remaining voluntary muscle control is variable and needs to be thoroughly assessed in each individual patient. Spasticity may also occur in muscles affected by upper motor neuron lesions. Distinction must be made between the poor production and regulation of voluntary movement and factors that cause spasticity. In addition, changes in the physical properties of muscle and other soft-tissue structures need to be considered.

In addition to muscle weakness, sensory abnormalities may interfere with motor recovery. TBI may also result in speech problems or bulbar dysfunction including dysphagia. Cerebellar disorders may occur and are notoriously difficult to rehabilitate. A variety of movement disorders have also been described including myoclonic jerks, parkinsonism, tremors, rigidity, and dystonia. Dystonia in particular may complicate the management of spasticity and may result in problems in differential diagnoses. Both peripheral and central injuries may be associated with dystonia. Another problem is pain, which is very common after a brain injury. Headache is the most common, followed by cervical pain. Many times myofascial sources are the cause of this pain although fractures, heterotopic ossification, dislocation, and radiculopathy need to be considered as possible sources of the pain. Seizures also complicate the management of TBI patients. Penetrating head injuries most typically result in a post-traumatic seizure disorder (12). With closed head injuries, less than 5% of patients experience a seizure within the first 2 wk of injury. The risk increases to 7% at 1 yr, with an 11% 5-yr risk of seizures in patients with contusions, hematomas, amnesia, or greater than 24 h of unconsciousness (13). Studies that have reviewed the natural history of post-traumatic seizures in a controlled setting found that the incidence of seizures can be reduced by 70% with anticonvulsants in the first week after a brain injury, but not beyond that point. These patients had a GCS of 10 or less, a hematoma on computed tomography (CT) scan, a penetrating skull wound, or a seizure within the first 24 h of injury and were treated with either prophylactic phenytoin or placebo (14). There is an overall rate of 25% for a first seizure regardless of anticonvulsant prophylaxis, and this has important implications because anticonvulsants, particularly phenytoin, phenobarbital, and carbamazepine, may impair motor and cognitive function.

At all stages during the recovery from TBI, a strong interdisciplinary approach is required in the management of these patients. In the acute stage of recovery from TBI, broad functional areas for improvement should be defined. These may include bed mobility, positioning, and reorientation. Subacutely, as the patient continues to improve, more specific skills and behavioral management needs to be addressed. Tasks may include transfers, dressing, or ambulation. It is important as a team to identify impairments in the patient that may improve, that may lead to disability if not managed, and that may have a reasonable expectation of responding to treatment. Occasionally, various disciplines may approach these impairments with different theoretical or clinical backgrounds and this may serve as a source of conflict for the team. However, it is important to remember that discipline-specific assessments need to be incorporated into a management plan that identifies patient-specific impairments, functional assessment, and patient-directed goals (15).

SPASTICITY IN ACUTE TBI

Spasticity is most commonly defined as a motor disorder characterized by velocity-dependent increase in tonic stretch reflexes with exaggerated tendon reflexes. Other components of spasticity include abnormal cutaneous and autonomic reflexes, lack of dexterity, motor paresis, fatigability, and typical patterns of overactivity (16,17). After TBI, spasticity may develop as a result of loss of cortical control over spinal-reflex centers. Typically this loss of control results in an increase in flexor tone in the upper extremities with a tendency toward extensor tone in the lower extremities. Hypertonicity may also occur in the trunk, facial, and oral-pharyngeal musculature. The approach to the management of spasticity after TBI will vary depending on the extent of injury, focal neurologic deficits, and the duration of time postinjury.

In the acute phase of a moderate-to-severe head injury, the patient may be comatose. Depending on the severity of the injury, that patient may develop spasticity within a few days to weeks after the cerebral trauma. Management of increasing limb tone is primarily preventive at this stage. Intervention should be considered when spasticity interferes with achievement of rehabilitation goals. In the severely injured comatose patient, these goals include prevention of the development of contractures, peripheral-compression neuropathies, management of fractures, and prevention of heterotopic ossification (HO). The mainstay of prevention is passive range of motion. Cryotherapy may be helpful in temporarily reducing spasticity and allow more extensive range of motion. The application of casts or splints to preserve or increase range of motion or prevent contractures has also shown the secondary beneficial effect of reducing spasticity (18). Proper positioning of the patient as well as frequent change of position is necessary to help decrease tone in spastic muscles.

If physical modalities alone do not significantly improve the tone or if spasticity is progressive despite these interventions, then pharmacological intervention may become necessary. Antispasticity medications must be carefully chosen and monitored to avoid negative effects on cognition and functional recovery. If these interventions fail to reduce spasticity,

Table 3
Treatment Options for Spasticity In Acute Traumatic Brain Injury

Goal in acute TBI: Prevention of spasticity	
Positioning	Treatment of factors that may worsen spasticity:
Changes of position	
Range of motion	Pain
Passive stretching	Fever
Passive lengthening	Decubitus ulcers
Splints and orthoses	Fractures
Casts	Seizures
Serial Casting	Metabolic dysfunction
Injectable drugs	Fecal impaction
Systemic drugs	Urinary retention

motor-point blocks, nerve blocks, or neuromuscular junction blocks may be considered (*see* Table 3).

It is important for the managing physician to consider non-neurologic factors that may contribute to the development or progression of spasticity. Tone may be increased by a number of factors that cannot be expressed by the nonverbal or aphasic patient. Pain, which may result from an occult fracture or heterotopic ossification, may increase tone. Urinary retention or fecal impaction may also increase tone, especially in the lower extremities. Decubitus ulcers, ingrown toenails, and intravenous (IV) infiltration may similarly adversely affect spasticity. The severely head-injured patient typically is at a higher metabolic state with a high degree of catabolism. Electrolyte or endocrine abnormalities as well as calcium and magnesium abnormalities may exacerbate spasticity. Fevers, with or without infection also have an adverse effect on muscle tone. Similarly, seizure activity may temporarily increase spasticity. The physician needs to be vigilant in recognizing, monitoring, and correcting any of these abnormalities in the severely brain-injured patient before considering primary treatment of the patients spasticity.

CONTRACTURES

In addition to spasticity, the TBI patient may exhibit abnormal limb posture or positioning for other reasons (*see* Table 4). Progressive increased tone in an extremity may lead to the development of dynamic contractures, and if left unattended, fixed contractures may develop. Other factors that

Table 4
Factors Contributing to Abnormal Limb Position In Traumatic Brain Injury

Paralysis
Immobilization
Soft-tissue contractures
Dynamic or static joint contractures
Fractures
Heterotopic ossification
Spasticity

may contribute to the development of contractures in the severely head-injured patient include prolonged mobilization as a consequence of orthopedic treatment, bed rest, or joint pain, as well as other associated musculoskeletal changes. The absence or reduction of normal mechanical stresses that are experienced during motor activities result in structural changes that cause joint stiffness. A joint contracture occurs when there is a loss of mobility of a joint and may originate in any components of the joint, including the soft tissue, tendons, intra-articular ligaments, or bony articulations (19). Joint contractures and limb deformities are sometimes initially neglected in acute TBI patients in favor of needed medical or surgical interventions. However, the surgical and hospital costs for correcting functionally significant joint contractures later in patients with brain injuries have been estimated to exceed $20,000 per surgical procedure (20). In patients with TBI, 84% of patients who progress to acute medical rehabilitation have significant contractures. These occur most frequently in the hips (81%), ankles (76%), and shoulders (76%) (21). Elderly patients, who have less-compliant soft tissue, patients with dementia, or those living in a nursing facility, are at a greater risk for the development of contractures.

The anatomic and pathologic changes that lead to the development of contractures have been well-studied. Immobilization itself produces progressive infiltration of fibrofatty connective tissue into the joint space (22). With prolonged immobilization, this connective tissue progressively covers the intra-articular soft-tissue structures such as the ligaments as well as the nonarticulating cartilage surfaces. Eventually adhesions develop between the exposed tissue surfaces. Pathological changes, which effect the articular cartilage, are similar. At first, the cartilage becomes fibrillated and later is replaced by a more mature fibrous tissue. This may extend to the subchondral bone with subsequent hyperemia and fibrovascular proliferation in the subadjacent marrow spaces. As the process progresses, mature fibrous tissue replaces the articular cartilage, causing joint ankylosis (23). Changes also occur in the periarticular fibrous connective tissue. Tendons, ligaments, and capsules consist primarily of organic collagen. Hyaluronic acid is the principal fibrous connective-tissue lubricant. With immobilization and stress deprivation, biochemical changes occur with a decrease in the water and hyaluronic acid content causing adhesions or cross-linking between adjacent collagen fibrils (24).

Structural changes are also noted in the skeletal muscle after immobilization. Clinically there is muscle atrophy, weakness, and a shift in fiber type from slow to fast twitch. Human studies have shown a 30% decrease in muscle cross-sectional area following 6 wk of immobilization (25). Animal studies have shown an increase in volume of intramuscular connective tissue with a decrease in the number of sarcomeres when a limb was immobilized in a shortened position. These muscles showed a significant decrease in extensibility. In patients with traumatic head injuries who are immobilized owing to coma, or medical or surgical complications, all of these pathological changes begin very early during the course of immobilization. Human studies have shown that the loss of muscle strength is greater than the degree of clinical atrophy. Some authors have suggested that a 50% loss in muscle strength can occur in as short as 6 wk after immobilization (26). If the brain-injured patient has, in addition, suffered an upper motor neuron lesion, an imbalance in muscle tone between agonist and antagonist muscle begin to develop across a joint. Functional contractures may develop as a joint is forced into a position or posture owing to a combination of muscle weakness and excessive muscle contraction secondary to spasticity. This leads to further immobilization of the joint in that position and the cascade of events described for the soft-tissue structures, combined with the spasticity, increase the risk of developing a fixed contracture. With spasticity, the upper extremities most commonly develop a predominantly flexor tone while the lower extremities are typically held in extension. The single most important factor for the development of a fixed contracture is lack of joint movement. Prevention is the cornerstone in managing contractures and positioning of the patient is a primary concern. In bed, the patient should be positioned to avoid extremity flexion. Splints, wedges, or weighted sandbags may assist in proper positioning. In the wheelchair, prolonged hip flexion and knee flexion should be avoided by frequent change of position. Daily or twice daily range of motion exercises must be performed either passively or with the patient's assistance. If the patient is developing hip-flexion contractures, prone positioning in bed may be necessary. Standing, either supported or unsupported, allows for stretch of the pelvis, hips, knees, and also the Achilles tendon. Repeated stretching of the hypertonic muscle may be more effective if heating of the connective tissue is done before stretching. Splinting, serial casting, and dynamic orthotics may also be considered in the management of the acute traumatic brain-injured patient who develops spasticity of a limb.

FRACTURES

Although many fractures may be recognized at the time of presentation in the severely brain-injured patient more subtle ones are often missed. The managing physician needs to be alert to these more occult fractures. Even patients who are semiconscious may wince or groan with passive limb movement or may resist active extremity movement. These signs, as well as any unexplained swelling or deformity, should prompt radiographic evaluation for occult fracture. Spasticity in a fractured limb may be increased owing to pain or swelling. In addition, there is a higher incidence of heterotopic ossification in a fractured limb. These fractures should be treated aggressively in the TBI patient to include open reduction and internal fixation when necessary, in order to promote early mobilization and decrease the likelihood of contracture formation (*27*).

HETEROTOPIC OSSIFICATION

HO may occur in up to 75% of patients who suffer a severe TBI. These primarily occur in the proximal joints of the limbs. Prolonged coma, spasticity, and associated fractures of the limb are additional risk factors for the development of HO (*27*). Clinical signs of HO may include swelling, pain or warmth at or near a joint, or the development of a contracture. However, this abnormal bony formation may also be occult and asymptomatic. Its presence may be indicated only by limited range of motion of the joint. Earliest diagnosis can be made by a triphasic bone scan, although later, ossification is visible on plain radiographs. Management of HO is difficult. Range of motion alone does not typically prevent or limit the development of the bony ossification. Diphosphonates (*28,29*), and indomethacin (*30*) have been used to arrest the early development of HO or to prevent its postoperative reoccurrence but consistent efficacy has not been established. Radiation therapy (*31*) has been used with variable success after total hip replacement. Surgery for removal of ectopic bone should be considered only to achieve a well-defined functional goal and should not be considered during the acute recovery stage from a TBI (*32*).

SPASTICITY IN SUBACUTE AND CHRONIC TBI

As one moves from the acute to subacute and chronic stages after a TBI, management of spasticity changes. Stretching, range of motion, and other

Table 5
Treatment Options for Spasticity In Subacute-Chronic Traumatic Brain Injury

Goal in subacute-chronic TBI: To achieve defined goals	
Positioning	Injectable drugs
Change of position	Systemic drugs
Range of motion	Intrathecal drugs
Passive stretch	Orthopedic surgical procedures
Passive lengthening	Neurosurgical procedures
Splint and orthoses	
Casts and serial casting	

physical modalities still serve as the initial foundation in the treatment of spasticity but are often inadequate. The managing physician may need to consider the use of medications, nerve blocks, motor-point blocks, or even surgical intervention (see Table 5).

Unlike the management of spasticity in the acutely brain-injured patient, the mere presence of spasticity in the subacute or chronic patient may not require therapeutic intervention. Spasticity may be beneficial in these patients. Increased tone in the lower extremities may allow the brain-injured patient to perform transfers, stand, or even walk owing to increased tone of antigravity muscles, or it may allow a paretic limb to withdraw from potentially dangerous stimuli. Spasticity may help prevent muscle atrophy, calcium loss from bone, and may decrease edema and the risk of deep venous thrombosis. It may also assist in cardiovascular conditioning. Negative features of spasticity are those that interfere with rehabilitation or activities of daily living. Spasticity may produce pain, result in fractures, and contribute to the development of decubitus skin ulcers. Spasticity may impair posture or produce an abnormal quality of movement of a limb or produce painful spasms, abnormal ambulation, and poor hygiene, and may interfere with nursing care (33,34). In patients with moderate to severe TBI the distribution of spasticity depends on the location and type of pathology of the initial injury. Spasticity may develop in a single limb or in both an upper and lower extremity on one side. Diffuse generalized spasticity may be seen in patients with severe diffuse axonal injury or bilateral cortical or subcortical damage. Patients who develop quadriparetic spasticity after TBI most typically have severe cognitive impairments or may remain in a persistent vegetative state (excluding the possibility of a concomitant spinal-cord injury). Patients who survive the initial brain injury, emerge from their coma, and become more physically functional will more likely suffer from focal extremity spasticity. In the postacute phase of the patient's recovery from TBI, spasticity treatment should be undertaken only to achieve clearly defined functional goals. In examining a patient with spasticity, both passive and active range of motion needs to be analyzed and recorded. Patient position, room temperature, and patient comfort must be taken into consideration during these measurements. In addition, the location or degree of spasticity may change when the patient is supine in bed vs sitting or standing. Detailed examination of muscle strength is also important. This should be recorded not only in the region of the spastic limb, but also more proximal and distal strength needs to be considered. A detailed sensory examination should also be included, as the patient's perception of pain, touch, and proprioception will play a role in deciding if a patient will tolerate casting or phenol injections. Balance problems and ataxia, if present, may limit functional success despite the reduction of spasticity in a limb. If the patient is ambulatory, careful observation of the swing and stance phases of gait will identify the distribution and extent of spasticity and whether an assistive device may aid in its treatment.

If available, gait analysis is extremely important in planning the treatment for focal spasticity in the lower extremities. Dynamic EMG, ground reaction-force analysis, and three-dimensional (3D) motion analysis of gait will help to further define which changes in the mechanics of gait will help with functional ambulation, and how these results might be achieved.

In addition to a detailed neurological examination, musculoskeletal and joint examination must also be performed. Both active and passive range of motion of the joints should be recorded by goniometric angle measurement. X-rays of bones and joints may be necessary if any focal areas of swelling or pain are identified. This will help exclude the possibility of occult fractures or heterotopic ossification. In addition, focal areas of muscle atrophy, weakness, or abnormal sensation may identify concomitant peripheral nerve injury or entrapment in this patient population. Finally, the cognitive and neurobehavioral aspects of the patient's TBI need to be taken into consideration. Many of the modalities to be discussed require patient cooperation and involvement in post-treatment rehabilitation. A confused, agitated, or language-impaired patient may be unable to understand or tolerate the placement of a cast, or the need for physical therapy after surgical intervention.

When should the treatment of increased muscle tone be considered? It should be considered when a patient is developing a contracture or progressing in abnormal posturing of a limb (*see* Table 6). It should also be considered when spastic muscles interfere with active movement of agonist or antagonist muscles. It is important to keep in mind that relief of spasticity

Table 6
Goals in the Treatment of Spasticity in Traumatic Brain Injury

Prevention of progressive limb contractures
Improved bed or wheelchair positioning
Decrease or control of pain
Better hygiene and nursing care
Ease of activities of daily living
Improved functional use of limbs for transfers and ambulation
To allow use of splints and orthoses
To allow residual voluntary muscle movement

may actually unmask underlying muscular weakness and fail to achieve this goal. Spasticity should be treated when it interferes with appropriate positioning or personal hygiene and if muscle spasms result in physical trauma to the patient. In addition, when physical modalities such as stretching or range of motion produce excessive pain or excessive therapy time is needed to simply prevent contracture rather than for allowing functional activities, then spasticity treatment should be considered.

THERAPEUTIC INTERVENTIONS FOR FOCAL SPASTICITY

Passive Stretch and Range of Motion

Professionals caring for patients with spasticity have long made the bedside observation that muscle resistance progressively diminishes as one continually ranges the limb and repeats this motion. A daily stretching regimen continues to be an integral part of any management program for spasticity. Passive stretch is a technique that moves the muscle through a range simulating normal patterns of movement. Passive stretch also tends to lengthen the muscle and is commonly used in the treatment of dynamic contractures. This technique involves prolonged holding of a desired position at the maximal point of tolerance. The physiologic basis for decreasing tone with passive stretch or passive lengthening is not clearly defined. This may be related to plastic changes within the CNS or mechanical changes at the muscle, tendon, and soft-tissue level. Spasticity reduction achieved by these modalities typically lasts only several hours, but may prevent the progression from a dynamic to a static contracture. Patients with spastic limbs with residual voluntary movement have shown improved finger extension movement but not force after manual stretch (35). The use of a mechanical leg-abductor device in patients with spastic paraparesis improved voluntary hip abduction lasting up to 16 h (36).

Muscle Strengthening

Controversy surrounds the use of muscle strengthening in treating spasticity. The physical therapeutic technique of proprioceptive facilitation developed by Kabat and Knott encouraged the training of weak muscles against the resistance of a therapist with the goal of increasing the strength in movement patterns opposing the spastic posture (*37*). In contrast, Bobath felt that resistive muscle strengthening increased tone. Her theory is based on the neurodevelopmental technique developed after observation of the normal neurophysiologic development of infants. Bobath concluded that regaining normal movements was impossible as long as muscle tone was increased. Her principles of therapeutic intervention are based on an attempt to inhibit the released tonic reflexes by passively bringing the patient into reflex-inhibitory postures (*38*).

These techniques, among others, have continued to be a source of conflict in choosing an appropriate physical therapy approach in the treatment of spasticity. However, recent studies in children and adolescents with spasticity from cerebral palsy (CP) have demonstrated that strength and gross motor ability improved with isokinetic training (*39*). In another study, programs aimed at improving quadriceps strength in children with CP with spastic diplegia resulted in improved walking without an apparent increase in tone (*40*).

Miscellaneous Physical Therapeutic Interventions

A variety of techniques have been used with the observation of a clinical decrease in spasticity. Vibration applied over tendons or muscles of an antagonistic muscle in a spastic limb causes sustained discharges in neural afferents (*41*). Vibration of wrist extensors results in passive contraction of those muscles in a wrist that is otherwise held in flexion. However, the studies addressing this technique do not distinguish between increased flexor tone and extensor muscle weakness. Topical cold (*42*) and topical anesthetics (*43*) may result in decreased tone presumably by decreasing sensitivity of cutaneous receptors and slowing nerve conduction. This may result in short periods of improved motor function. Although not scientifically proven, positioning the patient will temporarily clinically decrease spasticity and aid in the reduction of soft-tissue contractures (*44,45*). The effects of simple standing, especially in patients with spasticity of the lower extremities secondary to spinal-cord injury, have been evaluated. One study reported a decrease in the number of spasms (*46*), but others have shown no changes in spasticity, contractures, or bone density with this technique (*47*). Finally, there are a few reports of magnetic stimulation of the spinal cord (*48*) and acupuncture (*49*) resulting in reduced spasticity acutely. These techniques will however require more study to determine clinical efficacy.

Splints and Orthoses

There are several reasons to consider using splints and orthoses in patients with focal spasticity after TBI. They may be used to compensate for the paresis of a segment of a limb, by placing that limb in a more functional position. They may also reduce limb pain and prevent deformities secondary to contractures. These types of mechanical devices focus on the elastic components of increased muscle tone. Theoretically they act by reducing neuromuscular spindle reaction to stretch. Structurally, an orthoses may control joint instability, and biomechanically, it may alter the loading of a limb to keep the moment velocity below the threshold that must be reached before stretch-reflex activity appears in antagonist muscles. There are many types of splint designs. Because of lack of research and contradictory results in existing studies, questions remain whether splints should be used, and if so, which type is best (50). The original splint design, a resting volar splint, helps extend the spastic wrist and finger flexors. This type of splint places the spastic muscles under constant stretch. Textured dorsal splints may be used to facilitate extensor muscles of the forearm through cutaneous stimulation of the dorsal aspect of the forearm, thus inhibiting flexor muscles (50). Animal studies have shown that by facilitating the alpha-motor neuron firing of antagonist muscles and by facilitating gamma-motor neurons over extensor muscles, flexor spasticity can be improved. Studies comparing these two types of splints have shown reduced flexor spasticity in the hand independent of splint design (51). Clinical observation suggests that spreading of the fingers secondarily decreases flexor tone (52). Based on this theory, combination splints have been fabricated that incorporate a volar finger pan, wrist extension, as well as finger abduction (53). Although clinical observations suggest that tone is reduced with hand splinting, experimental evidence is scarce and no conclusions can be drawn about the most effective design. In addition, questions have been raised regarding the possibility that static splinting leads to joint stiffening, muscle atrophy, and fixed joint positioning (54).

Custom-fabricated orthoses are more consistently used in the treatment of lower extremity spasticity primarily because of gait requirements. With the assistance of biomechanical engineering, the ability to more exactly quantify abnormalities of gait, improvements in the understanding of flexion and extension moments, and the mechanical effects that an ankle foot orthoses (AFO) can exert on the more proximal knee and hip joints, improved AFOs have been designed. In an ambulatory TBI patient with lower extremity spasticity, typically plantar flexion and inversion positioning of the foot is seen. An AFO may help reduce the tone by placing the foot in a more neutral or dorsiflexed position. If the tone is severe, however, maintaining the position of the foot in the AFO may be difficult and skin irritation or breakdown may occur as a complication (55).

Casts

Theoretically, the use of a plaster cast on a spastic limb results in the autogenic inhibitory response of the Ib afferent fibers serving the Golgi tendon organs. An arm cast, for example, reduces tone of the spastic elbow flexors automatically every time the flexor tone is increased. The weight and warmth of the cast may also help to reduce spasticity. Casts may help in positioning of a limb and preventing the development of fixed contractures. In addition, casting can be used during the acute or subacute recovery stage after a TBI, as limb tone progresses despite physical modalities such as stretch and range of motion. A cast is typically applied at the point of maximum passive extension. Sometimes a local nerve block can be used prior to casting to obtain the maximal degree of extension. If residual voluntary movement is noted for example, in the triceps muscle, a forearm cast can be applied as a "dropout" cast that encircles the humerus but allows for extension at the elbow. In addition, the cast can later be bivalved, to allow for time out of the cast. Casting should be used in conjunction with aggressive physical therapy for stretching and range of motion between castings. Plaster casting is less irritating than plastic splinting, however, normal casting precautions need to be considered to prevent skin breakdown and neurovascular compromise (56). Casting may also allow for optimal joint positioning and in the lower extremity it may allow for better foot alignment by supporting the toes along with the longitudinal, peroneal, and metatarsal arches (57).

Serial casting decreases muscle tone and appears to be most effective in managing soft-tissue contractures that result from spasticity (58). This procedure involves positioning an extremity at the end of passive range of motion and casting in that position. The cast remains in place for 7–10 d and then is removed. The patient undergoes range of motion therapy between castings and is then re-casted at the new angle between four to five times. It is suggested that serial casting is most effective within 6 mo after an acute neurologic impairment in the TBI patient, while ongoing neurologic recovery is still possible. Serial casting extends on an average of 1–2 mo and has been shown to elongate the elastic component of the musculotendinous unit, increase the number of sarcomeres within the muscle fibers, and stretch the associated connective tissues (59).

Electrical Stimulation

Therapeutic electrical stimulation (ES) has been used for reduction of tone in antagonist muscles where stimulation of the afferent pathways results in inhibition of the agonist muscles, thus reducing their tone. This technique results in an immediate decrease in spasticity that may last from 15 min to 3 h with an average duration of 1 h after stimulation. The reappearance of spasticity is dependent on a number of factors, including the degree of spasticity and the patient's attempt to use the muscles after the electrical treatment. The suggested mechanisms for the immediate decrease in tone include activation of the extrafusal muscle fibers by orthodromic stimulation of the motor neuronal fibers, stimulation of Ia afferents that facilitate the contraction of weak target muscles, the inhibition of spastic angonists, stimulation of alpha-motor neurons via the Ia afferents, and stimulation of group II fibers of the weak muscles eliciting long-loop transcortical reflex mechanisms (60). Although one may speculate that spastic muscles should not be stimulated, studies have shown that electrical stimulation to these muscles may also result in decrease in spasticity (61). The effect is immediate but short-lived. Theories regarding the neurophysiologic effect of this type of stimulation include fatigue of muscles by repetitive stimulation or autogenic inhibition through increased response to the neurotendinous spindle. Cyclical use of electrical stimulation has been reported to decrease contractures, improve motor activity in agonist muscles, and reduce tone in antagonist muscle groups in both spastic hemiplegic and quadriplegic patients (60). However, the duration of the response is short and this technique appears to have limited long-term value in the treatment of spasticity in TBI patients.

Functional electrical stimulation (FES) is electrical stimulation applied to the peripheral nervous system (PNS) or CNS to achieve a functionally positive response. Animal studies in spinal-cord preparation cats have shown that FES may produce reciprocal flexor and extensor action in the lower extremities simulating stepping (62). Human studies involving peroneal nerve stimulation in spastic hemiparetic stroke patients showed some improvement in gait, presumably owing to stimulation of weak tibial anterior muscle, if not decreasing plantar flexor spasticity, allowing for dorsiflexion at the ankle and better gait mechanics (63,64). However, to date, this application is not practical for individual or home use. Muscles or nerves stimulated by FES need to be individualized and often multi-channel stimulation is required for optimal improvement in gait function and decrease in spasticity.

Another limited application for FES is that of stimulation of the extensor digitorum communis muscle and the ulnar nerve as a "hand opening" educational device in the spastic plegic upper extremity. Although hand opening can be achieved by this mechanism, it has not resulted in functional improvement (65). Relief of spasticity by electrical stimulation may be a nonspecific phenomena, not related to a specific group of afferent impulses, because purely cutaneous stimulation can also reduce spasticity. A mesh glove made of conductive wire has been used to stimulate cutaneous and muscle afferents as well as motor fibers of intrinsic hand muscles (66). This unit produces 50 Hz stimulation with a general decrease in overall hand spasticity. Biofeedback has also been used for many years for the treatment of spasticity, but the response is variable and does not always result in increased function. Reports have included evaluation of gait with biofeedback dorsiflexion assist (67), and arm spasticity in CP (68,69). In each of these studies, with training, patients could regulate spasticity and occasionally spasms. However, patient motivation was an important factor and, in general, biofeedback has not been demonstrated to have a definite usefulness in the treatment of spasticity.

Orthopedic Surgical Procedures

Orthopedic surgical intervention in the treatment of the traumatically brain-injured spastic patient is reserved for selected cases with specific indications. In general, orthopedic interventions may improve function, correct a deformity, or be done for cosmetic reasons. Tendon surgery is classified into three major categories: tenotomy, tendon transfer, and tendon lengthening.

Tenotomies should be reserved for the release of the tendon to severely spastic muscles in patients without voluntary movement. Tendon lengthening is performed to weaken spastic muscles and position joints at a more natural and useful angle. Tendon transfers may be undertaken so that muscles that remain at least partially functional can produce useful movement. Both tendon lengthening and tendon transfer are most useful if voluntary movement is preserved. They are also most successful in the lower extremity and do tend to improve borderline ambulation (70).

In the lower extremities, hamstring tendon sectioning or transfer of insertion may be performed for knee-flexion contractures. Achilles-tendon section or lengthening may help correct equinus foot deformity. Adductor-tendon section with or without obturator neurectomy may be performed for hip-adductor spasms. For hip-flexion spasms, the iliopsoas tendon or muscle section may be helpful. Toe-flexor tenotomies may help improve increased foot tone causing claw-foot deformity. Split posterior-tendon transfer may be indicated in varus hind-foot deformity during the stance phase of gait, with increasing varus deformity during the swing phase owing to spasticity of the posterior tibial muscle (71). This surgical procedure involves splitting the tendon and passing half of the tendon posterior to the tibia to insert on the peroneus brevis tendon. Alternately, half of the tendon may be transferred anteriorly through the interosseous membrane to the dorsum of the foot, but this has a failure rate of 10–60% in some studies, with the primary problem being secondary to a valgus over-correction.

The split anterior tibial transfer procedure is indicated for correction of equinovarus posturing, when excessive supination is present at the subtalar joint (72). In this procedure, the distal end of the split anterior tibial tendon is tunneled into the cuneiform and cuboid bones, creating an eversion force. This procedure is often combined with an Achilles tendon-lengthening procedure.

Orthopedic procedures in the upper extremity are more controversial and their outcome more variable. The most typical hand deformity is the thumb-in-palm. Orthopedically, these deformities have been classified into four types (73). Type 1 results from a weakness or paralysis of the extensor pollicis longus. Surgical treatment involves transfer of the palmaris longus or flexor carpi radialis tendon to the extensor pollicis longus. In the Type 2 deformity, there is spasticity or contraction of the adductor pollicis, flexor pollicis brevis, and abductor pollicis brevis. Release of the thenar muscles and the first dorsal interosseous has been advocated to enable the patient to produce a pinch movement. Type 3 deformity is represented by weakness or paralysis of the abductor pollicis longus. This is surgically treated by rerouting the muscle around the flexor carpi radialis and advancing its insertion distally. Finally, Type 4 deformity is seen with spasticity or contracture of the flexor pollicis longus (FPL). Z-lengthening of the FPL proximal to the transverse carpal ligament improves thumb positioning.

Another major problem with spasticity in the upper extremity is the unbalanced wrist. Abnormal positioning of the wrist may decrease the functional use of the hand by 60%. The wrist may be abnormally positioned in one of three fashions. First, flexion contracture of the wrist with hyperextension of the metacarpal-phalangeal joints and flexion of the proximal interphalangeal joints may be treated by dividing the flexor carpi radialis tendon and transferring it to the extensor radialis brevis. The second type of wrist deformity involves significant ulnar deviation of the wrist. In this condition, the radial extensors are weak and the extensor carpi ulnaris tendon is subluxed over the ulnar styloid, thus making the extensor carpi ulnaris a functional wrist flexor. Extensor carpi ulnaris-tendon transfer to the extensor carpi radialis brevis helps improve this condition. Finally, the wrist may be positioned in marked flexion with contracture of all three wrist flexors. In this condition, a Z-incision through the flexor carpi ulnaris, radialis, and palmaris longus tendons is done in an attempt to lengthen the tendons (74).

Orthopedic surgical intervention for spasticity should never be considered in the acute recovery phase from a TBI, while neurologic recovery may still be possible. Once the patient's neurologic status has stabilized, and spasticity continues to be a problem despite conservative modalities and pharmacological intervention, one may consider surgery. Orthopedic procedures in the lower extremities have been shown to improve functional gait. Procedures involving the upper extremities are not universally accepted in improving the patient's functional abilities. The complex actions required by the hand and fingers can be changed significantly by these procedures. For example, slight over-lengthening of the finger flexors may result in decreased grip strength. The complexity of the upper-extremity function often limits the use of tendon-transfer surgery in the limb and patients who do undergo these procedures for upper-extremity spasticity tend to continue to use their uninvolved upper extremity in performing activities of daily living.

Neurosurgical Procedures

Neurosurgical treatment of spasticity should be considered only when all other management approaches have failed. Stereotactic oblation of the globus pallidus, the thalamic nuclei, and cerebellum has been used for over 40 yr in the treatment of dyskinesia, rigidity, and less typically spasticity. In children with CP, dyskinetic movements have improved to some degree with this surgery, whereas spasticity in quadriplegic or diplegic patients has not improved (75). It is not clear that a specific area of the brain treated by electrocoagulation can relieve spasticity. Generally, stereotatic surgery results in poor outcome in the treatment of spasticity and is currently not recommended. Cerebellar stimulation has been used in an effort to decrease extensor hypertonia associated with spasticity (76). However, the initial positive response reported to decrease spasticity has not been substantiated by subsequent studies (77). Currently cerebellar stimulation has no proven role in treatment of spasticity.

For severe spasticity, one may consider transecting portions of the spinal cord or nerve roots. Selective posterior rhizotomy has been performed in the cervical and lumbosacral spinal cord. Posterior rhizotomy of C1-C3 has been performed in patients with CP with slight improvement in upper-extremity spasticity but this operation included significant potential for complications. Selective rhizotomy of L2-S2 is currently the most popular neurosurgical approach for severe spasticity in the lower extremities (78). Outcome is best in patients with minimal or no athetosis, good strength and motor control, minimal fixed contractures, and a high level of motivation and intelligence to allow for participation in intense physical therapy. A TBI patient with unilateral weakness such as hemiplegia would not be considered a candidate for surgical intervention. In addition, significant dystonia, ataxia, or fixed contractures would exclude this intervention. The results of posterior rhizotomy are variable but encouraging in appropriately selected patients. Decreased tone, improvement in gait dynamics, and a decreased need for assistive aids have been demonstrated (79).

Surgical neurectomy of peripheral nerves in the treatment of spasticity has also been advocated. Neurectomies have been performed for spastic gastrocnemius-soleus muscles, and for intractable ankle clonus (80). Although clonus and spasticity has been diminished after tibial-nerve neurectomy, there is often still a need for further orthopedic surgery such as tendon lengthening. In addition, neurectomies of mixed motor and sensory nerves may produce permanent, painful dysesthesias. Selective obturator neurectomy may lead to a loss of ambulation and result in abduction contractures. Owing to the variable response, high incidence of recurrent spasticity, and possible permanent painful dysesthesias, selective neurectomies are not recommended in the treatment of focal spasticity.

LOCAL PHARMACOLOGIC TREATMENT OF SPASTICITY

In the TBI patient with localized spasticity, specific muscle groups are often responsible for the increased muscle tone. In these circumstances, local treatments of those muscles where spasticity is most disabling may be considered by injection into a muscle or close to the nerve supplying the muscle. Local anesthetics such as lidocaine have a fully reversible action of short duration and alcohols such as ethanol and phenol have a longer duration of action. Botulinum toxin, which blocks the release of acetylcholine at the neuromuscular junction, may also be considered. Often, a combination of these agents is considered. For example, a local anesthetic may be injected for therapeutic testing or diagnostic procedures to help determine if a more long-lasting block will help improve function. It may help in deciding which muscle is contributing to pathological positioning, and the level of interference of antagonistic muscles. It may also be used in preparation for casting (*see* Table 7).

Anesthetics

Local anesthetics act by blocking nerve conduction when applied locally to the nerve or surrounding tissue. These agents act by increasing the membrane permeability to sodium ions. These agents also act on muscle tissue by similar ionic mechanisms. The gamma fibers supplying the muscle spindles are rapidly blocked by a local anesthetic (81). The onset of action typically occurs within minutes and depends on the rate of diffusion, degree of lipid solubility, and regional blood flow. Occasionally, vasoconstrictors may be used to increase the duration of action, but should not be injected into tissue supplied by end arteries, such as fingers and toes. Any time a local anesthetic is used, resuscitation equipment should be present for acute car-

Table 7
Local Pharmacological Treatment of Spasticity in Traumatic Brain Injury

	Onset	Duration	Indications
Lidocaine	Immediate	Hours	*Diagnositic block* Identify muscles causing abnormal position Identify muscles for longer-duration blocks Determine presence of soft-tissue contractures Determine presence of dynamic contractures Identify functional limitations produced by spastic muscles *Therapeutic block* Prior to casting to achieve maximal extension
Phenol	Immediate	Months	To improve range of motion Prevention of contractures As an adjunct to casting As an adjunct to orthopedic surgery To achieve functional goals For better positioning in splints and orthoses When spasticity does not respond to conservative management and treatments
Botulinum toxin	24–72 h	Months	Same as phenol

diopulmonary emergencies. These may occur if the anesthetic inadvertently enters the systemic circulation. Cardiac collapse, CNS depression, and respiratory failure may occur (*81*). Hypersensitivity ranging from an allergic rash to fatal anaphylaxis may occur. Caution needs to be used in patients with hepatic disease because most of the metabolism of local anesthetics occurs in the liver.

Local anesthetics are chosen depending on the desired duration of action. Short-acting anesthetics such as procaine last 20–40 min. Intermediate-acting anesthetics such as lidocaine may last 1–3 h, and long-acting bupivacaine may last for several hours. Overall, lidocaine produces a prompt and intermediately acting anesthesia and is often the drug of choice for the treatment of focal spasticity in the TBI patient. Lidocaine is available as lidocaine hydrochloride in dilutions from 0.5–4% with or without epinephrine. Bupivacaine hydrochloride is more potent than lidocaine and of longer duration. It may be preferred if a longer duration of action is needed to thoroughly assess whether functional improvement may result from long-term chemodenervation.

Local anesthetics may be injected intramuscularly in the vicinity of neuromuscular junction (*82*). Intramuscular blocks are reported to be more painful than nerve blocks and larger volumes of anesthetic may increase the likelihood of spread to nearby muscles. Local anesthetics may also be injected near a peripheral nerve. The anesthetic action depends on the diffusion of the agent from the epineurium to the central core of the nerve. For both intramuscular and nerve blocks, the tip of the injecting needle should be directed as closely as possible to the nerve trunk by searching for minimal stimulation required to produce the maximal muscle contraction or paresthesia. Repetitive monopolar stimulation of the targeted nerve or muscle helps the injector achieve proper positioning prior to injection of the anesthetic.

The injection of local anesthetics may be used diagnostically, to help determine whether a more long-term block of the same muscle or nerve could be functionally useful. Blocking a spastic muscle may help determine the role the spasticity is playing in the functional limitations of the limb, or whether a dynamic contracture is present. It may also help to determine which muscle is contributing to abnormal positioning and also whether the functional performance of a muscle is improved when it is free of antagonistic co-contraction. Because resistance to stretch of the joint is associated not only with spasticity but many of the soft-tissue changes described previously, temporarily relieving the spasticity with a local anesthetic may help determine the degree of soft-tissue involvement in an abnormal limb position.

Alcohols

Unlike local anesthetics, the alcohols act by producing structural damage to tissue. Although at low concentrations alcohol may act as a local anesthetic by decreasing sodium and potassium permeability, at higher concentrations alcohol acts nonselectively by denaturing proteins and causes cellular injury by dehydrating and precipitating proteins (*83*). Ethyl alcohol was the first alcohol compound studied experimentally and may block sensory and motor nerves, muscles, and the neuromuscular junction, at concentrations of greater than 10%. The onset of action is less than 1 h and the duration is 2–36 mo. Intramuscular injection of ethyl alcohol is painful and complications have included a burning sensation and local hyperemia usually of less than 36 h duration (*84*). Other occasional adverse effects have included phlebitis, permanent peripheral-nerve palsy, skin irritation if injected superficially, and systemic signs of intoxication. Overall, however, there are few reports of intramuscular or perineural adverse effects as compared to phenol. Most clinical trials in the treatment of spasticity have been done on children with CP. It appears that an intramuscular injection of 45% alcohol is safe, and acts by destruction of the muscle. In most cases, voluntary strength is not affected and the response may last from 6–12 mo and occasionally up to 3 yr (85). Alcohol appears most effective when injected close to the motor point.

Phenol is an alcohol that has been used as a neurolytic agent for over 50 yr. Like ethyl alcohol, phenol has some anesthetic properties, but acts primarily by chemical axonotomeses that occurs with destruction of the axons while the endoneural tubes are retained. It appears that all fiber types are affected by the chemical axonal loss (86).

Phenol is frequently administered during the recovery phase from CNS injury. In the TBI patient, relief of spasticity in the acute to subacute phase with phenol may improve range of motion and prevent contracture. Some studies indicate that this effect appears to be better in the traumatic brain-injured and spinal cord-injured patients rather than in stroke patients, owing to their longer recovery time. Phenol may be considered when severe spasticity does not respond to other usual conservative modalities. Its main advantages include more specific and complete ablation of tone and longer duration of action. It is also preferred over surgery during the period when neurologic recovery might be expected such as in the acute TBI patient. Later in the course of recovery from TBI, phenol may be considered in the treatment of spasticity when certain activities of the spastic limb are limited. For example, poor ambulation resulting from spastic ankle plantar flexion may be treated with injection into the gastrocnemius muscle or injection into the hip adductors help limit the spasms that interfere with hygiene and nursing care.

Phenol may be injected intramuscularly in aqueous solution. Initially, phenol was injected into the subarachnoid space, or epidurally, but complications were significant including nerve-root damage, arachnoiditis, meningitis, spinal-cord infarction, motor paralysis, saddle sensory loss, painful paresthesias, headaches, and even death (87). Perineural injections are now the technique of choice. At concentrations less than 3%, phenol has only local anesthetic properties. Clinically, most phenol is concentrated between 3 and 6%. Perineural injection of a nerve trunk has been reported to decrease spasticity on an average of 300 d (88). However, this technique results in a significant percentage of painful paresthesias and permanent muscle weakness. When a motor branch of a nerve can be identified with a neural stimulator, a closed motor-branch block may be considered. Injection of phenol by this mechanism prevents the numbness and paresthesias associated with a nerve-trunk injection. Nerves commonly approached by this method include the recurrent branch of the median nerve and the obturator nerve. The musculocutaneous nerve has also been approached by this technique, and even though it is a mixed motor and sensory nerve, it does respond well with few side effects (*89*). Open motor-point block requires surgical isolation of a motor-nerve branch. Phenol diluted at 3–5% in glycerin has been shown to decrease spasticity lasting between 2 and 8 mo. Nerves that may be approached by this technique include the motor branch of the median nerve and ulnar nerve in the forearm, the deep motor branch of the ulnar nerve at the wrist, the obturator nerve, the sciatic motor branch in the posterior thigh, and the posterior tibial nerve.

Finally, intramuscular motor-point block is a technique that directs the injection of phenol at the motor points within the muscle. This is done by using a surface stimulator over the skin, and an electrode placed in an area where the muscle can be maximally stimulated. A Teflon-coated needle connected to a stimulator is inserted to explore the area. The needle is maneuvered until a point of maximal muscle contraction is located. Phenol is then injected, and the procedure is repeated until multiple motor points have been identified and injected. Injection slightly proximal to the motor point appears to result in longer-lasting effect (*90*). The duration of action with intramuscular motor point blocks is shorter than an open motor-branch block, but is easier to administer, does not require surgery, and can be used in muscles whose nerve is difficult to isolate surgically.

Phenol can be prepared in aqueous or oil solution. It is more potent in oil than water, and is intermediately potent in glycerin. Aqueous solution of 3–5% is the dilution of choice for percutaneous injections, whereas 3% glycerin is recommended for open block. A volume of 2 cc is typical for percutaneous injection, and for open block, usually less than 0.5 cc per nerve branch is needed. The maximum safe dose of the drug has not been established. Phenol is excreted 80% by the kidneys and produces a smoky colored urine. Phenol injection should be limited to two nerves at a time. The most common immediate side effects are lightheadedness, nausea, and vomiting (*86*). Phenol should not be considered in patients with poor general health or severe contractures. Adverse effects include thrombophlebitis of the calf or thigh, which may be related to the number of injections and the volume of phenol use, and also peripheral-nerve injury. This is especially true in the forearm where the muscles are close to the median and ulnar nerves. If phenol is inadvertently administered systemically, complications may include tremors, seizures, respiratory failure, and direct myocardial suppression (86).

The advantage in using phenol is the ability to see an immediate response with near nerve injections, with small doses of the drug. The muscle contraction is seen to stop even though electrical stimulation continues. The drug is of low cost with relative ease of sterilization and preparation. Its longer duration of action is also an important consideration.

Botulinum Toxin

Botulinum toxin is a thermolabile exotoxin that has been used in the treatment of involuntary movement disorders. It has become increasingly popular for use in the treatment of muscle spasticity of CNS origin. Botulinum toxin type A is available in the United States and types B and F are currently under investigation for clinical use. Toxin type A binds to the synaptosome-associated protein (SNAP), and types B and F attach to the vesicular-associated membrane protein (VAMP) (91). Presently in the United States, the Food and Drug Administration (FDA) has approved botulinum toxin type A for the treatment of strabismus, blepharospasm, and hemifacial spasm. Off-label uses include focal dystonias including torticollis, laryngeal dystonia, oromandibular dystonia, and limb dystonia (92). The National Institutes of Health (NIH) (93) and the American Academy of Neurology (94) have published guidelines regarding the usefulness of botulinum toxin type A in the treatment of neurologic diseases. The American Academy of Neurology has also outlined its recommendations regarding guidelines for training for practitioners administering the toxin (95).

The toxin is frozen in a crystallized powder form in a vacuum bottle. It must be kept frozen at $-5°$ to $-20°$ centigrade until administration. At that time it is reconstituted with normal saline solution without preservatives. Appropriate mixing technique is required to insure potency of the toxin. The toxin is diluted to the desired concentration and a decision is made regarding the number of units to be used and the muscles to be injected. After aspiration to exclude a vascular puncture, the toxin is injected. Toxin placement may be enhanced by electromyography (EMG) guidance (96), and is especially important when injecting the forearm muscles, as well as locating fascicles of muscles for individual finger flexors.

The toxin acts by the attachment of the heavy sub-unit to the presynaptic neuron. The light chain is internalized within the neuron and interferes with the acetylcholine release from the vesicles (91). After injection of the toxin, a decline in motor endplate potentials can be electrically identified within a few hours. No changes are noted in the cell body and the storage and synthesis of acetylcholine remains normal. There is a delay in the onset of clinical effect between 24–72 h. Subjectively, the patient may not note a response for 7–10 d. The duration of response depends on the dose of the toxin administered, the muscle size, and the activity of the muscle. After injection, the muscle injected may become clinically atrophied, but over time there is nerve sprouting and reinnervation with a gradual wearing off of effect. The average duration is from 2–6 mo.

Botulinum toxin type A has been studied for the treatment of spasticity in multiple sclerosis (MS), spinal-cord injury, CP, stroke, and TBI. Among the original reports of clinical trials using botulinum toxin for spasticity was a study of six stroke patients with upper-limb spasticity who found relief of tone after the injection of toxin (*97,98*). Most of the trials have been open-label and nonblinded. However, a randomized, double-blind, crossover study of nine patients with leg adductor spasticity in nonambulating patients with MS showed a decrease in spasticity as well as increased ease of nursing care (*99*). Subsequent studies have shown an improvement in pain and painful spasms with the use of botulinum toxin. However, attempts to quantify functional improvement have been more difficult. In a recent double-blind, placebo-controlled, crossover trial, 12 patients with spasticity for MS, TBI, stroke, and hypoxic encephalopathy were treated in either the upper or lower extremities (*100*). These patients experienced no weakness or placebo effect but did have a decrease in the number of painful spasms and also decrease in tone by two grades on the Ashworth Scale. The duration of response was reported to average 2.4 months.

Several clinical multi-center trials examining the safety and efficacy of botulinum toxin Type A in the treatment of upper-limb spasticity after stroke have reported decreased spasticity with no serious adverse effects (*101,102*). There have, however, been only a few studies evaluating the treatment of spasticity with botulinum toxin in the TBI patient. Open-label studies specifically looking at limb spasticity have reported up to an 85% improvement in limb posture and range of motion, a significant decrease in pain (if present pretreatment) and a variable response in improved function ranging from 30–60% (*103*). Adults with either stroke or TBI who had spastic foot drop causing significant interference with stance and gait, shortening of the heel cord, ankle contractures, and difficulty with fitting an AFO were treated with botulinum toxin. EMG-guided injections of toxin in most patients showed improvement in several measures including ankle position at rest, range of passive movement, gait analysis, and ease of physical therapy (*104*). Another trial in adults with chronic lower-extremity spasticity has shown improvement in extensor spasticity after treatment with botulinum toxin. Improvements in gait velocity, stride length, stance symmetry, and length of the force point of action under the affected foot has been shown by measurement of ground-reaction forces (105). Improved ankle dorsiflexion, decreased ankle clonus, and decreased toe clawing has been demonstrated by kinematic electromyography (106).

Twenty-one patients with TBI and severe spasticity unresponsive to conservative management were treated with botulinum toxin in the wrist and finger flexors under EMG guidance. These patients received passive range of motion and casting if clinically indicated. It was reported that both range of motion of the wrist and the modified Ashworth Scale showed improvement after treatment with botulinum toxin type A, with no significant side effects (107).

In the traumatic brain-injured patient, botulinum toxin type A may be considered in the treatment of spasticity when the hypertonus has been unresponsive to conservative measures and typical pharmacological treatment. It may also be considered in patients who require an excessive frequency or duration of adjunctive treatments such as range of motion and stretching, or when spasticity interferes with functional activities and activities of daily living. Botulinum toxin type A may be used when the spasticity involves antagonist muscles that interfere with residual agonist muscle function and may be used adjunctively when casting or surgical procedures are anticipated. When continued postoperative spasticity may compromise the success of a surgical procedure, botulinum toxin may be helpful. Other indications for using botulinum toxin include pain relief from severe spasticity or spasms, to improve personal hygiene and nursing care, for better positioning to prevent skin breakdown, and to improve use of assistive devices such as AFOs.

Questions remain regarding comparative efficacy and safety of injectables in the treatment of focal spasticity. Although anesthetic agents may be used to help predict whether long duration blocks are warranted, without significantly weakening the targeted muscle, there may not be enough useful information to predict functional outcome. For each injectable drug, there is a need for placebo-controlled, randomized studies to reach definite conclusions on their safety and efficacy. This is true in comparing alcohol to phenol. Alcohol has been used primarily in children by intramuscular injection, while phenol has been chiefly used in adults by perineural injections. When comparing alcohol and phenol to botulinum toxin, the former agents have earlier onset of action and perhaps longer duration. They certainly cost less and have lack of antigenicity. However, their lack of selectivity on motor function, the tissue destruction, and chronic painful dysesthesias or vascular reactions may prompt one to choose botulinum toxin. In the severe TBI patient, where recovery of intact muscle and sensory perception is not expected, alcohol or phenol may prove to be more appropriate than botulinum toxin, where treatment of spasticity would be primarily performed for hygiene and comfort. Botulinum toxin, with its absence of histological destruction, may be preferable when there is hope for recovery of active function of the injected limb. In one study comparing phenol injections to botulinum toxin in lower-extremity spasticity, the Ashworth Scale for dorsiflexion tone improved significantly following treatment with either injectable, and by 12 wk improvement in both treatment groups returned to baseline. Dysesthesias and a peroneal-nerve paralysis limited the ambulation scores in the phenol group (*108*). More studies comparing botulinum toxin and phenol are needed.

SYSTEMIC PHARMACOLOGICAL TREATMENTS FOR SPASTICITY

Depending on the location of damage to the traumatically injured brain, spasticity may be focal or diffuse. Diffuse increased tone is typically seen in patients with diffuse axonal injury. Penetrating head injuries, or closed head injury with contusion or focal hemorrhage, may lead to focal spasticity. Oral pharmacological intervention is indicated for generalized spasticity, but it may also be required in the patient who develops focal spastic conditions, which are not responsive to conservative modalities of treatment.

In general, centrally acting antispasticity drugs act by either suppression of excitation of the glutamate system or by enhancing the inhibition of the gamma-amino butyric acid (GABA) and glycine systems. Peripherally, antispasticity drugs may act by affecting ion flux at the level of the muscle. Pharmacological management of spasticity in the TBI patient is a challenge because many of these patients suffer from coma, cognitive problems, or impaired behavior in addition to their spasticity. Studies of most of the major centrally acting antispastic agents have shown sedation and reduction of global performance as part of their side-effect profile. It may be preferable to use centrally acting drugs such as diazepam, baclofen, or tizanidine in patients with spasticity of spinal-cord origin such as MS or spinal-cord injury. Dantrolene sodium may be preferable in spasticity of cerebral origin like stroke or TBI patients, because the drug acts peripherally. Conventional wisdom suggests that the sedating effects of these drugs may have more adverse effects in the stroke or TBI patient, and may impede recovery. However, to date, there have been no clinical trials specifically looking at the TBI patient population with regard to long-term outcome when these antispasticity drugs are used. In the chronic TBI patient with severe spasticity, limited likelihood of further neurologic recovery, and severe cognitive deficits, it may be more acceptable to use oral agents that may produce sedation, and result in a global performance reduction. These side effects may not be acceptable in the patient who has modest cognitive impairment associated with a physical impairment that is not functionally limiting. However, if spasticity is significantly impeding functional recovery, one may find the use of antispasticity drugs necessary. Defining the goal of treatment of spasticity in each individual patient is extremely important. If relief of spasticity will improve patient comfort, hygiene, and permit better nursing care, systemic pharmacology should be used. However, if the goal in treating focal spasticity is to help improve function then these agents should be used with more caution.

Animal studies have shown that certain drugs influence behavior in animals with focal brain injury. These effects may either help or impede the recovery process. It is also important to remember that these drug effects may not be the same in humans. For example, animal studies showing that amphetamines improve motor and visual recovery in rats after focal TBI, led to the hypothesis that amphetamine-facilitated recovery is owing to effects of this drug on noradrenergic neurons (109). This suggests that drugs that enhance norepinephrine release would be helpful in neurologic recovery while those that impair the release would be harmful. Antispasticity drugs that act on monoamines such as clonidine and tizanidine may have therapeutic implications based on this theory. When amphetamines were tested on human stroke patients, initial studies seemed to show improvement of recovery, however, subsequent clinical trials have failed to do so. In addition to antispasticity drugs, anticonvulsants, antidepressants, and antihypertensive drugs have been considered to adversely effect cognitive function and perhaps functional outcome after TBI (110), but little consistent data is available to advocate the use or avoidance of specific drugs.

GABA-ergic System Drugs

Baclofen, diazepam, clorazepate dipotassium, ketazolam, and clonazepam are all agents that act through the GABA-ergic system, to reduce spasticity. Only ketazolam has been studied specifically in TBI (*see* Table 8). Baclofen is a structural analog of GABA. Its antispastic efficacy has been demonstrated in MS and spinal-cord injury. In double-blind studies of post-stroke spasticity, its antispastic effect was good, but side effects, specifically sedation, were problematic. Muscle weakness produced by this drug can also be a problem for the functional patient but not those disabled by severe spasticity (*111*). A lack of seizure control can also occur during treatment with or abrupt withdrawal of baclofen. To date there have been no studies using baclofen for treatment of spasticity in TBI.

The antispasticity effect of benzodiazapines is mediated by a functionally coupled benzodiazapine-GABA-A receptor chloride ionophore complex

Table 8
Results of the Pharmacological Treatment of Spasticity in Specific Diseases

	MS spasticity	Spinal cord-injury spasticity	Stroke spasticity	TBI spasticity
Baclofen	Decreased	Decreased	Decreased/sedation	*
Diazepam	Decreased	Decreased	Decreased/sedation	*
Clorazepate	Decreased	*	Decreased	*
Ketazolam	Decreased	*	Decreased	Decreased
Clonazepam	Decreased/sedation	*	*	*
Dantrolene	*	*	Decreased	*
Tizanidine	Decreased	Decreased	Decreased	*

* Not studied to date

(*112*). Diazepam and clonazepam are long acting benzodiazepines. Diazepam has been used both in patients with MS and spinal-cord injury. The efficacy in paraplegia has been demonstrated by several double-line protocols (*113*), with a dose-dependent antispastic effect. Sedation is the most common problem with diazepam and in studies of spastic hemiplegic stroke patients, this side effect overshadowed its antispastic effect. Clorazepate dipotassium is a benzodiazapine analog. Double-blind studies in MS and stroke demonstrate a reduction in spasticity (*114*). Although no recent studies regarding the use of clorazepate and spasticity have been published, prior literature suggests that unlike diazepam, this drug does not impair memory or learning (*115*). Like other benzodiazepines, ketazolam has anti-spasticity properties and has been reported to be equally effective and slightly less sedating than diazepam in patients with MS, stroke, and TBI (*116*). Another benzodiazapine, clonazepam has been compared to baclofen in the treatment of spasticity in MS (*117*). Although the antispastic effect was similar, clonazepam produced significant sedation and fatigue.

Drugs Effecting Ion Flux

Dantrolene sodium, lamotrigine, and riluzole all act on ion channels of neuronal membranes. Dantrolene acts peripherally on the muscle fiber by reducing the muscle action potential-induced release of calcium from the sarcoplasmic reticulum (*118*). Owing to its peripheral mode of action, dantrolene is recommended in the treatment of spasticity of cerebral origin. In the spastic hemiplegic stroke patient, its antispasticity effect has been demonstrated in double-blind studies and tolerance is good without significant sedation (*119*). Because dantrolene works peripherally, it may be a better choice than baclofen or benzodiazepines in patients with memory and cognitive problems associated with TBI. However, dantrolene can be mildly sedating.

Lamotrigine is thought to act at voltage-sensitive sodium channels. A recent clinical trial suggests that lamotrigine may have promise in the treatment of muscle spasticity (*120*). Riluzole blocks voltage-sensitive sodium channels also, and has been shown to reduce stiffness in patients with amyotrophic lateral sclerosis (ALS) (*121*).

Drugs Acting on Monoamines

Tizanidine and clonidine act as alpha$_2$-adrenergic receptor agonists. In studies of spasticity in MS, spinal-cord injury, and stroke, the efficacy and safety profile was similar to baclofen. In a study of patients with spasticity associated with hemiplegia from stroke and TBI, tizanidine was compared to diazepam (*122*). Patients treated with tizanidine who had lower-extremity spasticity improved functional walking distances when compared to diazepam, although sedation was a predominant side effect in both groups.

Clonidine acts similarly to tizanidine but has more of a cardiac effect and may produce bradycardia and hypotension. In addition, it has been shown to impair motor recovery in animal studies (*123*). To date, there have been no double-blind studies demonstrating its efficacy in the treatment of spasticity. Until further data is available, the use of clonidine for the treatment of spasticity in TBI is not recommended.

Other Agents with Antispasticity Properties

Cyproheptadine has anticholinergic, antiserotonergic, and antihistaminic effects. It has been reported to improve spasticity in MS and spinal cord-injury patients. In one study, cyproheptadine showed similar antispastic effects as baclofen in paraplegic patients (*124*). Orphenadrine citrate acts as a glutamate antagonist. When used intravenously in spinal cord-injured patients, it relieves spasticity rapidly and may be useful as adjunctive therapy in the acute treatment of spasticity in the TBI patient (*125*). Phenytoin historically had been used in the treatment of spasticity before other agents were available. But aside from patients who are already on it for the treatment of seizures, and because of its potential side effects, other drugs should first be considered in the treatment of spasticity, especially in TBI patients. Phenothiazines also have antispastic effects, which may be related to alpha-adrenergic block. Sedation, however, is a significant problem and should not be used in brain injured patients unless associated psychiatric disturbances are present that would warrant the use of this type of drug (*126*).

Intrathecal Antispasticity Drugs

Baclofen and morphine have been used for the treatment of intractable spasticity by intrathecal administration. This route of administration should be reserved for severe spasticity of the lower extremities, which has been intractable and unresponsive to oral pharmacological intervention. Initially used exclusively for spasticity from spinal-cord injury, it is now recognized as safe and efficacious in the treatment of spasticity of central origin, both in CP and TBI patients (*127*). The use of intrathecal baclofen (ITB) may be considered in the chronic TBI patient with uncontrolled lower-extremity spasticity or spasms.

CLINICAL PATTERNS OF SPASTICITY

When a patient develops spasticity from a TBI, characteristic patterns of joint positioning may be assumed (*see* Table 9). These positions depend on the degree of residual voluntary motor control, the degree of spasticity in agonist and antagonist muscles, and abnormalities of the joints and soft tissues around the joint that may lead to contractures. In attempting to treat focal spasticity, it is important to identify the specific muscles that may contribute to such an abnormal limb position. This is especially true if denervation techniques or surgical intervention is anticipated. For example, an injection of botulinum toxin or phenol into the biceps of a patient with a flexed elbow may not improve the position, if that position is owing to a fixed contracture of the biceps tendon.

A thorough clinical examination combined with radiographs of the limb, dynamic EMG evaluation, and possibly a diagnostic muscle or nerve block will help determine whether spasticity is responsible for the abnormal limb position, and if so, which muscles may be involved.

Upper Extremities

The Hand and Fingers

In the distal upper limb, the clenched fist with flexion of the fingers is the most typical spastic position seen clinically. This position may result in difficulty maintaining hygiene of the hand, skin breakdown, and tearing of the skin of the palm as the fingernails invade this area. If the patient has some degree of remaining voluntary control of finger movement, relief of spasticity may improve their ability to grasp and pinch. Not all fingers may be equally affected. The flexor digitorum profundus and flexor digitorum sublimis are the finger flexors most commonly responsible for this type of clenched fist positioning. However, it is important to remember that the intrinsic hand muscles may also demonstrate increased tone. Extension at the

Table 9
Clinical Patterns of Spasticity in Traumatic Brain Injury

Position	Muscles involved	Position	Muscles involved
Finger flexion	Flexor digitorum profundus Flexor digitorum sublimis Intrinsic hand muscles	Foot varus	Tibialis posterior Medial gastrocnemius Lateral gastrocnemius Soleus
Thumb-in-palm	Adductor pollicis		Tibialis anterior
	Flexor pollicis brevis Flexor pollicis longus	Foot valgus	Peroneus Longus/brevis Gastrocnemius Soleus
Wrist flexion	Flexor carpi ulnaris Flexor carpi radialis	Knee flexed	Hamstrings Quadriceps
Forearm pronated	Pronator quadratus Pronator teres	Knee extended	Rectus femoris Vastus medialis Vastus lateralis
Elbow flexed	Brachioradialis Biceps		Vastus intermedius Hamstrings
	Brachialis	Hip adducted	Rectus femoris
Shoulder adducted and internally rotated	Pectoralis major Latissimus dorsi Teres major Subscapularis	and internally rotated	Iliopsoas Adductor longus Pectineus

proximal interphalangeal joints may be seen with spasticity of the intrinsic dorsal interossei. The most typical abnormal positioning of the thumb is the thumb-in-palm deformity. This may result from increased tone in the adductor pollicis, flexor pollicis brevis, or flexor pollicis longus. In acute TBI, this type of hand flexion positioning can develop rapidly. Initially, splinting may be used to help limit the flexion position of the fingers and thumb but as the tone increases, it may no longer be possible to position the hand in the splint. Dynamic EMG and lidocaine blocks may be helpful in determining which muscles are contributing to the spastic positioning of the hand and fingers. Botulinum toxin treatment can be very effective when administered by EMG guidance to help identify not only the spastic finger flexors, but also individual fascicles of selected finger flexors.

The Wrist and Forearm

Wrist flexion and forearm pronation are the most common spastic deformities in this area. In the flexed wrist, the flexor carpi radialis is the most typically involved, although the flexor carpi ulnaris may also play a role in the wrist positioning. The flexed wrist positioning may inhibit hand function by as much as 60%, because it severely impairs the grasp and release functions of the hand. Acutely in the TBI patient, volar splints may help limit uncontrolled wrist flexion but if spasticity progresses, phenol motor-point blocks into the wrist flexors or botulinum toxin injections may be helpful. Serial casting may also be considered acutely while there is still potential for functional motor recovery.

Commonly, forearm pronation is seen in association with wrist flexion. Much more uncommonly, forearm supination may occur. Like the flexed wrist, the pronated forearm also interferes with functional use of the hand. Muscles typically responsible for this positioning include the pronator quadratus and pronator teres. In acute TBI, serial casting can be considered but typically these casts must also include the elbow joint, which may result in unwanted flexion at the elbow. X-ray of the wrist and forearm is important to exclude the possibility of an occult fracture or dislocation. In addition, heterotopic ossification between the radius and ulna needs to be excluded radiographically.

The Elbow

Typically, the elbow flexors are more spastic than the extensors and this position once again limits the use of the hand. If severe, it may produce skin breakdown in the antecubital fossa. This position also may markedly impair upper-extremity dressing. The three major elbow flexors are the biceps, brachioradialis, and brachialis. The flexed-elbow position is typically a combination of static and dynamic contracture deformities. Early in the course of TBI recovery, serial casts may be applied. This mechanism not only helps improve spasticity, but also serves to stretch the shortening soft-tissue structures. Once again, radiographs of the elbow should be taken to rule out bony abnormalities that may account for the abnormal flexion position. Phenol injection into the musculocutaneous nerve may be considered, but because dysesthesias may occur, this should be reserved for patients with a depressed level of awareness. Motor-point phenol blocks may be considered in the biceps or brachioradialis. Likewise, botulinum toxin injections may help relieve focal spasticity. In the chronic TBI patient, when no additional neurologic recovery is expected, surgical lengthening of contracted elbow flexors may be considered.

The Shoulder

Adduction and internal rotation is the typical position of the spastic shoulder. When present, the flexed elbow, wrist, and fingers are also typically seen. The arm is held tightly against the chest wall and this positioning severely restricts the use of the distal upper extremity. Skin breakdown, poor axillary hygiene, and difficulty dressing are significant functional consequences of this position. The pectoralis major is typically involved, but the latissimus dorsi, teres major, and subscapularis may be involved in this type of spastic positioning. Typically, the shoulder in this position is painful. However, keep in mind that multiple factors may play a role of production of pain, including capsulitis, tendonitis or bursitis, frozen shoulder, myofascial pain, brachial plexopathy, shoulder subluxation or dislocation, degenerative joint disease, and reflex sympathetic dystrophy. Diagnostic lidocaine blocks to the innervation of the pectoralis major, latissimus dorsi, and teres major may help determine which of these muscles is contributing to the spastic posturing of the shoulder, and if all are blocked, the contribution of the subscapularis will be determined. Dynamic EMG recordings may help distinguish voluntary motor control from spastic reaction of adductor muscles during attempted abduction by the patient. Radiographs in this area are essential to rule out fracture or dislocation. In addition, heterotopic ossification is seen in approx 10% of patients with TBI and the shoulder joint is involved in at least 25% of these cases. Early in the course of recovery from TBI, range of motion of the shoulder is essential in preventing pain and limited mobility. There is no practical way to splint or cast this joint. Once tightness of the shoulder occurs, nerve blocks to the various shoulder muscles may help determine how much of the limited range of motion is owing to soft-tissue contractures or adhesive capsulitis. Subscapular nerve block with phenol has been used to treat the painful hemiplegic shoulder. Injection of botulinum toxin into the pectoralis major may improve range of motion enough to allow access to the axilla for hygiene and dressing. Although technically difficult, the subscapularis muscle can be approached for phenol injection. Late in the course of recovery from TBI, surgical release of offending muscles may be considered, and bony excision of extensive heterotopic ossification may also be necessary.

Lower Extremities
The Foot

Equinovarus or valgus deformity are the most common patterns of abnormal positioning of the foot with spasticity. In equinovarus, the foot and ankle are plantar flexed and inverted. Curling or clawing of the toes may also occur. This abnormal foot positioning significantly limits normal gait. The forefoot, rather than the heel, typically touches down first during the stance phase of gait. In addition, weight is primarily distributed on the lateral border of the foot. During the swing phase of gait, the toes do not adequately clear the floor and secondary abnormal positioning of the knee and hip may occur. Muscles that may contribute to this deformity include the tibialis posterior, medial and lateral gastrocnemius, soleus, tibialis anterior, lateral hamstrings, extensor hallucis longus, and peroneus longus. Often clinical examination alone is not adequate in determining which of these muscles is contributing to the spastic positioning. Diagnostic lidocaine blocks and dynamic EMG may be helpful.

Early in recovery from an acute TBI, orthotic management may be adequate to control equinus foot positioning. As spasticity progresses, proper positioning of the foot within the orthosis may not be possible and percutaneous motor-point block of the muscles may be helpful. This should be combined with a stretching and range-of-motion therapy. The tibial nerve may be temporarily blocked with lidocaine as a diagnostic test, but should not be injected with phenol owing to painful dysesthesias. In chronic TBI patients with a persistent equinovarus positioning despite conservative therapy, surgical intervention may be necessary. This can include an Achilles-tendon lengthening or tendon-transfer procedure. Injection of botulinum toxin may help reduce the spasticity enough to promote improved gait mechanics and may allow proper foot positioning within an AFO.

In the valgus foot deformity, the ankle and foot are turned outward and toe flexion may be present. Muscles that may contribute to this deformity include the peroneus longus and brevis, gastrocnemius, and soleus. Weak tibialis anterior or long toe flexors may also contribute to this deformity. It is important to exclude the possibility of a pre-existing condition such as pes planus or congenital flexible flat feet. Comparison should be made with the uninvolved foot. Also, in the traumatically injured patient, rupture of the tibialis posterior tendon may contribute to this type of valgus deformity. In ambulatory patients, this foot deformity may lead to genu valgum deformity as well. Management of this deformity includes diagnostic lidocaine blocks to one or more muscles to help determine which is contributing to the deformity and then chemodenervation can be considered.

Persistent extension of the great toe may be seen with or without associated foot deformities of the valgus or varus types. This "hitchhikers" great toe may lead to an inability to wear a shoe owing to pain. Typically, the extensor hallucis longus (EHL) is the spastic muscle and may be treated with phenol motor-point block, botulinum toxin injection, or if necessary, surgical section of the tendon of the EHL.

The Knee

Either knee flexors or extensors may result in abnormal knee positioning. With knee-extensor spasticity, the knee remains extended throughout the gait cycle owing to an inability to flex the knee during the swing phase of gait. Limb clearance and advancement is a problem. Muscles contributing to this position may include the rectus femoris, vastus medialis, lateralis, or intermedius, and the hamstrings. Dynamic EMG (if available), gait analysis with 3D motion analysis, and ground reaction-force plate may help determine which spastic muscles are playing a role in the abnormal gait mechanics. If all heads of the quadriceps muscle are involved, percutaneous motor blocks with phenol may be considered. However, weakening the muscles may result in loss of ambulation or ability to transfer in the nonambulatory patient. Temporary lidocaine motor-point blocks may also be helpful in determining which muscles are involved in the spasticity and chemodenervation with botulinum toxin may be considered.

If spasticity is present in the hamstrings, a persistent flexed-knee positioning may be seen. The quadriceps group may also be overactive to compensate for the flexor forces and to help stabilize the knee to prevent collapse. In the nonambulatory patient, flexed-knee posturing may prevent proper positioning in the wheelchair. Early in acute TBI serial casting may help maintain the knee in the extended position or chemodenervation of targeted hamstring muscles may help reduce this deformity. Surgical section or lengthening of the hamstring tendon should be considered only in the chronically spastic patient.

The Hips and Thighs

When spasticity is present proximally in the lower extremities, hip flexion is the most typical abnormal position. This is frequently coupled with adduction of the thighs. Often, secondary knee-flexion positioning is also seen with this type of spasticity. Muscles that may contribute to the flexed-hip position include the rectus femoris, iliopsoas, adductor longus, and pectineus. Tight thigh adductors result in a scissoring type gait in the ambulatory patient and may produce tight hip adduction in the nonambulator. Muscles that contribute to this position include the adductor longus, adductor magnus, and the gracilis. Both hip flexion and adduction can interfere with positioning in bed or a wheelchair, perineal care, gait, and sexual activity.

Acute TBI patients with hip spasticity may be treated with stretch and range of motion. Foam triangles between the legs may also help. Occasionally, placing the patient in the prone position has also relieved hip-flexion spasticity. When neurologic recovery is still possible, temporary blocks with phenol or botulinum toxin can be considered. Radiographs to rule out fracture, hip dislocation, or heterotopic ossification are important. The hip is a common place for the development of HO after TBI. Diagnostic obturator nerve blocks may help establish whether fixed contractures are present. In the chronically spastic TBI patient, tendon section or lengthening may be necessary, and ITB may be considered.

SUMMARY

In addition to identifying which spastic muscles may be contributing to an abnormal limb posture, it is imperative to identify the goals in treating the spasticity. In general, during the acute phase of recovery from a TBI, spasticity should be treated aggressively with range of motion, stretching, and splinting as necessary. If the spasticity is focal, chemodenervation can be considered with or without associated serial casting. In addition to relief of spasticity, prevention of soft-tissue contractures and bony deformities is important. Oral pharmacological agents may be considered depending on the patient's level of awareness, cognitive function, and distribution and severity of the spasticity.

As the TBI patient emerges from coma, the treatment of spasticity should be aimed toward improving function. Goals in the treatment of spasticity may include relief of pain, better personal hygiene, ease of dressing or nursing care, improved positioning in a wheelchair or bed, better ambulation, or ease in using assistive devices such as splints and AFOs. In the severely brain-injured patients with severe cognitive impairment and diffuse spasticity, oral systemic pharmacological treatment may be considered as well as more invasive surgical treatment to allow for patient comfort, positioning, and better nursing care.

Although many of the treatment options discussed in this chapter may be used in the treatment of spasticity from any cause, the TBI patient offers a special challenge. The nature of the head injury, the location of the brain damage, and associated neurologic impairments such as cognitive and behavioral problems result in a special challenge to those caring for these patients. The managing physician must be keenly aware of the natural history of recovery from TBI and recognize that this is a dynamic process. Management of the acute TBI patient differs significantly from the more chronic patient. The management of the medical and surgical problems suffered during a TBI also plays a role in how patients are managed acutely. Later, the patient's memory or cognitive disabilities may interfere with their ability to participate in and cooperate with anticipated treatment of spasticity.

A number of questions remain in the pharmacological treatment of spasticity after TBI. Currently available and newly developed antispasticity drugs need to be studied specifically in TBI patients. Injectable agents such as phenol and botulinum toxin also need to be compared as to efficacy and safety.

REFERENCES

1. Sorensen, S. and Kraus, J. (1991) Occurrence, severity, and outcomes of brain injury. *J. Head Trauma Rehabil.* **6,** 1–10.
2. Frankowski, R. F. (1986) The demography of head injury in the United States, in *Neurotrauma,* vol. 1. (Miner, M. and Wagner, K. A., eds.) Butterworth, Boston, pp. 1–17.
3. Kraus, J., Black, M., Hessol, N., et al. (1984) The incidence of acute brain injury and serious impairment in a defined population. *Am. J. Epidemiol.* **119,** 186–201.
4. Povlishock, J. (1992) Traumatically induced axonal injury: pathogenesis and pathobiological implications. *Brain Pathol.* **2,** 1–12.
5. Ott, L., McClain, C., Gillespie, M., et al. (1994) Cytokines and metabolic dysfunction after severe head injury. *J. Neurotrauma* **11,** 447–472.
6. Lobato, R., Cordobes, F., Rivas, J., et al. (1983) Outcome from severe head injury related to the type of intracranial lesion: a computed tomography study. *J. Neurosurg.* **59,** 762–774.
7. Jennett, B., Teasdale, G., Braakman, R., et al. (1979) Prognosis in a series of patients with severe head injury. *Neurosurgery* **4,** 283–289.
8. Sparadeo, F. and Gill, D. (1989) Effects of prior alcohol use on head injury recovery. *J. Head Trauma Rehabil.* **4,** 75–82.
9. Najenson, T., Mendelson, L., Schechter, I., David, C., Mintz, N., and Groswasser, Z. (1974) Rehabilitation after severe head injury. *Scand. J. Rehabil. Med.* **6,** 5–14.
10. Multi-Society Task Force on PVS. (1994) Medical aspects of the persistent vegetative state. *N. Engl. J. Med.* **330,** 1572–1579.
11. Bond, M. R. and Brooks, D. N. (1976) Understanding the process of recovery as a basis for investigation of rehabilitation for the brain injured. *Scand. J. Rehabil. Med.* **8,** 127–131.
12. Salazar, A., Jabbari, B., Vance, S., et al. (1985) Epilepsy after penetration head injury: clinical correlates. *Neurology* **35,** 140–141.
13. Annegers, J., Grabow, J., Groover, R., et al. (1980) Seizures after head trauma: a population study. *Neurology* **30,** 683–689.
14. Temkin, N., Dikmen, S., Wilensky, A., et al. (1990) A randomized, double-blind study of phenytoin for the prevention of post-traumatic seizures. *N. Engl. J. Med.* **323,** 497–502.
15. Jozefczyk, P. B. (1994) Interdisciplinary team approach to rehabilitation, in *Handbook of Neurorehabilitation* (Good, D. C. and Couch, J. R. eds.), Marcel Dekker, New York, pp. 153–164.
16. Young, R. R. (1987) Physiologic and pharmacological approaches to spasticity. *Neurolog. Clin.* **5(4),** 529–539.
17. Young, R. R. (1994) Spasticity: a review. *Neurology* **44(Suppl 9),** S12–S20.
18. Barnard, P., Dill, H., Eldredge, P., et al. (1984) Reduction of hypertonicity by early casting in a comatose head-injured individual. *Phys. Ther.* **64,** 1540–1542.
19. Thaxter, T., Mann, R., and Anderson, C. (1965) Degeneration of immobilized knee joints in rats. *J. Bone Joint Surg.* **47A,** 567–569.

20. Kaplan, M., Yablon, S., Ivanhoe, C., et al. (1995) Surgical correction of contracture: the casting of failed joint management in acquired brain injury. *Arch. Phys. Med. Rehabil.* **76,** 1082–1085.
21. Yarkony, G. M., Sahgal, V. (1987) Contractures: a major complication of craniocerebral trauma. *Clin. Orthop.* **219,** 93–96.
22. Salter, R. and Field, P. (1960) The effects of continuous compression on lining articular cartilage. *J. Bone Joint Surg. Am.* **42A,** 31–36.
23. Enneking, W. and Horowitz, M. (1972) The intra-articular effects of immobilization on the human knee. *J. Bone Joint Surg. Am.* **42A,** 973–975.
24. Amiel, D., Akeson, W., Harwood, R., et al. (1980) Effect of immobilization on the types of collagen synthesized in periarticular connective tissue. *Conn. Tiss. Res.* **8,** 27–32.
25. Hather, B., Adams, G., Tesh, P., et al. (1992) Skeletal muscle responses to lower limb suspension in humans. *J. Appl. Physiol.* **72,** 1493–1498.
26. Veldhuizen, J., Verstappen, F., Vroemen, J., et al. (1993) Functional and morphological adaptions following four weeks of knee immobilization. *Int. J. Sports Med.* **14,** 283–287.
27. Garland, D. E. (1988) Clinical observations on fractures and heterotopic ossification in spinal cord and traumatic brain injured populations. *Clin. Orthop.* **233,** 86–101.
28. Mital, M. A., Garber, J. E., and Stinson, J. T. (1987) Ectopic bone formation in children and adolescents with head injuries: its management. *J. Pediatr. Orthop.* **7,** 83–90.
29. Stover, S. L., Hahn, H. R., and Miller, J. M. (1976) Disodium etidronate in the prevention of heterotopic ossification following spinal cord injury. *Paraplegia* **14,** 146–156.
30. Ritter, M. A. and Sieber, J. M. (1985) Prophylactic indomethocin for the prevention of heterotopic bone formation following total hip arthroplasty. *Clin. Orthop.* **196,** 217–225.
31. Coventry, M. B. and Scanlon, P. W. (1981) The use of radiation to discourage ectopic bone. *J. Bone Joint Surg. Am.* **63,** 201–208.
32. Garland, D. E., Hanscom, D. A., Keenan, M. A., et al, (1985) Resection of heterotopic ossification in the adult with head trauma. *J. Bone Joint Surg. Am.* **67,** 1261–1269.
33. Young, R. R. (1995) Spastic paresis, in *Diagnosis and Management of Disorders of the Spinal Cord* (Young, R. R. and Woolsey, R. M. eds.), Saunders, Philadelphia, pp. 363–376.
34. Little, J. W. and Massagli, T. L. (1993) Spasticity and associated abnormalities of muscle tone, in *Rehabilitation Medicine: Principles and Practice,* 2nd ed. (DeLisa, J. A., ed.), Lippincott, Philadelphia, pp. 666–680.
35. Carey, J. R. (1990) Manual stretch: effect on finger movement control and force control in stroke subjects with spastic extrinsic finger flexor muscles. *Arch. Phys. Med. Rehabil.* **71,** 888–894.
36. Odeen, I. (1981) Reduction of muscular hypertonus by long-term muscles stretch. *Scand. J. Rehabil. Med.* **13,** 93–99.
37. Kabat, H. and Knott, M. (1954) Proprioceptive facilitation therapy for paralysis. *Physiotherapy* **40,** 171.

38. Bobath, B. (1990) Adult hemiplegia: Evaluation and Treatment, 3rd ed. Butterworth-Heinemann, Toronto, Canada.
39. MacPhail, H. E. and Kramer, J. F. (1995) Effect of isokinetic strength-training on functional ability and walking efficiency in adolescents with cerebral palsy. *Dev. Med. Child Neurol.* **37**, 763–775.
40. Damiano, D. L., Vaughn, C. L., and Abel, M. F. (1995) Muscle response to heavy resistance exercise in children with spastic cerebral palsy. *Dev. Med. Chlid Neurol.* **37**, 731–739.
41. Hagbarth, K. E. and Eklund, G. (1969) The muscle vibrator: a useful tool in neurological therapeutic work. *Scand. J. Rehabil. Med.* **1**, 26–34.
42. Miglietta, O. (1973) Action of cold on spasticity. *Am. J. Phys. Med.* **52**, 198–205.
43. Sabbahi, M. A., DeLuca, C. J., and Powers, W. R. (1981) Topical anesthesia: a possible treatment for spasticity. *Arch. Phys. Med. Rehabil.* **62**, 310–314.
44. Carr, E. K. and Kenney, F. D. (1992) Positioning of the stroke patient: a review of the literature. *Intl. J. Nurs. Studies* **29(4)**, 355–369.
45. Myhr, U. and vonWendt, L. (1993) Influence of different sitting positions and abduction orthoses on leg muscle activity in children with cerebral palsy. *Dev. Med. Child Neurol.* **35(10)**, 870–880.
46. Bohannon, R. W. (1993) Tilt table standing for reducing spasticity after spinal cord injury. *Arch. Phys. Med. Rehabil.* **74(10)**, 1121–1122.
47. Kunkel, C. F., Scremin, A. M., Eisenbreg, B., Garcia, J. F., Roberts. S., and Martinez, S. (1993) Effect of "standing" on spasticity, contracture, and osteoporosis in paralyzed males. *Arch. Phys. Med. Rehabil.* **74(1)**, 73–78.
48. Nielsten, J. F. (1995) A new treatment of spasticity with repetitive magnetic stimulation in multiple sclerosis. *J. Neuro. Neurosurg. Psychiatry* **58(2)**, 254–255.
49. Yu, Y. H., Wang, H. C., and Wang, Z. J. (1995) Effect of acupuncture on spinal motor neuron excitability in stroke patients. *Chin. Med. J.* **56(4)**, 258–263.
50. Langlois, S., MacKinnon, J. R., and Pederson, L. (1989) Hand splints and cerebral spasticity: a review of the literature. *Can. J. Occup. Ther.* **56(3)**, 113–119.
51. McPherson, J. J., Kreimeyer, D., Aalderks, M., and Gallagher, T. (1982) A comparison of dorsal and volar resting hand splints in the reduction of hypertonus. *Am. J. Occup. Ther.* **36(10)**, 664–670.
52. Langlois, S., Pederson, L., and MacKinnon, J. R. (1991) The effects of splinting on the spastic hemiplegic hand: Report of a feasibility study. *Can. J. Occup. Ther.* **58(1)**, 17–25.
53. Snook, J. H. (1979) Spasticity reduction splint. *Am. J. Occup. Ther.* **33**, 648–651.
54. Mathiowetz, V., Bolding, D., and Trombly, C. (1983) Immediate effects of a positioning device on the normal and spastic hand measured by electromyography. *Am. J. Occup. Ther.* **37(4)**, 247–254.
55. Sankey, R. J., Anderson, D. M., and Young, J. A. (1989) Characteristics of ankle-foot orthoses for management of the spastic lower limb. *Dev. Med. Child Neurol.* **31**, 466–470.

56. King, II, TI. (1982) Plaster splinting as a means of reducing elbow flexor spasticity: a case study. *Am. J. Occup. Ther.* **36(10),** 671–673.
57. Hinderer, K. A., Harris, S. R., Purdy, A. H., Chew, D. E., Staheli, L. T., McLaughlin, J. F., and Jaffe, K. M. (1988) Effects of "tone-reducing" vs. standard plaster casts on gait improvement of children with cerebral palsy. *Dev. Med. Child Neurol.* **30,** 370–377.
58. Booth, B. J., Doyle, M., and Montgomery, J. (1983) Serial casting for the management of spasticity in the head-injured adult. *Phys. Ther.* **63(12),** 1960–1966.
59. Conine, T. A., Sullivan, T., Mackie, T., and Goodman, M. (1990) Effect of serial casting for the prevention of equinus in patients with acute head injury. *Arch. Phys. Med. Rehabil.* **71,** 310–312.
60. Alfieri, V. (1982) Electrical treatment spasticity. *Scand. J. Rehabil. Med.* **14,** 177–182.
61. King, II, TI. (1996) The effect of neuromuscular electrical stimulation in reducing one. *Am. J. Occup. Ther.* **50(1),** 62–64.
62. Grillner, S. and Zangger, P. (1979) On the central generation of locomotion in the low spinal cat. *Exp. Brain Res.* **34,** 241–261.
63. Larsson, L. E. (1994) Functional electrical stimulation. *Scand. J. Rehabil. Med.* **(Suppl. 30),** 63–72.
64. Liberson, W. T., Holmquest, H. J., Scot, D., and Dow, M. (1961) Functional electrotherapy: stimulation of the peroneal nerve synchronized with the swing phase of the gait of hemiplegic patients. *Arch. Phys. Med. Rehabil.* **42,** 101–105.
65. Hines, A. E., Crago, P. E., and Billian, C. (1993) Functional electrical stimulation for the reduction of spasticity in the hemiplegic patient. *Biomed. Sci. Instrum.* **29,** 259–266.
66. Dimitrijevic, M. M. (1994) Mesh glove: a method for whole-hand electrical stimulation in upper motion neuron dysfunction. *Scand. J. Rehabil. Med.* **26,** 183–186.
67. Basmajian, J. V., Kukulka, C. G., Narayan, M. G., and Takebe, K. (1975) Biofeedback treatment of foot-drop after stroke compared with standard rehabilitation technique: effects on voluntary control and strength. *Arch. Phys. Med. Rehabil.* **56,** 231–236.
68. Neilson, P. D. and McCaughey, J. (1982) Self-regulation of spasm and spasticity in cerebral palsy. *J. Neurol. Neurosurg. Psychiatry* **45,** 320–330.
69. Nash, J., Nielson, P. D., and O'Dwyer, N. J. (1989) Reducing spasticity to control muscle contracture of children with cerebral palsy. *Dev. Med. Child Neurol.* **31,** 471–480.
70. Bleck, E. (1987) *Orthopedic Management in Cerebral Palsy.* MacKeith Press, London.
71. Kagaya, H., Yamada, S., Nagasawa, T., Ishihara, Y., Kodama, H., and Endoh, H. (1996) Split posterior tibial tendon transfer for varus deformity of the hindfoot. *Clin. Orthop. Rel. Res.* **323,** 254–260.
72. Waters, R. L., Frazier, J., Garland, D. E., Jordan, C., and Perry, J. (1982) Electromyographic gait analysis before and after operative treatment for hemiplegic equinus and equinovarus deformity. *J. Bone Joint Surg.* **64A,** 284–288.

73. Sakellarides, H. T., Mital, M. A., Matza, R. A., and Dimakopoulos, P. (1995) Classification and surgical treatment of thumb-in-palm deformity in cerebral palsy and spastic paralysis. *J. Hand Surg.* **20(3),** 428–431.
74. Sakellarides, H. T. and Kirvin, F. M. (1995) Management of the unbalanced wrist in cerebral palsy by tendon transfer. *Ann. Plast. Surg.* **35,** 90–94.
75. Speelman, D. and Van Mann, J. (1989) Cerebral palsy and stereotactic neurosurgery: long term results. *J. Neurol. Neurosurg. Psychiatry* **52,** 23–30.
76. Cooper, I. S., Riklan, M., Amin, I., Waltz, J. M., and Cullinan, T. (1976) Chronic cerebellar stimulation in cerebral palsy. *Neurology* **26,** 744–753.
77. Gahm, N. H., Russman, B. S., Cerciello, R. L., et al. (1981) Chronic cerebellar stimulatioin for cerebral palsy: a double-blind study. *Neurology* **31,** 87–90.
78. Peacock, W. J. and Staudt, L. A. (1990) Spasticity in cerebral palsy and the selective posterior rhizotomy procedure. *J. Child Neurol.* **5,** 179–185.
79. Peacock, W. J. and Staudt, L. A. (1991) Functional outcomes following selective posterior rhizotomy in children with cerebral palsy. *J. Neurosurg.* **74,** 380–385.
80. Sindou, M. and Mertens, P. (1988) Selective neurectomy of the tibial nerve for treatment of the spastic foot. *Neurosurgery* **23,** 738–744.
81. Ritchie, J. M. and Greene, N. M. (1980) Local anesthetics, in *The Pharmacological Basis of Therapeutics,* 6th ed. (Goodman, L. S. and Gilman, A. eds.), MacMillan, New York, pp. 300–320.
82. Koman, L. A., Mooney, J. F., and Patersen Smith, B. (1996) Neuromuscular blockade in the management of cerebral palsy. *J. Child Neurol.* **11(Suppl. 1),** S23–S28.
83. Ritchie, J. M. (1980) The Aliphatic Alcohols, in *The Pharmacologic Basis of Therapeutics,* 6th ed. (Goodman, L. S. and GIlman, A., eds.), MacMillan, New York, pp. 376–390.
84. Carpenter, E. B. and Seitz, D. G. (1980) Intramuscular alcohol as an aid in the management of spastic cerebral palsy. *Dev. Med. Child Neurol.* **22,** 497–501.
85. Tardieu, C., Tardieu, G., Hariga, J., and Gagnard, L. (1968) Treatment of spasticity by injection of dilute alcohol at the motor point or by epidural route: clinical extension of an experiment on the decerebrate cat. *Dev. Med. Child Neurol.* **10,** 555–568.
86. Felsenthal, G. (1974) Pharmacology of phenol in nerve blocks: a review. *Arch. Phys. Med. Rehabil.* **55,** 13–16.
87. Botte, M. J., Abrams, R. A., and Bodine-Fowler, S. C. (1995) Treatment of acquired muscle spasticity using phenol peripheral nerve blocks. *Orthopedics* **18(2),** 151–159.
88. Khalil, A. A. and Betts, H. B. (1967) Peripheral nerve block with phenol in the management of spasticity. *JAMA* **200(13),** 1155–1157.
89. Keenan, M. A., Tomas, E. S., Stone, L., and Gersten, L. M. (1990) Percutaneous phenol block of the musculocutaneous nerve to control elbow flexor spasticity. *J. Hand Surg.* **15A,** 340–346.
90. Awad, E. A. and Dykstra, D. (1990) Treatment of spasticity by neurolysis, in *Krusen's Handbook of Physical Medicine and Rehabilitation,* 4th ed. (Kottke, F. J. and Leahmann, J. F., eds.), W.B. Saunders, Philadelphia, pp. 1154–1161.

91. Hambleton, P. (1992) Clostridium botulinum toxins: a general review of involvement in disease, structure, mode of action and preparation for clinical use. *J. Neurol.* **239,** 16–20.
92. Hughes, A. J. (1994) Botulinum toxin in clinical practice. *Drugs* **48(6),** 888–893.
93. National Institutes of Health. (1991) Consensus Development Conference Statement, November 12–14, 1990. Clinical use of botulinum toxin. *Arch. Neurol.* **48,** 1294–1298.
94. Therapeutics and Technology Assessment Subcommittee of the American Academy of Neurology. (1990) Assessment: the clinical usefulness of botulinum toxin-A in treating neurologic disorders. *Neurology* **40,** 1332–1336.
95. Therapeutics and Technology Assessment Subcommittee of the American Academy of Neurology. (1994) Assessment: training guidelines for the use of botulinum toxin for the treatment of neurologic disorders. *Neurology* **44,** 2401–2403.
96. Comella, C. L., Buchman, A. S., Tanner, C. M., Brown-Thoms, N. C., and Goetz, C. G. (1992) Botulinum toxin injection for spasmodic torticollis; increased magnitude of benefit with electromyographic assistance. *Neurology* **42,** 878–882.
97. Das, T. K. and Park, D. M. (1989) Effect of treatment of botulinum toxin on spasticity. *Postgrad. Med. J.* **65,** 209–210.
98. Das, T. K. and Park, D. M. (1989) Botulinum toxin in treating spasticity. *BJCP* **43(11),** 401–403.
99. Snow, B. J., Tsui, J. K., Bhatt, B. H., Varelas, M., Hashimoto, S. A., and Calne, D. B. (1990) Treatment of spasticity with botulinum toxin: a double-blind study. *Ann. Neurol.* **28,** 512–515.
100. Grazko, M. A., Polo, K. B., and Jabbari, B. (1995) Botulinum toxin A for spasticity, muscle spasms, and rigidity. *Neurology* **45,** 712–717.
101. Simpson, D. M., Alexander, D. N., O'Brien, C. F., Tagliati, M., Aswad, A. S., Leon, J. M., et al. (1996) Botulinum toxin type A in the treatment of upper extremity spasticity: A randomized double-blind placebo-controlled trial. *Neurology* **46,** 1306–1310.
102. Childers, M. K., Brashear, A., Jozefczyk, P. B., et al. (1999) A multi-center, double-blind, placebo-controlled dose response trial of Botulinum Toxin Type A in upper limb spasticity post-stroke. *Neurology* **52(6),** S2.
103. Dunne, J. W., Heye, N., and Dunne, S. L. (1995) Treatment of chronic limb spasticity with botulinum toxin A. *J. Neurol. Neurosurg. Psychiatry* **58,** 232–235.
104. Dengler, R., Neyer, U., Wohlfarth, K., Bettig, U., and Janzik, H. H. (1992) Local botulinum toxin in the treatment of spastic foot drop. *J. Neurol.* **239,** 375–378.
105. Hesse, S., Lucke, D., Maezic, M., Bertelt, C., Friedrich, H., Gregoric, M., and Mauritz, K. H. (1994) Botulinum toxin treatment for lower limb extensor spasticity in chronic hemiparetic patients. *J. Neurol. Neurosurg. Psychiatry* **57,** 1321–1324.
106. Hesse, S., Krajnik, J., Luecke, D., Jahnke, M. T., Gregoric, M., and Mauritz,

K. H. (1996) Ankle muscle activity before and after botulinum toxin therapy for lower limb extensor spasticity in chronic hemiparetic patients. *Stroke* **27**, 455–460.
107. Yablon, S. A., Agana, B. T., Ivanhoe, C. B., and Boake, C. (1996) Botulinum toxin in severe upper extremity spasticity among patients with traumatic brain injury: an open-labeled trial. *Neurology* **47**, 939–944.
108. Kirazli, Y., Yagiz, D. A., Kismali, B., and Aksit, R. (1998) Comparison of phenol block on botulinum toxin type A in the treatment of spastic foot after stroke: A randomized, double-blind trial. *Am. J. Phys. Med. Rehabil.* **77**, 510–515.
109. Fuxe, K. and Ungerstedt, U. (1970) Histochemical, biochemical and functional studies on central monoamine neurons after acute and chronic amphetamine administration, in *Amphetamines and Related Compounds* (Costa, E. and Garattini, S. eds.), Raven Press, New York, pp. 257–288.
110. Goldstein, L. B. (1994) Pharmacologic enhancement of recovery, in *The Handbook of Neurorehabilitation* (Good, D. C. and Couch, J. eds.), Marcel Dekker, New York, pp. 343–369.
111. From, A. and Heltberg, A. (1975) A double-blind trial with baclofen and diazepam in spasticity due to multiple sclerosis. *Acta. Neurol. Scand.* **51**, 158–166.
112. Costa, E. and Guidotti, A. (1979) Molecular mechanisms in the receptor action of benzodiazepines. *Ann. Rev. Toxicol.* **19**, 531–545.
113. Corbett, M., Frankel, H. L., and Michaelis, L. (1972) A double-blind cross over trial of valium in the treatment of spasticity. *Paraplegia* **10**, 19–22.
114. Lossius, R., Dietrichson, P., and Lunde, P. K. M. (1985) Effect of clorazepate in spasticity and rigidity: A quantitative study of reflexes and plasma concentrations. *Acta Neurol. Scand.* **71**, 190–194.
115. Scharf, M. B., Hirschowitz, J., Woods, M., et al. (1985) Lack of amnestic effects of clorazepate on geriatric recall. *Clin. Psychiatry* **46(2)**, 518–520.
116. Basmajan, J. V., Shandarkass, K., and Russell, D. (1986) Ketazolam once daily for spasticity: double-blind, crossover study. *Arch. Phys. Med. Rehabil.* **67**, 556–557.
117. Cendrowski, W. and Sobczyk, W. (1977) Clonazepam, baclofen, and placebo in the treatment of spasticity. *Eur. Neurol.* **16**, 257–262.
118. Pinder, R. M., Brogden, R. N., Speight, T. M., and Avery, G. S. (1977) Dantrolene sodium: a review of its pharmacological properties and therapeutic efficacy in spasticity. *Drugs* **13**, 3–23.
119. Katrak, P. H., Cole, A., Poulos, C. J., McCauley, J. C. K. (1992) Objective assessment of spasticity, strength and function with early exhibition of dantrolene sodium after cerebrovascular accident: a randomize double-blind study. *Arch. Phys. Med. Rehabil.* **73**, 4–9.
120. Bonicalzi, V. and Canavero, S. (1996) Lamotrigine effects of chronic pain: an open-label pilot study (abstract). Proceedings of the 8th World Congress on Pain, p. 173.
121. Bensimon, G., Lamcomblez, L., Meininger, V. (1994) A controlled trial of riluzole in amyotrophic lateral sclerosis. *N. Engl. J. Med.* **330(9)**, 585–591.

122. Bes, A., Eyssette, M., Pierrot-Deseilligny, E., Rohmer, T., and Warter, J. M. (1988) A multi-centre, double-blind trial of tizanidine as antispastic agent in spasticity associated with hemiplegia. *Curr. Med. Res. Opin.* **10(10),** 709–718.
123. Goldstein, L. B. and Davis, J. N. (1990) Clonidine impairs recovery of beam waking in rats. *Brain Res.* **508,** 305–309.
124. Nance, P. (1994) A comparison of clonidine, cyproheptadine, and baclofen in spastic spinal cord injured patients. *J. Am. Paraplegia Soc.* **17,** 151–157.
125. Casale, R., Glynn, C., and Buonocore, M. (1995) Reduction of spastic hypertonia in patients with spinal cord injury: a double-blind comparison of intravenous orphenadrine citrate and placebo. *Arch. Phys. Med. Rehabil.* **76,** 660–665.
126. Cohan, S. L., Raines, A., Panagakos, J., et al. (1980) Phenytoin and chlorpromazine in the treatment of spasticity. *Arch. Neurol.* **37,** 360–364.
127. Albright, A. L., Barron, W. B., Fasick, M. P., Polinko, P., and Janosky, J. (1993) Continuous intrathecal baclofen infusion for spasticity of cerebral origin. *JAMA* **270,** 2475–2477.

20
Spasticity in Spinal Cord Injury
A Clinician's Approach

Kurt Fiedler and Douglas R. Jeffery

INTRODUCTION

This chapter reviews the current understanding and management of spasticity following spinal-cord injury (SCI). Attempts to formally define the term "spasticity" vary with the physiological prejudices of the definer, but patients and their caregivers alike often lump together the spasms, the variable stiffness of muscles, the consequent further reduction in dexterity, and the associated pain into a single clinical problem for which treatment is demanded. The first section in this chapter presents an approach to the clinical differentiation of the contributing factors; the second section specifically outlines potential anatomical problem areas; and the third section offers a clinician's approach to sequential intervention.

FACTORS CONTRIBUTING TO SPASTICITY

Owing to the ambiguity of precise definition and the obvious difficulties in quantification, the incidence and prevalence of spasticity following SCI has not been well-studied. "Spasms" have been described in 15–42% of various cohorts (*1,2*). More inclusive studies cogently find significant signs of spasticity in approx 80% of patients with upper motor neuron lesions, and argue that "treatment was warranted" in about two-thirds of these individuals (*3*). Follow-up studies suggest increasing need for treatment over time (*4*), but do not distinguish between the effects of duration of injury and the effects of comorbidity associated with increasing age. In occasional cases, spasticity as the single subtle presenting clue of otherwise occult incomplete cervical SCI has been noted (*5*).

So far, attempts at quantification of spasticity appear either idiosyncratic or simply too subjective; they will not be addressed here beyond bluntly noting that most clinicians find little use in the Ashworth scale or other

From: *Current Clinical Neurology: Clinical Evaluation and Management of Spasticity*
Edited by: D. A. Gelber and D. R. Jeffery © Humana Press, Inc., Totowa, NJ

published scales or grading systems of muscle tone. A recent extensive meta-analysis of putative functional outcome measures to assess interventions for spasticity found multiple confounding factors in most protocols, as well as in data reporting and analysis (6). Rehabilitation nurses, occupational and physical therapists, and physicians, if they have sufficient physical contact with their patients, will be acutely aware of the degree to which spasticity affects the patient as well as its day-to-day variability. Equally, response to treatment will be evident in terms of reduction in both disability (functional limitations) and handicap (societal impact).

Accrediting agencies and third-party payors can be appeased with sequential documentation of progress charted by the widely used Functional Independence Measure (FIM) (7). However, it should be noted that clinicians whose practices principally focus on persons with SCI note the consistent failure of this measure to adequately reflect either significant gains or, perhaps more importantly, subtle losses in the course of the labor and resource-intensive rehabilitation of this population (8). In the unhealthy setting of adult-onset spasticity following SCI, the loss of normal descending neural modulation at multiple levels results in apparently ineffective movement, caused by "senseless" responses to afferent stimuli, such as changes in position or posture, ambient temperature, or visceral sensations. These supraspinal modulations include both inhibitory effects on stretch reflexes mediated through the dorsal reticulospinal tract, and facilitory effects on extensor (antigravity) tone, mediated through the medial reticulospinal and vestibulospinal tracts; these modulators in turn are further affected by segmental propriospinal mechanisms (9).

Superimposed on the increased tone owing to loss of, or imbalance in, descending control, is the variable stiffness that develops in muscles that are relatively unexercised (10,11). This stiffness is an often overlooked contributor to the development of "contracture," usually ascribed to loss of anchoring-tendon length and elasticity. The electrically active increased muscular tension attendant on spasticity is sometimes characterized as exercise itself, but in contrast to natural or trained exertion, it is obviously neither graduated nor interrupted by periodic relaxation in response to antagonistic movement. The viscoelastic mechanical changes in disused tissues bring about so-called "thixotropic" added changes in tone that are truly passive, i.e., electromyographically silent (12,13). Both passive and active increases in muscle tone predominantly present as clinical muscle pain (14), and are often combined with the undesired movements by the patient into complaints of "spasms."

Previous efforts to differentiate the spasticity owing to SCI from that owing to cerebral lesions contrasted the relative amounts of hypertonia in flex-

Spasticity in SCI 355

ion or extension, reflex hyperexcitability, and weakness or loss of dexterity. No consistent picture has emerged when these factors have been used as criteria by which to differentiate these sources of spasticity. A recent study showed a similar divergence of patterns of spasticity even in a group of relatively homogeneous patients following cerebrovascular accidents (15). The clinician's need for awareness of underlying diagnoses persists, not so much as to the level of the lesion as with regard to the contributions of co-morbid illness and pain to the intensity of spastic signs and symptoms. Excess spasticity has been defined as that owing to superimposed afferent stimuli, over and above the basic spasticity owing to the spinal lesion itself (16). The distinction between spasticity of spinal cord vs cerebral origin is less important than the recognition that neural changes, both helpful and detrimental, continue to evolve as time passes following SCI (17).

Investigation and patient education regarding causative factors intrinsic and extrinsic to the nervous system is warranted (18). Intrinsic factors include physiologic facilitators and inhibitors, such as posture, ambient temperature, nature of the lesion, and direct pharmacological effects on the central nervous system (CNS). Influential factors extrinsic to the nervous system include infection anywhere; genito-urological irritants (retention; stones or other masses; reflux; penile, epididymo-orchitic, or vaginal lesions); bowel problems (constipation, impaction, hemmorhoids, rectal prolapse); skin (pressure sores, warts, burns, infestations, nail problems); muscle, bone, and joint lesions (contracture, tears, sprains, occult fractures, heterotopic ossification, etc.); and other sequelae of relative immobility, especially deep venous thrombosis; and the effects of constricting garments, wheelchairs, and bedding. Of these, the most likely causes of an acute episode of excess spasticity are constipation or urinary-tract infection. In such acute episodes, in addition to increased spasticity, the elevated blood pressure, headache, piloerection, and focal vasomotor signs of autonomic dysreflexia may be present, signaling a potential life-threatening emergency unique to persons with SCI (19).

Emotional factors must always be addressed: consideration of pre-morbid as well as reactive anxiety, depression, and the pervasive stress endemic to such a disastrous event as SCI. In addition, somatic signs including spasticity are affected by personality traits. The influence of individual coping styles and attribution of locus of control is a significant factor having the potential to affect the severity of spasticity (20).

SPECIFIC ANATOMICAL PROBLEM AREAS RELATIVE TO SPASTICITY

Because of the clinician's expectation that muscular disuse will inevitably lead to postural abnormalities, there may be failure to adequately focus on the most common chronic cause of excess spasticity: contracture. Contracture are semi-fixed abnormal postures brought about by intrinsic changes in joint-related musculoskeletal tissues held in relative immobility and under nonphysiologically sustained tension.

Like many other practices in SCI medicine, the emphasis on containment of spasticity "within tolerable—and even useful—limits," owes much to the insight of Dr. Ludwig Guttmann, based on his clinical experience following his founding the now world-renowned Stoke Mandeville SCI Centre Hospital at Aylesbury, UK. His approach to prevention is based on two interrelated components: 1) regular periodic passive range of motion of all joints below the level of the lesion; and 2) careful positioning of the patient's limbs during the time between regular ranging (*21*).

The following specific anatomical areas, with the most likely potential contracture identified, are highly susceptible to the vicious cycle of "spasticity leads to contracture which leads to further spasticity." The consequent increase in tone is likely to be generalized not merely to the whole limb, but the entire area affected by the SCI. This might be regarded as an instance of "mass reflex" referring to the spread of upper motor neuron (UMN) lesion effects.

This list is largely based on the classic summary presented by Michaelis, who noted that "Guttmann's precept warrants a joint by joint description" (*16*). In all cases, regular passive range of motion and avoidance of pressure from bedding or garments are needed, and in selected instances, splinting is indicated. If orthotics are used, appropriate monitoring to avoid pressure sores is mandatory.

- Toes: Flexion-contracture generally; extension-contracture of the great toes.
- Ankles: Drop-foot, with either pronation or supination.
- Knees: Hyperextension and flexion-contracture. When supine, the knee should be in full extension; when the patient is side-lying, in about 20° flexion. Avoid placing pillows beneath the knees, but wedging between them is important to avoid pressure sores.
- Hips: Similar to knees. Avoidance of flexion-contracture, involving iliopsoas, is of major importance to subsequent positioning in bed and/or chair, as well as preventing excess spasticity. Hyperextension should be avoided as well, with its sequelae of exaggerated lumbar lordosis and abdominal muscle stretching. In all positions, the lower limbs should be about 10° abducted. This ensures that the adductors, naturally stronger as anti-gravity muscles than the abductors, are kept on stretch, while the gluteus medius is allowed to shorten to counteract over adduction.
- Fingers: Depending on the exact level of injury, extension- and flexion-contracture of metacarpals and phalangeal joints. Care to splint the thumb in opposition is worthwhile though difficult to maintain.

- Wrists: "Cocked-up" at 20° extension. Avoid radial or ulnar deviation.
- Elbows: Maintain in extension. Note that in the not-uncommon C5-6 lesion, biceps will be preserved, but triceps paralyzed, which will promote a tendency towards flexion-contracture.
- Shoulders: Similarly, note the common loss of pectoral-adductor function with preservation of the predominantly abducting deltoid in lesions as varied as C4-7. Accordingly, the upper arm should be positioned alongside the chest when supine or prone; in forward extension when side-lying. When it occurs, excessive shoulder abduction, which is usually close to the "endzone" at the level of injury, is often very painful, and triggers mass reflex responses. Of pertinence to the afferent aspects of induced excess spasticity at this level, is the little-noted predominance of sensory input from the shoulders; this is in fact secondary only to the face and hands. (An intriguing correlate is the high density of so-called premonitory urges from the shoulder girdle in persons with Tourette syndrome [22].)

A recent study points out probable cognitive aspects of contracture avoidance, as well as the potential for multi-level tonic somatic effects. Acute SCI patients with co-existent or suspected head injury were more likely to develop contracture (15%) than patients without that comorbid complication (7.4%) (23).

Although not traditionally included in topographic considerations of spasticity, the neuropathic effects of SCI on the urinary bladder may be usefully characterized by the familiar models of UMN and lower motor neuron (LMN) lesions, which will perhaps also permit abandoning the unfortunate use of the inaccurate term "neurogenic." The characteristic picture of decreased or absent tendon stretch reflexes and muscle atrophy owing to a LMN lesion is seen in the state of flaccid distention and potential trabeculation of the urinary bladder detrusor muscle following conus or cauda equina injuries, i.e., LMN lesions. On the other hand, the lack of compliance of the irritable, tautly-shrunken detrusor, parallels the classic UMN lesion picture of a hyperactive stretch reflex and spastic musculature. Cystometric studies show nonphysiologic pressure/volume relationships in both cases (24). In the case of LMN damage, the absence of detrusor reflex contraction results in failure to elevate bladder pressure sufficient to overcome the pressure of the tonically closed urethral sphincter, with consequent urinary retention until "overflow incontinence" occurs. In contrast, the frequent small-volume micturition pattern of the UMN-lesioned individual reflects the rapid recurrence of detrusor-generated pressures overcoming the urethral closure pressure. Both pictures can be further complicated by neuropathic failure of normal reflex relaxation of the sphincter which is normally triggered by detrusor contraction; this condition is termed detrusor-sphincter dyssynergia (DSD). The clinical sequelae of DSD include ureteral reflux, development of so-called hydroureters, and the full range of renal complications associated with infection and stone-formation.

A CLINICIAN'S GUIDE TO SEQUENTIAL INTERVENTION FOR SCI-ASSOCIATED SPASTICITY

The prevention of deformities is an important aspect in the treatment of SCI. Because deformities are often the result of sustained increases in muscle tone, the reduction in muscle tone is important in preventing deformities. Inhibition of tone, avoidance of muscle fiber and tendon shortening, loss of elasticity, and minimization of associated pain may be achieved through proper bed and wheelchair positioning as discussed in the previous section. The use of conventional positioning splints (25) and/or inhibitory orthoses, which provide prolonged active stretch across an affected joint, may also be helpful in the prevention of contracture resulting from increased muscle tone (26).

The actual utility of moderate spasticity is self-evident, as anyone who has attempted to move (or dress) a truly flaccid person can attest. Accordingly, maintenance physical therapy is a second line of treatment. This utilizes physiatric measures from routine application of stretch, hot and cold "modalities," mat, balance, sitting, standing, and respiratory training, and gait practice with various supports, suspension, work-hardening exercise, sport, and assistive/augmented communication-device involvement. Modulating the neurogenic components of spasticity including supraspinal, propriospinal, and segmental aspects of spasticity alleviates the thixotropic changes discussed earlier.

Beyond this initial physical training, advanced kinesiology and functional stimulation (both electrical and magnetic), show the most promise in psychomotor/behavioral treatment of spasticity. The early conceptual work of Dimitrijevic (27) and Barbeau (28) focusing on computer-assisted training has been recently applied to selected subpopulations of persons with SCI. Progress, not surprisingly, has been most significant in those with "incomplete" lesions (12), and for those with appropriate lifestyle, potential commitment, and occupation (29). But the clinical reality that locomotion demands high energy expenditure, particularly in patients additionally constrained by excess spasticity, and the anecdotal feelings of deafferented patients that they are "being moved" rather than moving themselves, continue to limit patient and provider enthusiasm for this approach.

The choice of a surgeon (16) to write the chapter on SCI spasticity for the authoritative multi-volume *Handbook of Neurology* 25 years ago, is significant in retrospect. Phenolic and other chemical neural ablations, myotomies, tenotomies and tendon lengthening, capsulotomies, neurectomies, and even myelotomies and cordectomies were accepted treatment modalities. With regard to the still current use of rhizotomy for the congenital spasticity of cerebral palsy (CP), although assiduous long-term follow-up documents improvements lasting 10 years or more (*30*), its popularity is waning. This is probably owing to a reduction in indications for any subsequent orthopedic surgery in such patients, who are increasingly treated with long-term intrathecal baclofen (ITB) infusions (*31*).

APPROACH TO THE TREATMENT OF SPASTICITY IN SCI

There are several important principles of treatment worthy of statement prior to discussion of treatment modalities. The first principle is that the goal of spasticity treatment is to improve quality of life. More clearly stated, it is not the phenomena of spasticity that requires treatment, but the consequences of spasticity and the associated deficits brought about by increased muscle tone that are the targets of therapy. The presence of spasticity alone is not a reason to treat. Treatment of spasticity should be undertaken when it interferes with function or when it becomes painful or exacerbates other painful syndromes seen in SCI.

The second principle of treatment calls for flexibility in the treatment regimen. Treatment should be targeted to the timing of the symptoms. The point to be made is that the timing of the symptoms is an important consideration in the schedule of drug administration. Dosage is also an important issue. Often in clinical practice doses are not titrated to effect and the flexibility is not brought into the regimen. For effective treatment, the dose must be titrated to maximize functional ability. Doses above that level may produce increased weakness or sedation. Doses below the desired level are subtherapeutic. As pointed out earlier, the severity of spasticity may vary over time and even within the course of the day. As a result, it is sometimes useful to use additional doses on an as-needed basis. This allows the patient more control over their symptoms and can be useful when spasticity is exacerbated as a result of pain or other environmental factors.

As in any clinical situation, individual patient characteristics, including the available support system as well as idiosyncratic pharmacological responses, guide the choice of treatments. This is particularly true as one progresses from manipulative therapy to invasive procedures, such as the placement of ITB pumps.

This leads to the most important modern modality in the treatment of spasticity in patients with traumatic SCI: pharmacological. A variety of new and old treatments are now available. Importantly, there are better pharmacologic modalities for the treatment of spasticity in SCI than ever before. Tizanidine, baclofen, diazepam, botulinum toxin, and dantrolene are the mainstays of therapy. Each has its own advantages and disadvantages depending on the severity of spasticity, co-existant medical regimen, and individual patient characteristics. Each of these modalities is discussed in detail in previous chapters in this volume. The following pages will provide a clinical guideline for their use in the treatment of spasticity in patients with SCI.

Baclofen

A first-line agent in the treatment of spasticity owing to SCI is baclofen. Often the severity of spasticity in SCI is far greater than that seen in inflammatory diseases involving the spinal cord such as multiple sclerosis (MS) or transverse myelitis. Baclofen may be used in doses ranging from 10 mg t.i.d. to 240 mg daily in divided doses. Because most SCI patients lack any significant motor control, the fact that baclofen decreases muscle strength has little effect on functional abilities in most patients with SCI. Nevertheless, in SCI patients with partial injuries who are ambulatory with assistive devices, baclofen may result in a deterioration of functional abilities, particulary gait. The use of oral baclofen is discussed in detail in this volume. Baclofen is well-tolerated in the majority of patients and leads to significant reductions in tone and spasms. The doses required to control spasticity in SCI often produce considerable side effects including fatigue and sedation. In addition, the abrupt discontinuation of baclofen may be associated with a withdrawal that can include seizures as well as hallucinations. Suffice it to say that in spasticity owing to SCI, oral baclofen alone is usually insufficient to control spasticity. Often combination therapy with other pharmacologic agents is required.

Tizanidine

Another first-line therapy is tizanidine. Tizanidine is an alpha-adrenergic agonist similar to clonidine, but with much less of an effect on blood pressure. It is discussed in detail in this volume. Tizanidine has several advantages over baclofen, particularly in patients with partial injuries who remain ambulatory with assistive devices or in those who have some preservation of functional muscle strength. The starting dose is 1 mg to 2 mg t.i.d. to q.i.d. with 4 mg at H.S. The half-life of tizanidine is quite short at 2.5 h. Consequently, dosing on a q.i.d. schedule is probably more appropriate. The dose is then titrated upward to achieve the desired level of muscle tone. The maximal dose studied in patients with SCI was 32 mg daily or 8 mg q.i.d, although in practice, tizanidine may be titrated upwards to doses exceeding 48 mg daily. Tizanidine has been shown to significantly reduce the frequency of painful spasms and clonus as well as substantially reduce spasticity scores on the Ashworth scale (*32*). Among its primary advantages is that it has little or no effect on muscle strength at doses that markedly decrease muscle tone. This is important in patients with partial injury and retained mobility. In those patients who are ambulatory with assistive devices, this becomes an important issue because any decrease in muscle strength could result in a further impairment in ambulation and possible falls with resulting injury. Consequently, in patients with partial or incomplete SCI who remain ambulatory, tizanidine is often the preferred drug. Other advantages over baclofen include its lack of a withdrawal syndrome and its relative lack of effect on mental status. Baclofen tends to have a greater effect on mental status in doses that are required to relieve spasticity in patients with SCI. In addition, tizanidine may have significant antinociceptive effects. Because 60% of patients with SCI suffer from neurologic pain syndromes, tizanidine may be of use in the control of both spasticity and pain. Again, in SCI spasticity is often quite severe and multiple oral agents may be required to have even a minimal impact of spasticity. One potential drawback to the use of tizanidine in patients with SCI is its effect on blood pressure. In patients with cervical SCI, baseline blood pressures may be quite low. The tendency of tizanidine to decrease blood pressure is usually minimal but in this population tizanidine may have significant effects on blood pressure and therefore caution should be exercised when using this agent in these patients.

Benzodiazepines

Benzodiazepines have also been proven to be useful in the treatment of spasticity of spinal-cord and cerebral origin (33). The prototype agent is diazepam, which has been in use since the 1960s for treatment of spasticity of spinal-cord origin. Other agents such as clonezepam are acceptable alternatives. The benzodiazepines act pre- and postsynaptically to enhance the affinity of gamma-amino butyric acid (GABA) receptors for their endogenous ligand. Diazepam is effective in the treatment of spasticity in SCI but suffers from several important drawbacks compared to newer agents. It increases weakness at doses that relieve painful spasms. As pointed out earlier, this is important for those patients with partial injuries requiring unilateral or bilateral assistance for ambulation. Increasing weakness in that group of patients will predispose them to falls, which can result in serious injury. In addition, it suffers from abuse potential and is associated with a withdrawal syndrome that may involve anxiety, agitation, irritability, and seizures. Finally, it clouds consciousness and may bring about significant confusion.

In rare instances when patients are unable to tolerate first line agents such as tizanidine or baclofen, diazepam may be a useful alternative. In such instances it should be introduced at doses of 2 mg b.i.d. or t.i.d. and titrated to effect. It may also be dosed in the evening for patients suffering from nocturnal spasms. It suffers from the same drawback as seen with baclofen in that strength is adversely effected and gait may be more impaired as a result.

Dantrium

Dantrium has also been shown effective in the treatment of spasticity. Its mechanism differs from other agents in that it acts directly on muscle. Dantrium blocks the release of calcium from the sarcoplasmic reticulum and effectively interferes with excitation-contraction coupling (34). As a result, it decreases spasticity by interfering with muscle contraction. In disease states such as SCI where weakness is owing to lesions of the CNS, dantrium will significantly increase weakness. Dantrium suffers from other major drawbacks, the most important of which is hepatotoxicity. The overall risk of hepatotoxicity is 1.8% and fatal reactions occur in 0.3%. Those at the greatest risk are women over the age of 30 taking more than 300 mg/d for over 2 mo. Those patients taking other agents that are metabolized by the liver are also at higher risk. Given the variety of agents that have proven efficacy in spasticity in SCI, the risk associated with dantrium and its deleterious effect on muscle strength outweigh the potential benefit in the majority of cases.

ALTERNATIVE AND ADJUNCT THERAPIES FOR SPASTICITY IN SCI

A wide variety of adjunctive agents have a useful role in the treatment of spasticity in MS. These include gabapentin, clonidine, clonezepam, cyclobenzaprine, cannabinoids, and opiates have been shown in smaller studies to reduce muscle tone and decrease the frequency of painful spasms and clonus (35–43). Alternative and adjunct therapies are discussed in detail in this volume (see Chapter 14). Each of these agents may prove useful as adjunct therapy but none has the efficacy required of a first-line agent. Gabapentin deserves mention because of its beneficial effect on central pain syndromes seen in MS patients. Pain syndromes characterized by dysthesthetic burning sensations in the extremities may worsen spasticity and increased muscle tone may exacerbate pain. Gabapentin is effective in the treatment for chronic-pain syndromes in SCI and in MS and in doses greater than 900 mg daily it may bring about relief from painful spasms and clonus (35,36). The other agents mentioned previously find use as adjuncts when first-line agents are not tolerated at fully therapeutic doses or when first-line agents fail to bring the manifestations of spasticity under sufficient control.

Intrathecal Baclofen

When patients with SCI develop spasticity that cannot be controlled with oral medication at maximal doses, the baclofen pump becomes a possible therapeutic alternative. Refractory spasticity tends to occur in SCI. ITB should not be considered in those with spasticity of only moderate severity. In those with severe spasticity owing to SCI, the baclofen pump may be a very effective alternative. The ITB pump is discussed in detail in this volume (see Chapter 15). Briefly, when a patient with intractable spasticity has failed oral medication, a test dose of ITB is administered. A baseline measure of tone is obtained and a test dose of 50–100 µg is administered intrathecally over a period of 5 min. The patient is then observed for 8–12 h and measurements of spasticity are made periodically. The Ashworth scale is the recommended measure. The effect of ITB is usually quite impressive and brings about a dramatic reduction in muscle tone within an hour. In patients who do not show a reduction in tone or in those who develop increased weakness, the baclofen pump may not be appropriate. If the test dose is successful, pump implantation can proceed.

A variety of reports have confirmed the efficacy of ITB in spasticity of cerebral and spinal origin (44–52). Significant reductions in the Ashworth score as well as decreases in the frequency of spasms and clonus have been confirmed. In SCI patients, functional independence measures were also improved with ITB (50,51). In patients with advanced disability, it can also improve quality of life and ease the burden care for caretakers as well as nursing staff. Following pump implantation, an inpatient stay in a rehabilitation facility is appropriate to adjust the dose and to facilitate adjustment to the decrease in tone so that functional independence is maintained or improved. During the first year after implantation, some tolerance occurs and the dose of baclofen must be adjusted upward to maintain therapeutic effect in the desired range. After the first year, there is little additional tolerance that takes place.

While the ITB pump has proven to be an invaluable aid in the treatment of severe spasticity, several words of caution are in order. First, the baclofen pump is only appropriate for those patients with intractable spasticity whose quality of life and functional abilities are severely impaired owing to spasticity. There are a number of other potential problems and pitfalls. Overdosage can occur quite easily and this may be seen in the early stages after pump implantation. Mechanical failure of the pump and catheter kinks and dislodgment may also be problematic and can precipitate baclofen-withdrawal syndromes (53). This can result in hallucinations, psychosis, and seizures. Further, it may be difficult to distinguish between overdose and withdrawal. A test dose of physostigmine may be helpful in this regard because it will block some of the toxic effects of overdose. Nevertheless, the problem of abrupt withdrawal necessitates the availability of personnel familiar with pump operation 24 h a day. In addition, patients who are not reliable are poor candidates for the baclofen pump because they are more likely to miss refill appointments and run the risk of abrupt withdrawal. It is useful for patients to have oral baclofen to prevent withdrawal should a pump malfunction or catheter kink occur. Despite its potential pitfalls, in patients with intractable generalized spasticity there is no better therapeutic option.

Botulinum Toxin and Nerve Blocks

In patients with focal spasticity, the use of botulinum toxin may be of benefit when used in conjunction with other approaches. The use of botulinum toxin is discussed in greater detail in this volume. Isolated spasticity rarely occurs in SCI but some muscle groups may exhibit an increase in tone out of proportion to other muscle groups, for example, in patients with severe hip-adductor spasticity that interferes with hygiene. It is in these instances where botulinum toxin may be useful. It acts directly on muscle and results in the inhibition of acetylcholine release from presynaptic terminals. The major drawback of botulinum toxin is that it weakens the muscle and is not rapidly reversible. In the majority of patients with SCI, this represents only a minor drawback because there may not be functional use of muscle strength. Although functional abilities of the involved limbs do not usually improve, but it may have beneficial effects on pain and ease of care.

Nerve blocks are another alternative in the treatment of focal spasticity. The same indications and limitations that apply with botulinum toxin are also applicable to nerve blocks. They are discussed in detail elsewhere in this volume. The most commonly used agent is phenol. Alternative agents include ethanol and lidocaine. Phenol is a neurolytic agent that destroys axons and myelin but leaves the endoneurial sheath intact. Muscle weakness brought about by phenol block has a duration of 1–12 mo. Phenol blocks have the ability to reduce focal spasticity and may be beneficial in targeting muscle groups whose tone is increased out of proportion to the rest of the body. They produce muscle weakness and would not be expected to improve function but may improve comfort and ease of care. When compared with botulinum toxin, there is no specific advantage of phenol block over toxin injection. In fact, botulinum toxin injection is less complicated and does not require surgical intervention as does open motor-point blocks.

Orthopedic Procedures

Patients with severe spasticity owing to SCI are prone to develop contractures, which may impair range of motion and predispose to decubitus-ulcer formation. This occurs when a contracture produces a pressure point. For example, a patient with a severe flexion contracture at the ankle would be highly susceptible to decubitus-ulcer formation on the heel. Similarly, a patient with flexion contractures at the hip is susceptible to a decubitus-ulcer formation on the posterior aspects of the hips and at the heels. In these patients with severe spasticity and fixed contractures, orthopedic procedures may be used to advantage to achieve normal position and to allow for improved range of motion. Used alone, they are of little benefit, but when used in conjunction with a coordinated plan to treat severe spasticity they may have significant benefit in the treatment of severe spasticity owing to SCI. Orthopedic procedures are discussed in detail in this text. Briefly, tenotomies and tendon lengthenings are among the most commonly employed procedures. These are generally performed on muscles in which there is no voluntary movement. Examples include Achilles-tendon lengthening to allow for extension of the ankle and release of the hamstrings tendon to correct flexion contracture at the knee. These procedures are usual employed to prevent tertiary complication of advanced disability including the prevention of decubitus ulcers and to ease nursing care. Occasionally they can be employed in patients with less-advanced disability to improve function. An example can be found in an Achilles tendon-lengthening procedure, which would allow for the use of an ankle foot orthotic (AFO) to improve ambulation.

In closing, one may hope for further conceptual as well as observational studies, which will permit a greater understanding of the altered physiology that results in spasticity following SCI, and corresponding new varieties of treatment. The treatment available for the modification of increased muscle tone and its consequences in SCI have improved dramatically over the past decade. A careful and well-thought-out approach using physical therapy, pharmacologic modalities, and adjunctive measures provides the optimal approach to management, which must be individualized according to patient needs and characteristics.

REFERENCES

1. Zankel, H. T., Sutton, B. B., and Burney, T. E. (1954) A paraplegic program under physical medicine and rehabilitation: one year experience. *Arch. Phys. Med.* **35,** 296–302.
2. Young, R. R. (1994) A review. *Neurology* **44(Suppl. 9),** S12–S20.
3. Kaplan, L. I., Grynbaum, B. B., Lloyd, K. E., and Rusk, H. A. (1962) Pain and spasticity in patients with spinal cord dysfunction: results of a follow-up study. *JAMA* **182,** 918–925.
4. Maynard, F. M., Karunas, R. S., and Waring, W. P. (1990) Epidemiology of spasticity following traumatic spinal cord injury. *Arch. Phys. Med. Rehabil.* **71,** 566–569.

5. Bicknell, J. M. and Fiedler, K. (1992) Unrecognized incomplete cervical spinal cord injury: review of nine new and 28 previously reported cases. *Am. J. Emerg. Med.* **10,** 336–343.
6. Hinderer, S. R. and Gupta, S. (1996) Functional outcome measures to assess interventions for spasticity. *Arch. Phys. Med. Rehabil.* **77,** 1083–1089.
7. Forer, S., et al. (1987) Task Force for Development of a Uniform Data System for Medical Rehabilitation. *Guide for Use of the Uniform Data Set for Medical Rehabilitation (FIM).* Research Foundation SUNY, Buffalo, NY.
8. Catz, A., Tamir, A., et al. (1997) SCIM - Spinal cord independence measure: a new disability scale for patients with spinal cord lesions. *Spinal Cord* **35,** 850–856.
9. Brown P. (1994) Pathophysiology of spasticity. *J. Neurol. Neurosurg. Psychiatry* **57,** 773–777.
10. Hufschmidt, A. and Mauritz, K-H. (1985) Chronic transformation of muscle in spasticity: a peripheral contribution to increased tone. *J. Neurol. Neurosurg. Psychiatry* **48,** 676–685.
11. Walsh, E. G. (1993) A review of some measurements of muscle wasting, tone and clonus in paraplegia. *Paraplegia* **31,** 75–81.
12. Dietz, V., Wirz, M., Curt, A., and Colombo, G. (1998) Locomotor pattern in paraplegic patients: training effects and recovery of spinal cord function. *Spinal Cord* **36,** 380–390.
13. Hagbarth, K. E. (1994) Evaluation of and methods to change muscle tone. *Scand. J. Rehabil. Med. Suppl.* **30,** 19–32.
14. Simons D. G. and Mense, S. (1998) Understanding and measurement of muscle tone as related to clinical muscle pain. *Pain* **75,** 1–17.
15. O'Dwyer, N. J., Ada, L., and Neilson, P. D. (1996) Spasticity and muscle contracture following stroke. *Brain* **119,** 1737–1749.
16. Michaelis, L. S. (1976) Spasticity in spinal cord injuries, in *Injuries of the Spine and Spinal Cord, Part II. Handbook of Clinical Neurology,* vol 26. (Vinken, P. J., Bruyn, G. W., and Braakman, R., eds.), American Elsevier, New York, pp. 477–487.
17. Little, J. W., Ditunno, J. F., Stiens, S., and Harris, R. M. (1999) Incomplete spinal cord injury: neuronal mechanisms of motor recovery and hyperreflexia. *Arch. Phys. Med. Rehabil.* **80,** 587–599.
18. Ragnarsson, K. T. (1992) Functional electrical stimulation and suppression of spasticity following spinal cord injury. *Bull. NY Acad. Med.* **68,** 351–364.
19. Bok, Y. L., Karmakar, M. G., et al. (1995) Autonomic dysreflexia revisited. *J. Spinal Cord Med.* **18,** 75–87.
20. Frank, R. G., Umlauf, R. L., Wonderlich, S. A., et al. (1987) Differences in coping styles among persons with spinal cord injury: a cluster analytic approach. *J. Consult. Clin. Psychol.* **55,** 727–731.
21. Guttmann, L. (1973) *Spinal Cord Injuries: Comprehensive Management and Research.* Blackwell, Oxford, UK, pg. 21.
22. Leckman, J. F., Pauls, D. L., Peterson, B. S., et al. (1992) Pathogenesis of Tourette syndrome: clues from the clinical phenotype and natural history. *Adv. Neurol.* **58,** 15–24.

23. Daylan, M., Sherman, A., and Cardenas, D. D. (1998) Factors associated with contractures in acute spinal cord injury. *Spinal Cord* **36,** 405–408.
24. Massey, J. A. (1988) Urodynamic and neurophysiological assessment of the neuropathic bladder, in *Spinal Cord Dysfunction: Assessment* (Illis, L.S., ed.), Oxford University Press, Oxford,
25. Zorowitz, R. D., Hughes, M. B., et al. (1996) Shoulder subluxation and pain after stroke: correlation or coincidence? *Am. J. Occup. Ther.* **50,** 194–201.
26. McPherson, J. J., Beck, A. H., and Franszcak, N. (1985) Dynamic splint to reduce the passive component of hypertonicity. *Arch. Phys. Med. Rehabil.* **66,** 249–252.
27. Dimitrijevic, Faganel, J., and Young, R. R. (1981) Underlying mechanisms of the effects of spinal cord stimulation in motor disorders: a review of the discussion. *Appl. Neurophysiol.* **44,** 133–140.
28. Barbeau, H. and Fung, J. (1992) New experimental approaches in the treatment of spastic gait disorders, in *Movement Disorders in Children* (Forssberg, H. and Hirschfeld, H., eds.) *Med. Sports Science* Karger, Basel.
29. Rushton, D. N., Barr, F. M. D., Donaldson, N de N, et al. (1998) Selecting candidates for a lower limb stimulator implant programme: a patient-centered method. *Spinal Cord* **36,** 303–309.
30. Subramanian, N., Vaughan, C. L., Peter, J. C., and Arens, L. J. (1998) Gait before and ten years after rhizotomy in children with cerebral palsy spasticity. *J. Neurosurg.* **88,** 1014–1019.
31. Gerszten, P. C., Albright, L., and Johnstone, G. F. (1998) Intrathecal baclofen infusion and subsequent orthopedic surgery in patients with spastic cerebral palsy. *J. Neurosurg.* **88,** 1009.
32. Nance, P. W., Bugaresti, J., Shellenberger, K., Sheramata, W., Martinez-Arizala, A., and the North American Tizanidine Study Group. (1994) Efficacy and safety of tizanidine in the treatment of spasticity in patients with spinal cord injury. *Neurology* **44(Suppl. 9),** S44–S52.
33. Davidoff, R. A. (1985) Antispasticity drugs: mechanism of action. *Ann. Neurol.* **17,** 107–116.
34. Pinder, R. M., Brogden, R. J. N., Speight, T. M., and Avery, G. S. (1997) Dantrolene sodium: a review of its pharmacological properties and therapeutic efficacy in spasticity. *Drugs* **13,** 3–23.
35. Gruenthal, M., Mueller, M., Olson, W. L., Priebe, M. M., Sherwood, A. M., and Olson, W. H. (1997) Gabapentin for the treatment of spasticity in patients with spinal cord injury. *Spinal Cord* **35,** 868–869.
36. Priebe, M. M., Sherwood, A. M., Graves, D. E., Mueller, M., and Olson, W. H. (1997) Effectiveness of gabapentin in controlling spasticity: a quantitative study. *Spinal Cord* **35,** 171–175.
37. Barbeau, H., Richards, C. L., and Bedard, B. J. (1982) Action of cyproheptadine in spastic paraparetic patients. *J. Neurol. Neurosurg. Psychiatry* **45,** 923.
38. Nance, P. (1994) A comparison of clonidine, cyroheptadine and baclofen in spastic spinal cord injured patients. *J. Am. Paraplegia Soc.* **17,** 151–157.
39. Weingarden, S. I. and Belen, J. G. (1992) Clonidine transdermal system for treatment of spasticity in spinal cord injury. *Arch. Phys. Med. Rehabil.* **73,** 876–877.

40. Erickson, D. L., Blacklock, J. B., Michaelson, M., Sperling, K. B., and Lo, J. N. (1985) Control of spasticity by implantable continuous flow morphine pump. *Neurology* **16,** 215–217.
41. Donovan, W. H., Carter, R. E., Rossi, C. D., and Wilkerson, M. A. (1988) Clonidine effect on spasticity: a clinical trial. *Arch. Phys. Med. Rehabil.* **69,** 193–194.
42. Meinck, H. M., Schönle, P. W., and Conrad, B. (1989) Effect of cannabinoids on spasticity and ataxia in multiple sclerosis. *J. Neurol.* **236,** 120–122.
43. Mueller, M. E., Gruenthal, M., and Olson, W. L. (1997) Gabapentin for relief of upper motor neuron symptoms in multiple sclerosis. *Arch. Phys. Med. Rehabil.* **78,** 521–524.
44. Coffey, R. J., Cahill, D., Steers, W., and Park, T. S. (1993) Intrathecal baclofen for intractable spasticity of spinal origin: results of long-term multicenter study. *J. Neurosurg.* **78,** 226–232.
45. Nance, P., Schryvers, O., Schmidt, B., Dubo, H., Loveridge, B., and Fewer, D. (1995) Intrathecal baclofen therapy for adults with spinal spasticity: therapeutic efficacy and effect on hospital admissions. *Can. J. Neurol. Sci.* **22,** 22–29.
46. Lazorthes, Y., Sallerin-Caute, B., Verdie, J., Bastide, R., and Carillo, J. (1990) Chronic intrathecal baclofen administration for control of severe spasticity. *J. Neurosurg.* **72,** 393–402.
47. Rifici, C., Kofler, M., Kronenberg, M., Kofler, A., Bramanti, P., and Saltuari, L. (1994) Intrathecal baclofen application in patients with supraspinal spasticity secondary to severe traumatic brain injury. *Funct. Neurol.* **9,** 29–34.
48. Penn, R. D., Savoy, S. M., Corcos, D., Latash, M., Gottlieb, G., Parke, B., and Kroin, J. S. (1989) Intrathecal baclofen for severe spinal spasticity. *N. Engl. J. Med.* **320,** 517–521.
49. Latash, M. L., Penn, R. D,, Corcos, D. M., and Gottlieb, G. L. (1990) Effects of intrathecal baclofen on voluntary motor control in spastic paresis. *J. Neurosurg.* **72,** 388–392.
50. Loubser, P. G., Narayan, R. K., Sandin, K. J., Donovan, W. H., and Russell, K. D. (1991) Continuous infusion of intrathecal baclofen: long-term effects on spasticity in spinal cord injury. *Paraplegia* **29,** 48–52.
51. Ochs, G., Struppler, A., Meyerson, B. A., Linderoth, B., and Gybels, J. (1989) Intrathecal baclofen for long-term treatment of spasticity; a multicentre study. *J. Neurol. Neurosurg. Psychiatry* **52,** 933–939.
52. Meythaler, J. M., DeVivo, M. J., and Hadley, M. (1996) Prospective study on the use of bolus intrathecal baclofen for spastic hypertonia due to acquired brain injury. *Arch. Phys. Med. Rehabil.* **77,** 461–466.
53. Reeves, R. K., Stolp-Smith, K. A., and Christopherson, M. W. (1998) Hyperthermia, rhabdomyolysis, and disseminated intravascular coagulation associated with baclofen pump catheter failure. *Arch. Phys. Med. Rehabil.* **79,** 353–356.

Index

A

Ablative intrathecal sclerosing agents, 261
Acetylcholine, 8
Achilles tendon
   lengthening, 235, 299, 323, 365
   vibration, 7
Acupuncture, 62–63
Acute traumatic brain injury spasticity, 311–312
Adducted/internally rotated shoulder, 211–212
   muscles contributing to, 71
Adducted thighs
   muscles contributing to, 71
Adolescents
   education plan, 268
AFO. *See* Ankle foot orthoses
Alcohol blocks
   vs. botulinum toxin, 333
   vs. phenol blocks, 333
Alpha$_2$-adrenergic agonists, 151–153
Alpha adrenergic blocking agents, 153
Aminoglycosides
   botulinum toxin, 182
Amyotrophic lateral sclerosis
   baclofen, 111
Anesthetics
   local, 162, 326–328
   topical, 319
Angular stiffness
   mechanical recordings, 35

Ankle
   plantar flexion spasticity
      tibial nerve blocks, 166
   SCI, 356
Ankle foot orthoses (AFO), 67
   articulated, 81–82
   floor reaction, 85–86
   hinged, 81–82
   hinged clamshell closure, 85
   solid-ankle, 85
   thermoplastic, 80
   types, 79–86
Anterior horn cell, 288–289
Anticonvulsants, 153–154
Anxious, 24
Appearance
   UMN syndrome, 20
Arthrodesis
   shoulder, 210
   wrist, 219
Articulated ankle foot orthoses, 81, 82
Ashworth Scale, 23, 31, 190

B

Babinski sign, 4
Baclofen, 9, 24, 25, 103–121
   absorption, 105
   adverse effects, 112–113
      withdrawal, 118
   amyotrophic lateral sclerosis, 111
   chemistry, 103
   clinical effects, 106–107

clinical studies, 108–109
vs. clonazepam, 112
CP, 111, 275
vs. diazepam, 112
distribution, 105
dosage, 118, 120
elimination, 105–106
future, 120–121
intrathecal. *See* Intrathecal baclofen
mechanism of action, 104–105
metabolism, 105–106
MS, 294–295
vs. diazepam, 140
pharmacokinetics, 105–112
SCI, 110–111, 360
side effects, 114–115, 119, 295
stroke, 111
structure, 104
tardive dyskinesia, 113
TBI, 335–336
vs. tizanidine, 128
toxicity, 113, 116–117, 118, 121
Barthel Index (BI), 40
Becker splint, 74
Benzodiazepines, 137–143
administration, 142–143
adverse effects, 142
clinical trials, 139–142
CP, 274–275
GABA, 139
history, 137–138
mechanism of action, 138–139
MS, 295–296
pharmacology, 139
SCI, 361–362
traumatic brain injury, 141
Berman Movement Scale
CP, 272

BI, 40
Biofeedback, 58
Biomechanical Analysis system, 69
Bi-valved foam block wrist hand finger orthosis, 75
Bladder sphincter dyssynergia
tizanidine, 131
Blocking, 15
Blocks
alcohol
vs. botulinum toxin, 333
vs. phenol, 333
ethyl alcohol, 328–329
intramuscular, 328
motor point, 330
nerve. *See* Nerve blocks
Bobath approach, 50
Bobath splint, 74
Botox, 173
Botulinum toxin, 9, 25, 173–183
vs. alcohol blocks, 333
clinical trials, 182
contraindications, 182
CP, 277
dosage, 179
electrical stimulation, 178–179
EMG, 176–178
future research, 183
injection techniques, 175–179
mechanism of action, 173–175
MS, 298–299
muscle selection, 179
outcome, 181
vs. phenol blocks, 179, 333
pregnancy, 182
SCI, 364
sedation, 22
TBI, 331–334
treatment objectives, 179–182

Index

Botulinum toxin type A
  injection preparation, 175
  stroke, 96–97
Boutonniere deformities, 225–226
Bracing
  CP, 277–278
Bupivacaine, 162
  TBI, 328

C

Calf paresis
  flexor digitorum longus to os calcis transfer, 242–243
Cannabinoids, 156
Carpal tunnel release, 223
Casts, 59–60
  cost, 59
  inhibition, 59–60
    ankle orthoses, 82
    cerebral palsy, 273
  plaster
    TBI, 321
  progressive serial, 59–60
  serial, 74
    cerebral palsy, 273
    stroke, 76–77
    TBI, 321
Cavus deformities
  Steindler stripping, 240–241
  triple arthrodesis, 241
Central pain syndromes, 23
  stroke, 14
Cerebellar stimulation
  chronic, 94
  TBI, 325
Cerebral lesions, 4
Cerebral palsy (CP), 267–281
  adaptive equipment, 273–274
  educational planning, 267–269
  electrical stimulation, 99–100, 273
  evaluation tools, 271–272
  functional activities, 273
  future, 281
  inhibition casting, 273
  neurodevelopmental training, 272–273
  obturator nerve blocks, 166
  orthopedic surgery, 277–280
  pharmacotherapy, 111, 128, 141, 274–277
  physical and occupational therapy, 270–271
  selective dorsal rhizotomy, 280–281
  serial casting, 273
  splinting, 274
  strengthening/stretching, 273
Cerebral shock, 16–17
Children. *See also* Cerebral palsy
  dantrolene dosing, 148
  diazepam dosing, 142–143
  education plan, 268
  physical and occupational therapy
    CP, 271
  tizanidine
    dosing, 130
Chronic cerebellar stimulation, 94
Chronic traumatic brain injury
  spasticity, 315–318
Clasp-knife phenomenon, 15, 31
Classrooms
  CP, 271
Claw foot
  toe flexor release, 241–242
Clenched fist, 220–222
  medial nerve block, 220–221
  muscles contributing, 221–222
  muscles contributing to, 71
Clonazepam
  vs. baclofen, 112

dosage, 143
  TBI, 335–336
Clonidine, 151–153
  CP, 275
  intrathecal, 193
  TBI, 337
Clonus, 16
Clorazepate
  TBI, 335–336
Co-contraction, 16
Cold compresses, 24
Coma
  TBI, 308–309
Cone splint, 74
Confusion, 22
Contractures, 18, 23, 72–73
  prevention, 59
  TBI, 312–315
Cooling, 57
Corticosteroids
  intrathecal, 188
Cost
  casting, 59
  intrathecal baclofen, 22
CP. *See* Cerebral palsy
Creep, 72
Cutaneous electrotherapy
  spinal cord injury, 97–98
Cyclical electrical stimulation
  hemiplegia, 95–96
Cyclobenzaprine, 155
Cyproheptadine, 10, 155
  TBI, 337

D

Dantrium
  MS, 296
  SCI, 362
Dantrolene, 9, 24, 147–149
  adverse effects, 148

CP, 275
dosage, 147–148
indications, 147–148
mechanism of action, 147
pediatric dosing, 148
sedation, 22, 147
side effects, 22
TBI, 334, 336–337
urinary dribbling, 23
usage, 147–148
weakness, 147
Decubitus ulcer
  heel, 365
Deep tendon reflexes
  grading, 30–31
Denervation, 208–209
Diazepam, 9, 24
  administration, 142–143
  vs. baclofen, 112
  cerebral palsy, 141
  history, 137
  mechanism of action, 138–139
  MS, 296
    vs. baclofen, 140
  paraplegics, 141–142
  pediatric dosing, 142–143
  SCI, 139–140, 361–362
  stroke, 140–141
  TBI, 335–336
  vs. tizanidine, 128, 131–132
Diffuse axonal injury, 307
Disuse atrophy, 18
Dorsal column stimulation
  multiple sclerosis, 98–99
Dorsal rhizotomy, 262–263
  selective, 280–281
Dorsal root entry zone lesions, 4
Dynamic multichannel
    electromyography, 205–206

Index

Dynamic orthoses
  elbow, 78–79
Dynamic splinting, 59
Dynamic stiff knee gait
  extension deformity, 232–234
Dysesthesia, 163
Dysport, 173
Dystonia, 14

E

Elbow
  flexed
    muscles contributing to, 71
  flexion deformity, 206–207
  functional lengthening, 212–213
  nonfunctional release, 213–214
  orthoses, 77–79
    types, 77–79
  SCI, 357
  spastic extension, 214
  spastic flexion, 212
    musculocutaneous nerve
      blocks, 167–168
  TBI, 340
  triceps lengthening, 214
  ulnar neuropathy, 214
Electrical stimulation, 57–58, 93–100.
  See also Transcutaneous
  electrical nerve stimulation
  botulinum toxin, 178–179
  cerebral palsy, 99–100, 273
  cyclical, 95–96
  functional, 322
  hemiplegia, 95–97
  history, 94–95
  shoulder, 210
  stroke, 96
  super threshold
    hemiplegia, 96
  TBI, 321–323

Electromyography (EMG)
  botulinum toxin, 176–178
  dynamic multichannel, 205–206
  surface, 37
Electrotherapy
  cutaneous
    spinal cord injury, 97–98
EMG. *See* Electromyography
Enkephalin, 8
Environmental factors
  spasticity measurement, 29
Epidural spinal cord stimulation, 98
Equinovarus foot deformity, 207
  extensor hallucis lengthening, 238
Equinovarus posturing
  TBI, 324
Equinus deformities
  Achilles tendon lengthening, 235
Equinus foot deformity
  TBI, 323
Ethanol nerve blocks, 161–162, 164
Ethyl alcohol blocks
  TBI, 328–329
Etidocaine, 162
Extended knee
  muscles contributing to, 71
Extensor hallucis longus, 238

F

Family
  education
    CP, 268
Fatigue, 17
  spasticity measurement, 29
Femoral nerve blocks
  patient selection, 167
  range of motion evaluation, 203
Finger. *See also* Wrist hand finger
    orthoses
  abduction splint, 74

flexors
    fractional lengthening, 222–223
    orthoses, 73–77
        treatment approach, 73
        types, 73–77
    SCI, 356
    TBI, 338–339
Flaccidity, 17
Flexed elbow
    muscles contributing to, 71
Flexed hip
    muscles contributing to, 71
Flexed knee
    muscles contributing to, 71
Flexed wrist
    muscles contributing to, 71
Flexor carpi radialis, 216–219
Flexor carpi ulnaris, 216–219
Flexor digitorum profundus, 216–219
Flexor digitorum sublimis, 216–219
Flexor pronator origin
    release, 215
Flexor spasms
    control, 20
Floor reaction ankle foot orthoses, 85–86
Foot
    deformities
        equinovarus, 207
        equinus, 323
        nonambulatory patient, 243
    TBI, 341–342
Forearm
    pronated
        muscles contributing to, 71
    spastic pronation, 215
    spastic supination, 216
    TBI, 339–340
Fractional lengthening, 208–209

Fractures
    TBI, 315
Fugl-Meyer scale, 40
Functional electrical stimulation
    TBI, 322
Functional Independence Measure, 40, 354
Functionally based therapies, 54–55
F-waves, 40

G

GABA. *See* Gamma amino butyric acid
Gabapentin, 153–154
    MS, 153, 297
    SCI, 153–154, 362
Gait-lab technology, 37
Gamma amino butyric acid (GABA), 8, 289
    agonists
        sedation, 22
    benzodiazepines, 139
    TBI, 334
Gegenhalten, 18
Glasgow Coma Scale, 305–306
Glutamate, 8
Glycine, 8
Goniometer
    CP, 271
Grade school children
    education plan, 268
    physical and occupational therapy
        CP, 271
Gross motor functional measure
    CP, 271
Guyon's Canal, 223

H

Habituation, 142
Hallucinations, 129

Index

Hand. *See also* Wrist hand finger orthoses
  finger flexors
    fractional lengthening, 222–223
    functional procedures *vs.* hygiene procedures, 220–221
    intrinsic minus deformities, 226–227
    intrinsic spasticity, 225–226
    spastic clenched fist, 220–222
    spastic thumb-in-palm deformity, 224–225
    superficialis to profundus tendon transfer, 223–224
  TBI, 338–339
Headaches
  tension
    tizanidine, 132
Heat, 57
Heel
  decubitus ulcer, 365
Hemiballismus, 201
Hemiplegia, 4
  electrical stimulation, 95–97
Hemiplegic dystonia, 4
Hepatotoxicity, 22
Heterotopic ossification
  TBI, 315
Hind foot deformities
  TBI, 323–324
Hinged ankle foot orthoses, 81–82
Hinged clamshell closure ankle foot orthoses, 85
Hip
  adduction deformity, 227–228
    obturator neurectomy, 227
    tenotomy, 227–228
  adductor spasms
    TBI, 323
  extension deformity, 230–231
    proximal hamstring release, 230–231
  flexed
    muscles contributing to, 71
  flexion deformity, 228–230
    complete hip release, 229–230
    pectineus release, 228–229
  flexion spasms
    TBI, 323
  flexor spasticity
    paravertebral lumbar spine nerve blocks, 167
  orthoses, 88–89
  SCI, 356
  TBI, 343–344
Hitchhiker's great toe, 238
H/M ratio, 39
Hoke technique, 236
H reflex, 37–39, 55
Hyperactive stretch reflexes, 6
Hypertonia, 14
  degree, 15
  differential diagnosis, 18–19
  non-neurological exacerbators, 24
Hypertonicity, 70–72
Hypoxic ischemic injury, 307

I

Ibuprofen
  vs. tizanidine, 131
Ice bags, 24
Incontinence, 22
Infants
  physical and occupational therapy CP, 270–271
Infection, 23
Inflatable wrist hand immobilization orthosis, 74–75

Inhibition casting, 59–60
  ankle orthoses, 82
  cerebral palsy, 273
Instrumented hammers, 34
Intraabdominal infections, 23
Intramuscular blocks
  TBI, 328
Intramuscular motor point blocks
  TBI, 330
Intrathecal baclofen, 25
  clinical trials, 188–189
  cost, 22
  CP, 276–277
  MS, 297–298
  patient selection, 189–190
  pump implantation protocol, 190–192
    complications, 191–192
  SCI, 362–363
  TBI, 338
Intrathecal clonidine, 193
Intrathecal corticosteroids, 188
Intrathecal medications, 187–188
  history, 188
Intrathecal methylprednisolone, 188
Intrathecal morphine, 188, 192–193
  TBI, 338
Intrathecal tizanidine, 193

J, K

Joint
  compression, 56
  contraction, 56
KAFO, 87
Ketozolam
  TBI, 335–336
Knee
  extended
    muscles contributing to, 71
  extension deformity, 232–235
    quadriceps lengthening, 234–235
    rectus femoris to gracilis transfer, 232–234
  extensor spasticity
    femoral nerve blocks, 167
  flexed
    muscles contributing to, 71
  flexion contractures
    TBI, 323
  flexion deformity, 231–232
    distal hamstring lengthening, 231–232
    distal hamstring release, 232
  flexor spasms
    sciatic nerve blocks, 166–167
  muscles
    spasticity measurement, 33
  SCI, 356
  TBI, 342–343
Knee ankle foot orthosis (KAFO), 87
Knee orthoses (KOs), 86–87

L

Lamotrigine
  TBI, 336–337
Lap trays, 61
Lead pipe rigidity, 18
Lidocaine, 162
Local anesthetics
  nerve blocks, 162
  TBI, 326–328
Low back pain
  tizanidine, 131
Lower extremities
  TBI, 341–344
Lower extremity nerve blocks
  patient selection, 166–167
L-threonine, 10

Index

Lumbar spine nerve blocks
  paravertebral
    patient selection, 167

M

Manual pressure, 55
Marijuana, 156
Medial nerve blocks
  patient selection, 168
  spastic clenched fist, 220–221
Medical Research Council scale, 30
Memantine, 10
Methylprednisolone
  intrathecal, 188
Microcomputer-based systems
  pendulum test, 33
Modified Ashworth scale, 31–32
  CP, 271
Morphine
  intrathecal, 188, 192–193, 338
Motions
  facilitation, 52
Motor control
  clinical evaluation, 202–205
  clinical scale, 204
  grading, 204–205
  laboratory assessment, 205–208
Motor evoked potentials, 206
Motor neurons
  activated, 7–8
  excitability, 7
Motor point blocks
  intramuscular, 330
  nerve, 164, 168
Motor unit potentials, 176
Multiple sclerosis (MS), 17, 287–300
  alternative therapies, 296–299
  botulinum toxin, 298–299
  dorsal column stimulation, 98–99
  functional consequences, 289–291

nerve blocks, 298–299
orthopedic procedures, 299
spasticity origins, 288–289
treatment, 107–110, 127, 140, 153, 291–297
Muscle contractions
  electrophysiological evaluation, 37–40
Muscles
  contraction, 4
  tone
    quantifying, 204
    testing, 31
  torque
    mechanical recordings, 35
Muscle tendon units
  lengthening, 208–209
Musculocutaneous nerve blocks
  patient selection, 167–168
Myasthenia gravis
  botulinum toxin, 182
Myelotomy, 260
Myobloc, 175
Myotonia, 19

N

Naloxone, 58
NDT, 49–51
Nerve blocks, 159–169. *See also*
    Blocks
  adverse effects, 162–163
  aftercare, 168–169
  benefits, 160
  ethanol, 161–162, 164
  femoral
    patient selection, 167
    range of motion evaluation, 203
  lower extremity
    patient selection, 166–167

medial
  spastic clenched fist, 220–221
median
  patient selection, 168
motor point, 164, 168
MS, 298–299
musculocutaneous
  patient selection, 167–168
obturator
  patient selection, 166
open, 165
paravertebral lumbar spine
  patient selection, 167
patient selection, 165–168
phenol, 161, 163–164
  MS, 299
  subscapularis muscle, 168
phenol motor point, 168
SCI, 364
sciatic
  patient selection, 166–167
  range of motion evaluation, 203
TBI, 326–328
tibial
  patient selection, 166
timing, 160–161
types, 163–165
upper extremity
  patient selection, 167–168
Nerve trunk blocks
  percutaneous closed, 163–164
Neuroablative procedures, 258
Neurodevelopmental therapy (NDT), 49–51
Neuromodulators, 8
Neuro-orthopedic surgery, 197
  indications, 199–201
  philosophy, 199

Neurosurgical management, 257–263
  ablative intrathecal sclerosing agents, 261
  dorsal rhizotomies, 262–263
  myelotomy, 260
  percutaneous neurotomy, 257–258
  selective open neurotomy, 258–259
  selective spinal cordectomy, 260–261
  stereotaxic ablative procedures, 261–262
Neurotransmitters, 8–9
Nicotine, 10
Noradrenergic pathways, 8
Nyquist plots, 35

O

Obturator nerve blocks
  patient selection, 166
Occupational therapy
  cerebral palsy, 270–271
Open nerve blocks, 165
Open neurotomy
  selective, 258–259
Opiates, 10
Orphenadrine, 155
  TBI, 337
Orthopedic surgical techniques, 208–209
Orthoses
  ankle foot. *See* Ankle foot orthoses
  description, 67–68
  dynamic
    elbow, 78–79
  function
    description, 68
  functional controls, 68
  inflatable wrist hand
    immobilization, 74–75

Index

knee, 86–87
knee ankle foot, 87
nomenclatures, 67–68
prefabricated
   ankle, 85–86
static, 67–68
static progressive, 67–68
   elbow, 77–78
   wrist, 73–77
wrist hand, 67
wrist hand finger. *See* Wrist hand finger orthoses
Orthotic devices, 59–60
Orthotic intervention
   clinical basis, 70–73
Orthotic management, 67–89
Orthotic prescription, 69
Orthotic principles
   tissue mechanics, 72
Oswestry scale, 32
Overflow patterns, 50

P

Pain, 4, 23
Palmaris longus, 216–219
Paradoxical agitation, 22
Paraplegics
   diazepam, 141–142
Paravertebral lumbar spine nerve blocks
   patient selection, 167
Paresis
   cause of, 5
   vs. spasticity, 3
Parkinson's disease, 28
Passive stretching
   spasticity measurement, 29
Peabody Developmental Motor Scales
   CP, 272

Pediatric Evaluations of Disability Inventory (PEDI)
   CP, 272
Pendulum test, 33
   experimental setup, 34
Percutaneous closed nerve trunk blocks, 163–164
Percutaneous neurotomy, 257–258
Peripheral neuropathy, 201–202
Persistent vegetative state
   TBI, 309
Pes equinovarus
   muscles contributing to, 71
Phasic reflexes, 14
Phenol nerve blocks, 25, 161, 163–164
   adverse effects, 330–331
   vs. alcohol blocks, 333
   vs. botulinum toxin, 179, 333
   motor point, 168
   MS, 299
   subscapularis muscle, 168
   TBI, 329–330
Phenothiazines, 155–156
   TBI, 337
Phenytoin
   TBI, 337
Physical medicine, 24
Physical therapy
   cerebral palsy, 270–271
Piracetam, 154
Plantar-flexed ankle, 83
Plaster casting
   TBI, 321
Plastic deformation
   soft tissue, 72
Pneumonia, 23
PNF, 51–52
Positioning, 24
   skin breakdown, 18

spasticity
  measurement, 29
  reduction, 60–62
Posterior rhizotomy
  selective, 325
Prefabricated orthoses
  ankle, 85–86
Pregnancy
  botulinum toxin, 182
  tizanidine, 131
Pressure points, 18
Presynaptic inhibition
  reduction, 8
Primitive patterning reflexes
  unmasking, 203–204
Procaine
  TBI, 327–328
Progabide, 154–155
Progressive serial casting
  ankle orthoses, 82
Progressive stretching
  ankle orthoses, 82–83
Pronated forearm
  muscles contributing to, 71
Pronator quadratus
  lengthening, 215
Pronator teres
  lengthening, 215
Prone lying, 62
Proprioceptive facilitation
  TBI, 319
Proprioceptive neuromuscular
  facilitation (PNF), 51–52

Q, R

Quality of life, 40
Quanfacine
  CP, 275
R_2, 33–34
  calculation, 35

Range of motion
  assessment, 203
  exercises, 20
  skin breakdown, 18
Rebound spasticity, 118
Reciprocal inhibition
  reduction, 8
Reflexes
  testing, 31
Refractory spasticity
  MS, 297
Renshaw activity, 8
Resting volar splints
  TBI, 320
Rigidity
  vs. spasticity, 28, 31
Riluzole
  TBI, 336–337
Rocking, 56

S

School children
  education plan, 268
  physical and occupational therapy
    CP, 271
SCI. *See* Spinal cord injury
Sciatic nerve blocks
  patient selection, 166–167
  range of motion evaluation, 203
Sclerosing agents
  ablative intrathecal, 261
Sedation, 21–22
  dantrolene, 147
Selective dorsal rhizotomy
  cerebral palsy, 280–281
Selective open neurotomy, 258–259
Selective posterior rhizotomy
  TBI, 325
Sensory deprivation, 53
Sensory integration, 52–54

Index

Sensory motor integration, 53
Serial casting, 59–60, 74
  cerebral palsy, 273
  progressive
    ankle orthoses, 82
  stroke, 76–77
  TBI, 321
Serotonin, 7
Shoulder
  adducted/internally rotated, 211–212
    muscles contributing to, 71
  adhesive capsulitis, 209
  arthrodesis, 210
  inferior subluxation, 209–210
    electrical stimulation, 210
  SCI, 357
  spastic abduction, 210
  supraspinatus slide, 210–211
  TBI, 340–341
Sinusoidal analysis, 35
Skin
  breakdown, 18
Slow rolling, 56
Slow spinning, 56
Snook splint, 74
Solid-ankle ankle foot orthoses, 85
Somatosensory evoked potentials, 206
Spasm frequency scale, 33
Spasms
  painful, 15
  pattern, 15–16
Spasm score, 32
Spastic brachioradialis
  decreasing tone, 213
Spastic catch, 14–15, 31
Spastic elbow flexion deformity, 206–207
Spastic hyperreflexia
  cause, 6

Spasticity
  biomechanical evaluation, 33–34
    problems, 35–36
  clinical consequences, 17–18
  clinical evaluation, 30–33
  clinical features, 25
  clinical physiology of, 3–5
  complications, 14, 17–18, 198
  definition, 13–14
  development
    temporal evolution, 5
  measurement, 27–41
    complicating factors, 29–30
    other outcome measures, 40
    rationale, 30
    timing, 29
  vs. paresis, 3
  pathophysiology, 5–6
  pharmacology, 8–10
  physical approach, 47–48
  reduction
    positioning, 60–62
  vs. rigidity, 28, 31
  therapeutic exercise, 47–63
  treatment, 21–25
    contraindications, 21–22
    cost, 22
    goals, 19
    systemic *vs.* local, 21
    team approach, 21
    timing, 21
  usefulness, 22–23
Spastic limb deformities
  evaluation, 201–202
Spastic paresis, 3
Spastic valgus foot, 207
Spinal cordectomy, 260–261
Spinal cord injury (SCI), 8, 353–365
  alternative therapy, 362–365

central pain syndromes, 14
cutaneous electrotherapy, 97–98
obturator nerve blocks, 166
spasticity
 anatomical problems, 355–358
 contributing factors, 353–355
TENS, 97–98
treatment, 110, 139–140, 153–154, 358–362
Spinal cord stimulation, 58
 epidural, 98
 transcutaneous, 97
Spinal lesions, 4
Spinal reflexes
 increased, 7
Spinal shock, 16–17, 29
SPLATT, 235–238
Splint, 24
 Becker, 74
 Bobath, 74
 cerebral palsy, 274
 cock up wrist, 223
 cone, 74
 dynamic, 59
 facilitation, 20
 finger-abduction, 74
 resting volar, 320
 Snook, 74
 static, 59
 TBI, 320–321
 textured dorsal, 320
 thumb spica, 225
Splinter skills, 53
Split anterior tibial tendon transfer (SPLATT), 235–238
Static orthoses, 67–68
Static progressive orthoses, 67–68
 elbow, 77–78
Static splinting, 59

Steindler stripping
 cavus deformities, 240–241
Stereotaxic ablative procedures, 261–262
Stiff knee gait, 207–208
Strength
 measurements, 272
 testing, 30, 31
Stress relaxation, 72
Stretching, 24
Stretch reflexes
 hyperactive, 6
Striatal toe
 muscles contributing to, 71
Stroke, 53
 baclofen, 111
 botulinum toxin type A, 96–97
 central pain syndromes, 14
 diazepam, 140–141
 electrical stimulation, 96
 serial casting, 76–77
 tizanidine, 127
Strychnine poisoning
 acute, 8
Subacute traumatic brain injury
 spasticity, 315–318
Subscapularis muscle
 phenol nerve blocks, 168
Substance P, 8
Super threshold electrical stimulation
 hemiplegia, 96
Supine lying, 62
Supraspinal lesions, 8
Surface electromyography, 37
Sustained stretch, 56
Swan neck deformities, 225–226
Synergy, 16
Systemic infections, 23

T

Tachyphylaxis, 142
Tardive dyskinesia
   baclofen, 113
TBI. *See* Traumatic brain injury
Temperature
   spasticity measurement, 29
Tendon jerk
   standardization, 34
TENS, 58
   hemiplegia, 96
   spinal cord injury, 97–98
Tension headaches
   tizanidine, 132
Tetrabenazine
   CP, 275
Textured dorsal splints
   TBI, 320
Thenar muscles
   proximal release, 223–224
Therapeutic exercise
   spasticity, 47–63
Thermoplastic ankle foot orthoses, 80
Thermoplastic wrist hand finger
     orthoses, 75–76
Thighs
   adducted
     muscles contributing to, 71
   TBI, 343–344
Thumb-in-palm deformity, 224–225
   muscles contributing to, 71
   TBI, 324
Thumb spica splint, 225
Tibial nerve blocks
   patient selection, 166
Timing
   spasticity measurement, 29
Tiredness, 24

Tizanidine, 9–10, 24, 125–132
   administration, 130
   vs. baclofen, 128
   bladder sphincter dyssynergia, 131
   clinical use, 131–132
   CP, 128, 275
   vs. diazepam, 128, 131–132
   drug interactions, 130–131
   efficacy studies, 126–128
   hepatotoxicity, 131
   vs. ibuprofen, 131
   intrathecal, 193
   low back pain, 131
   MS, 127, 292–294
   pediatric dosing, 130
   pharmacokinetics, 126
   pharmacology, 125–126
   pregnancy, 131
   SCI, 360–361
   side effects, 128–129, 294
   stroke, 127
   TBI, 337
   tension headaches, 132
Toddlers
   physical and occupational therapy
     CP, 270–271
Toes
   SCI, 356
Tone-reduction wrist hand finger
     orthoses, 74
Tonic head deviation, 61
Tonic reflexes, 14–15
Topical anesthetics
   TBI, 319
Topical cold
   TBI, 319
Transcutaneous electrical nerve
     stimulation (TENS), 58
   hemiplegia, 96
   spinal cord injury, 97–98

Transcutaneous spinal cord
    stimulation, 97
Transfers
    leg extensor spasms, 23
Traumatic brain injury (TBI), 305–344
    acute, 311–312
    benzodiazepines, 141
    casts, 321
    chronic, 315–318
    contractures, 312–315
    electrical stimulation, 321–323
    equinovarus posturing, 324
    equinus foot deformities, 323
    fractures, 315
    heterotopic ossification, 315
    hind foot deformities, 323–324
    hip adductor spasms, 323
    hip flexion spasms, 323
    knee flexion contractures, 323
    muscle strengthening, 319
    neurosurgical procedures, 325–326
    obturator nerve blocks, 166
    orthopedic surgical procedures,
        323–325
    orthoses, 320–321
    outcome indicators, 308–309
    passive stretch, 318
    pathophysiology, 307–308
    pharmacologic treatment, 326–338
    range of motion, 318
    recovery patterns, 309–312
    spasticity
        clinical patterns, 338–344
    splints, 320–321
    subacute, 315–318
    thumb-in-palm, 324
    unbalanced wrist, 324
Tremor, 14

Trihexyphenidyl
    CP, 275
Triple arthrodesis
    cavus deformities, 241

U

Ulnar nerve
    neurectomy, 223
UMN syndrome. *See* Upper motor
    neuron (UMN) syndrome
Unbalanced wrist
    TBI, 324
United Cerebral Palsy Association,
    268
Upper extremities
    nerve blocks
        patient selection, 167–168
    TBI, 338–341
Upper motor neuron (UMN)
    syndrome, 13–14, 27
    appearance, 20
    clinical features, 70
    deformities, 198
    negative symptoms, 16–17
    orthopedic interventions, 197–243
    positive symptoms, 14–16
    signs, 14–19
    symptoms, 288
Urinary dribbling
    dantrolene, 23
Urinary tract infections, 23

V

Valgus foot deformities
    peroneal lengthening, 239
    peroneus longus transfer, 239–240
Valproic acid, 154
Varus deformities
    SPLATT, 235–238
    tibialis anterior lengthening, 238
    tibialis posterior lengthening, 238

Index 385

Vibration, 56–57
　TBI, 319
Vigabatrin, 10
Voluntary movements
　incoordination, 17

W

Waxy flexibility, 18
Weakness, 16, 22
　dantrolene, 147
Wheelchair, 24
WHFO. *See* Wrist hand finger orthoses
WHO, 67
Wounds, 23
Wrist
　arthrodesis, 219
　cock up splint, 223
　spastic extension, 219–220
　　myotendinous lengthening, 219–220
　spastic flexion, 216–219
　　laboratory examination, 217
　　myotendinous lengthening, 217–218
　　wrist flexor release, 218–219
　TBI, 339–340
Wrist extensor tenodesis, 223
Wrist hand finger orthoses (WHFO)
　bi-valved foam block, 75
　thermoplastic, 75–76
　tone-reduction, 74
Wrist hand orthosis (WHO), 67
Wrist orthoses, 73–77
　treatment approach, 73
　types, 73–77
Wrists
　SCI, 357